Contents

Introduction 5
How to Use This Book 7

Chapter 1 Needling Considerations 11
Precautions to be Taken Before Needling 11
Needling Depth 11
Needling Angles 12
Needle Sizes 12
Needle Quality 12
Needling Contraindications 12
Dangerous Areas for Needling 13
Dangerous Points for Puncture 13
Untoward Reactions and Accidents 14

Chapter 2 Manual Techniques Considerations 15
Pressure Techniques 15
Friction Techniques 15
Stretching and Opening Techniques 15
Other Manual Techniques 15
Manual Techniques Contraindications 16

Chapter 3 Moxibustion Considerations 17
General Cautions 17
Points Contraindicated for Moxibustion 18
First Aid for Burns 18

Chapter 4 Cupping Considerations 19
Functions of Cupping 19
Guidelines and Precautions 19
After Cupping 20
Methods of Cupping 20

Chapter 5 Deqi 21
The Importance of Deqi 21
Specific Therapeutic Deqi 22

Chapter 6 Classification of Points 25
The Top Most Commonly Used Points 25
The Back-Shu and Front-Mu Points 26
The Source-Yuan Points 26
The Accumulation Cleft-Xi Points 26
The Connecting-Luo Points 26
The Four and Six Command Points 27
The Eight Gathering Hui Points 27
The Five Transporting Shu Points 27
Five Phase Point Selection 29
The Window of Heaven Points 30
The Nine Points for Returning Yang 30
The Thirteen Ghost Points 30
The Twelve Heavenly Star Points 30
The Points of the Four Seas 30
The Eight Extraordinary Vessels 30
The Eight Opening and Coupled Points 31
The Six Divisions 32
The Chinese Clock 32

Chapter 7 Principles of Point Selection 33
How to Choose Points 33
Selecting Points According to Area
(Local and Distal Points) 34
Selecting Points According to Syndromes 34
Selecting Points According to Diseases and
Conditions from Empirical Knowledge
and Clinical Practice 34

Chapter 8 Cun Measurements 41
General Guidelines 41
Cun Measurements According to Body Area 42

Chapter 9 Considerations, Cautions and Contraindications 45
General Contraindications 45
Considering Sensitive, Dangerous
and Contraindicated Points 46

Chapter 10 **Points of the Lung Channel**   47

Chapter 11 **Points of the
Large Intestine Channel**   59

Chapter 12 **Points of the Stomach Channel**   77

Chapter 13 **Points of the Spleen Channel**   115

Chapter 14 **Points of the Heart Channel**   135

Chapter 15 **Points of the
Small Intestine Channel**   145

Chapter 16 **Points of the Bladder Channel**   159

Chapter 17 **Points of the Kidney Channel**   201

Chapter 18 **Points of the
Pericardium Channel**   215

Chapter 19 **Points of the Sanjiao
(Triple Burner) Channel**   225

Chapter 20 **Points of the
Gallbladder Channel**   239

Chapter 21 **Points of the Liver Channel**   271

Chapter 22 **Points of the Ren Mai
(Conception Vessel) Channel**   287

Chapter 23 **Points of the Du Mai
(Governing Vessel) Channel**   303

**Chapter 24 Extraordinary
(Miscellaneous) Non-channel Points**   321

Resources   345
Index of Points   347

Introduction

Stimulation of specific points on the body surface with the intention of obtaining particular/specific therapeutic effects has been used for thousands of years in many traditional healing systems. There are numerous ancient and modern techniques that have been applied to these points for the purpose of influencing the functional capacity of the body to correct physical and energetic dysfunctions. The application of physical pressure (acupressure), the insertion of needles (acupuncture) and the use of suction cups, magnets, or special herbs and oils, are all traditional methods commonly employed in Eastern therapeutic systems. This text presents clinically useful, practical information for a wide range of specialists including acupuncturists, shiatsu practitioners, physiotherapists and massage therapists.

It describes the common techniques that can be applied to the major acu-points, such as acupuncture, moxibustion, guasha, cupping, magnet therapy and manually applied techniques, as well as describing the different therapeutic effects that can be achieved via those treatment methods.

The various techniques are clearly delineated in headed subsections. It is recommended that all the sections on the different modes of treatment are studied, even if the intention is to use some, but not all, of those methods. This will facilitate a deeper understanding of each point. For example, shiatsu practitioners, tuina practitioners and other bodywork therapists will improve their understanding of the different layers and depths associated with pressure by studying the needling section. Acupuncturists will greatly benefit from using manual techniques, either in the clinic or as self-treatment recommendations for their patients. Most practitioners of Eastern healing systems will benefit from the moxibustion, cupping, guasha and magnet therapy guidelines offered in the text. Furthermore, physiotherapists, nurses and many medical specialists will benefit from the manual techniques section.

Chris Jarmey and Ilaira Bouratinos, 2008

How to Use This Book

Introduction to the Text Format

The text for each point begins with a clear title giving its name and number, followed by a calligraphic image of the Chinese ideogram. Below the title, the classification of the point is mentioned (where relevant). The main text outlines a comprehensive description of the location of the point.

The remaining text is presented in different sections, discussing the treatment and applications. They include the following:

- **Best treatment positions**
- **Needling**
- **Manual techniques and shiatsu**
- **Moxibustion**
- **Cupping**
- **Guasha**
- **Magnets**
- **Stimulation sensation**
- **Actions and indications**
- **Synopsis of the main functions and areas affected**

Title Format

Point name-numbers
The Standard International Acupuncture Nomenclature is used throughout the text. Each point's name consists of the name of the channel and the number of the point from the beginning of the channel, e.g. Lu-9.

Chinese point names
The Chinese point names are written in Pinyin, e.g. Taiyuan.

Chinese characters
E.g. 魚際. The traditional ideograms have been chosen.

English translation
These 'interpretations' of the Chinese point names are those the authors understand as most representative of their meaning, e.g. Great Deep Pool.

Main Text Format

Classification
Classification terms are given in English, followed by the Chinese term. For example, Source-*Yuan* point. For more details, see Chapter 6. For points of the Five Phase categories, the Tonification, Sedation and Horary nature is mentioned in brackets.

Location description
Classical Chinese locations have been used throughout the text. Where there are in effect two or more locations for a point, this is clearly described in the text. Variations of location according to other systems and the authors' own experiences are also mentioned where relevant.

This section also mentions useful tips for locating the point. Every effort has been made to be as anatomically precise as possible and thus resolve the contradictions sometimes found in existing point location descriptions.

The described locations mention the relevant bones, muscles and soft tissues, as well as the superficial anatomical landmarks. The major blood vessels and nerves are mentioned in the *needling cautions* section (marked with an exclamation mark [!]).

The precision of anatomical description does not, however, relieve the practitioner of the responsibility for careful observation and palpation of the area to be treated, so that underlying structures such as blood vessels are protected and the most therapeutically reactive sites are located precisely. The fundamental importance of the role of palpation in point location must not be neglected.

Best treatment positions
This section discusses the best choice of treatment positions to ensure that the point is effectively accessed. Furthermore, it gives special tips in relation to the above.

At the end of this section, the general sensitivity levels of the point are specified, plus general cautions and contraindications in relation to all treatment methods, where relevant. For more information, see the section on sensitive, dangerous and contraindicated points, page 13.

Cautionary notes are marked with an exclamation mark [!]. Text marked with a double exclamation mark [!!] denotes potentially dangerous techniques and contraindications.

Needling
This section details the main needling techniques, including the *minimum and maximum depths, angles* and *directions* for insertion.

The text marked with an exclamation mark [!] cautions the acupuncturist to avoid the blood vessels, nerves and other sensitive structures found at the needling site. Furthermore, text marked with a double exclamation mark [!!] denotes dangerous techniques and contraindications. For more details, see Chapter 1.

Manual techniques and shiatsu
Most points can be treated by manual techniques, whether it is sustained or moving pressure, superficial or deep friction, oil massage or other useful physical manipulation methods such as stretching and mobilisation.

This section details the most effective ways to apply a choice of manual techniques to points where these methods are applicable. Variations and different techniques are discussed in relation to their therapeutic effect and the desired outcome.

The text marked with an exclamation mark [!] mentions the relevant cautions, whereas a double exclamation mark [!!] indicates dangerous techniques and contraindications, accordingly. For more details, see Chapter 2.

Moxibustion
This section details the points indicated for moxibustion and those contraindicated. As a general rule, where there is no mention of it at all, moxibustion should not be used. The times, quantities and types of moxa mentioned are based mainly on Chinese recommendations. Where 'indirect' moxa is mentioned, both traditional moxa poles and other more modern methods of moxa application are intended for use. For more details, see Chapter 3.

Cupping
Cupping is mentioned only where applicable. Where it is not mentioned, it should not be used. For more details, see Chapter 4.

Guasha
The basic guasha method is mentioned where considered most useful and applicable. Where it is not mentioned, it should not generally be used.

Magnets
This section mentions basic usage of magnets and certain point combinations.

Although there are many different points of view on the subject of magnet usage, it is important to understand that the mechanism via which they work is still not fully understood.

Although there are differing opinions on which pole of the magnet is more tonifying or sedating, it is taken in this text that the North Pole is more tonifying and the South more dispersing, when in the Earth's Northern Hemisphere (the opposite applies in the Southern Hemisphere). Throughout the text, it is taken that the treatment is applied in the Northern Hemisphere.

Stimulation sensation
This section discusses the most common manifestations of *deqi* acquired from stimulating the point. It details the quality, intensity, direction and areas the sensation should reach depending on the required therapeutic results. It also mentions other manifestations of deqi such as changes in the pulse, or breathing rate.

Although *deqi* is mostly relevant to the application of acupuncture and manual techniques such as massage and shiatsu, it may also apply to magnet therapy and moxibustion. This section is based on the major acupuncture texts as well as the authors' experience. For more details, see Chapter 5.

Actions and indications
This section discusses the applications for each point. It requires that the reader have an understanding of Traditional Chinese Medicine (TCM) diagnosis and differentiation of syndromes. The main actions (functions) are clearly presented and accompanied by the relevant indications (including signs, symptoms and diseases). The major functions are emphasised in *italic* text. They are based mainly, but not exclusively, on classical Chinese medical theory. Furthermore, there are numerous comments mentioning various interesting and important facts relating to the point.

At the end of the text for each point* there is a quick reference section (synopsis), clearly defined in a text box, highlighting the body areas, organs and functions that are deemed of most use in the clinic.

* Except for a small number of less commonly used points.

Main Areas: Mentions the main body areas, tissues, organs, systems and Zangfu affected by the point.

Main Functions: Mentions the main functions of the point to complement and re-emphasise the italicised functions in the actions and indications section.

The main functions listed in the synopsis text box are often the same as the major functions that are italicised in the section on actions and indications. This means that these repeated functions are of most clinical relevance. In some cases, the synopsis of functions differs from the italicised text. This means that those functions mentioned in the text box are the most clinically relevant. The reason for this is that the italicised functions in the main text are mostly major traditional Chinese functions. For example, *regulating qi and Blood* is a traditional function, whereas *lowering blood pressure* is not (see St-9). Therefore, the italicised functions in the main text and synopsis box must be compared.

The reader must note, however, that because Eastern medicine is an 'art' rather than a precise 'science', there is immense variation in the actions of the points, both in terms of the different traditional schools of thought and the individual practitioner. Therefore, the synopsis of main functions and italicised text serves as a general guide only. Furthermore, the functions that are emphasised, have been chosen as those deemed most clinically applicable according to the authors' own experience and understanding. In this sense, they can be altered or substituted by each practitioner, as he/she considers most appropriate. Every effort has been made to include the most accurate information from principal traditional and contemporary sources.

For example, the synopsis for point Lu-9:

Main Areas: Chest. Lungs. Blood vessels.

Main Functions: Tonifies chest qi. Strengthens the breath and voice. Nourishes Lung yin. Transforms phlegm. Benefits the vessels and improves circulation.

About the Illustrations

These illustrations aim to be as anatomically precise as possible and to show the relevant structures.

The needle insertion site is illustrated with a dot. A broader area around this dot is illustrated with light blue shading. This area displays the site where manual techniques, moxibustion, guasha and cupping can be applied (where relevant). Most of the point illustrations have the shaded area, except where, for reasons of clarity, it was excluded. Also, where there is more than one illustration for any given point, the shaded area is not always repeated.

These shaded areas may also illustrate other possible sites for needling, acupressure and other treatment methods. Possible reasons for treating outside the main point as illustrated with the dot include:

- If deqi cannot be achieved at the specified point, the practitioner must palpate this area carefully to ascertain a more reactive location to insert the needle or apply the pressure, magnet, moxibustion, etc.

- If there is distortion of the main needling site (for example: swelling, skin eruptions, scar tissue, extreme tightness, distended blood vessels), then the practitioner must insert the needle at a different site.

Also, the shaded area may illustrate the area the needle shaft may reach at a deeper level, particularly when applying oblique or transverse needling. For example, the large shaded area between the middle and anterior fibres of the deltoid muscle for the point LI-15 not only illustrates the manual techniques region, but also the area where the needle will be located when using the second needling method mentioned (i.e. needle up to 2 cun at a transverse angle distally, between the anterior and medial fibres of the muscle).

The reader may also notice that some of the dots illustrating a point appear to be slightly smaller (or larger) than others. This is because points do vary somewhat in size. For example, the Well-Jing points at the tips of the fingers are smaller than large fleshy points such as Sp-6 or GB-30.

Chapter 1
Needling Considerations

Precautions to be Taken Before Needling

After carefully assessing the patient's history and current condition, and ruling out any specific or general contraindications (see Chapter 9), the following factors must be taken into account:

- Particularities of the needling sites, including inherent and acquired variations;

- Proximity to vital organs, vessels and other sensitive areas;

- Characteristics of the needles, including size and gauge;

- Angle of needle insertion;

- Depth of needle insertion;

- Manipulation technique(s) used;

- Intensity of stimulation given.

Other precautions to be taken into account:

- The patient should be in a comfortable position, adequately supported by cushions before needling;

- Ensure that the patient remains still and does not change position during needle retention;

- Apply aseptic needling techniques conscientiously;

- Take environmental factors into account, particularly temperature and moisture.

Needling Depth

	Shallow insertion	Deep insertion
Body type	Thin, weak	Robust, obese
Age	Elderly, children	Middle years

The needle depths recommended throughout the text are considered for adults of varying body type within the norm. They do not take into account the following cases, for which the practitioner will have to modify the needling depth accordingly:

- Obesity (deeper needling required);

- Emaciation (more superficial needling required, or only subcutaneous or transcutaneous needling applicable);

- Dwarfism and other genetic variations;

- Extreme deformity (acquired or inherited).

The **minimum depths** are recommended to obtain deqi. Nevertheless, in a substantial proportion of cases, deqi is, or can be, obtained more superficially, subcutaneously or even transcutaneously. However, in general, the minimum depths are too superficial for large body types.

The **maximum depths** are recommended to obtain deqi in large build body types. This means that in a small body type, these depths should NOT be reached (use the minimum depths).

The importance of NOT surpassing the maximum depths cannot be emphasised enough. Surpassing these depths poses CONSIDERABLE RISK OF INJURY.

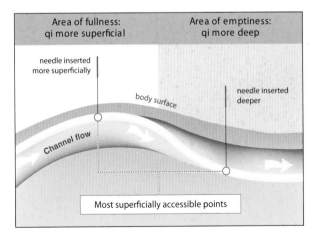

Figure 1.1: Needle depth variation in area of fullness and emptiness along the course of the channel.

Furthermore, it is important to gauge depth by feeling the qi reaction at the needle. If there is no reaction superficially after manipulating, progressively increase depth in order to achieve deqi. Sometimes deqi can be achieved more superficially and sometimes more deeply (see note on deqi stimulation sensation, page 22).

! The maximum depths have been chosen to be on the cautious side of some traditional Chinese needling recommendations that prescribe deeper needling. For example, certain Chinese doctors needle thoracic and upper back points (much) more deeply and at more dangerous angles than is recommended throughout this text. In practice, this means that one can, albeit extremely cautiously, and only after adequate experience, needle more deeply in specific cases.

Needling Angles

The relevant angle and depth of needling must be carefully determined after analysis of the following: the physiological anatomy of the area to be treated and any observable distortions or pathological changes at the needling site, the desired result, and the underlying condition of the patient. Additionally, emotional or environmental factors that could have a bearing on the treatment must be taken into account.

There are three main angles of needle insertion that should be modified according to the treatment requirements.

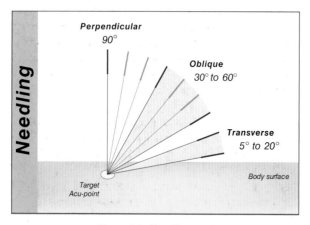

Figure 1.2: Needling angles.

1. Perpendicular insertion (90 degrees)
The most common insertion angle. Especially suitable for thick fleshy areas. More tonifying.

2. Oblique or slanted insertion (30 to 60 degrees)
Suitable where the flesh is thin or where an internal organ or vessel lies deep to the location. Effective to move qi in a particular direction. More dispersing.

3. Transverse insertion (5 to 20 degrees)
Suitable for thin areas with little flesh, and for subcutaneous or transcutaneous needling. Most of the head, face and neck points are needled transversely. Transverse needling is also used to join points.

! The correct needling angle is extremely important because it also indicates to the practitioner not to exceed the correct depth. For example, points on the scalp can be needled to a depth of up to 0.2 cun, BUT at a transverse angle, the needle may be inserted up to 1.5 cun.

Needle Sizes

The size of needles varies by manufacturer. Common needle sizes are listed in the following chart:

Chinese Gauge	Japanese Gauge	Actual Size (mm)
40	0	0.14
38	1	0.16
36	2	0.18
34	3	0.20
32	**5**	**0.25 standard size**
30	8	0.30
28	10	0.32

Figure 1.3: Needle sizes.

Needle Quality

Good quality needles are flexible, have a very sharp tip, and pierce the skin painlessly. It is recommended that only CE certified needles are used.

While needles have been made from a variety of metals, stainless steel is the material of choice for the modern practice. Even unused, new needles can on occasion be bent or blunt and should therefore be carefully inspected before use.

Needling Contraindications

General needling contraindications
Needling should not be applied into scar tissue, wounds, swellings such as cysts, lipomas, skin growths, moles, eruptions, boils, lesions, infections, or lymphoedema. Instead, other points are chosen either along the same channel pathway, or adjacent to the problem area.

Areas not to be punctured
Certain areas should not be punctured; e.g. the fontanelle in babies, the external genitalia, nipples, tongue, gums,

the umbilicus and the eyeball. Clearly nerves, blood vessels and internal organs should not be punctured.

! Needling should be applied with great caution or not at all in patients with bleeding and clotting disorders, or who are taking drugs with an anticoagulant effect, depending on each individual case.

Points contraindicated for needling
St-17, Ren-8.

Dangerous Areas for Needling

Facial points
Points on the face are very sensitive and bruising can easily occur. Nerves, glands and blood vessels are very superficial, especially in thin patients. Take care not to puncture them!

Circulatory system
Puncturing vessels holds the risk of internal bleeding or clot formation (especially in predisposed patients). Care should be taken when needling areas of poor circulation and vascular disease because there is an increased risk of infection or accidental puncturing of an artery (sometimes aberrant). This may lead to bleeding and haematoma formation, as well as to arterial spasm or more serious complications, particularly when pathological change is present, e.g. aneurysm or atherosclerosis.

Bleeding due to puncture of a superficial blood vessel may be stopped by direct pressure.

Thorax, abdomen and back
Deep needling of abdominal, thoracic and back points has the potential danger of puncturing the pleura or peritoneum and injuring vital organs. Cautious needling, preferably obliquely or horizontally, is of utmost importance. Great attention should be paid to the direction and depth of needle insertion. Puncturing organs can cause severe damage and requires emergency medical intervention.

Lung and pleura
In thin patients, 0.5 cm may be enough to puncture the pleura! Injury to the lung and pleura caused by too deep an insertion of a needle into points on the chest, back or supraclavicular fossa may cause traumatic pneumothorax. Cough, chest pain and dyspnoea are the usual symptoms and occur abruptly during the manipulation, especially if there is severe laceration of the lung by the needle. However, symptoms may develop gradually over several hours after the acupuncture treatment.

Intestines
Puncturing the intestines holds substantial risk of severe infection.

Liver, spleen and kidneys
Puncture of the liver or spleen may cause a tear and internal bleeding. Symptoms include local pain and tenderness, and rigidity of the abdominal muscles. Puncturing a kidney may cause lumbar pain and haematuria. If the damage is minor, the bleeding will stop spontaneously but if the bleeding is serious, a decrease of blood pressure and shock may ensue.

Central nervous system
Inappropriate manipulation at points between or beside the upper cervical vertebrae, such as GB-20 (Fengchi), Du-15 (Yamen) and Du-16 (Fengfu) may puncture the medulla oblongata, causing headache, nausea, vomiting, sudden slowing of respiration and disorientation, followed by convulsions, paralysis or coma. Between other vertebrae above the first lumbar, excessively deep needling may puncture the spinal cord, causing lightning electric pain perceived in the limbs or the trunk below the level of puncture.

Dangerous Points for Puncture

The following list contains the most dangerous points for needling, although only eight points are mentioned in the *Guidelines on Basic Training and Safety in Acupuncture* (WHO traditional medicine guidelines, Cervia, Italy, 2001), as being potentially dangerous and requiring special skill and experience in their use. Most of these points are also dangerous in the application of acupressure treatment. Some of these points are also contraindicated for moxibustion.

Dangerous points mentioned in the WHO guidelines on training in acupuncture are: Bl-1, St-1, Ren-22, St-9, Sp-11, Sp-12, Lu-9, Du-15, -16, Lu-1, St-12, and GB-20.

However, many other points discussed in this text are potentially equally dangerous. These include St-12–18, Sp-17–21, LI-17, -18, He-1, SI-14, -15, SI-17, Bl-11–23, -41, -51, Kd-25, -26, SJ-17, GB-3, -24, -25, Liv-13, -14, Ren-2, -3, -12, -17, -23, and Du-20.

Untoward Reactions and Accidents

Accidents and untoward reactions are generally avoidable if all aspects of the treatment are properly considered and adequate precautions are taken (see also previous sections). However, the practitioner should be able to effectively manage such a situation should it occur.

Accidental injury to important organs requires urgent medical or surgical help.

Stuck needle

In certain, albeit rare cases, it is possible for the needle to get stuck in the tissues, making it difficult to remove. It may be difficult or impossible to rotate, lift and thrust, or even to withdraw the needle. This is due to muscle spasm, rotation of the needle with too wide an amplitude, rotation in only one direction causing muscle fibres to tangle around the shaft, or to movement by the patient.

The patient should be asked to relax. If the cause is excessive rotation in one direction, the condition will be relieved when the needle is rotated in the opposite direction. If the stuck needle is due to muscle spasm, it should be left in place for a while, then withdrawn by rotating or massaging around the point, or another needle inserted nearby to divert the patient's attention. If the stuck needle is caused by the patient having changed position, the original posture should be resumed and the needle withdrawn.

Broken needle

Breaks may arise from poor quality manufacture, erosion between the shaft and the handle, strong muscle spasm or sudden movement of the patient, incorrect withdrawal of a stuck or bent needle, or prolonged use of galvanic current.

If a needle becomes bent during insertion, it should be withdrawn and replaced by another. Excessive force should be avoided when manipulating needles, particularly during lifting and thrusting. The junction between the handle and the shaft is the part that is prone to break. Therefore, when inserting the needle, one-quarter to one-third of the shaft should always be kept above the skin.

If a needle breaks, the patient should be told to remain calm and still, to prevent the broken part of the needle from going deeper into the tissues. If part of the broken needle is still above the skin, remove it with forceps. If the needle is at the same level as the skin, press around the site gently until the broken end is exposed, and then remove it with forceps. If the needle is completely under the skin, ask the patient to resume their previous position and the end of the needle shaft will often be exposed. If this is unsuccessful, surgical intervention may be necessary.

Local infection

Negligence in using strict aseptic techniques may cause local infection. When such infection is found, appropriate measures must be taken immediately, or refer the patient for medical treatment. Needling should be avoided in areas of lymphoedema.

Fainting

During acupuncture treatment, the patient may feel faint. The needling procedure and the sensations it may cause should therefore be carefully explained before the treatment. For those about to receive acupuncture for the first time, a lying position with gentle manipulation is preferred. The complexion should be closely watched and the pulse frequently checked to detect any untoward reactions as early as possible. Particular care should be taken when needling points that may cause hypotension (e.g. Liv-3 and LI-4) and points around the neck that may cause excessive sympathetic stimulation (e.g. GB-20 and GB-21).

Symptoms of impending faintness include feeling unwell, a sensation of dizziness, movement or swaying of surrounding objects, and weakness. An oppressive feeling in the chest, palpitations, nausea and vomiting may ensue. The complexion usually turns pale and the pulse is weak.

In severe cases, there may be coldness of the extremities, cold sweats, a fall in blood pressure, and a loss of consciousness. Such reactions are often due to nervousness, hunger, fatigue, and extreme weakness of the patient, an unsuitable position, or too forceful manipulation.

If warning symptoms appear, remove the needles immediately and make the patient lie flat with the head down and the legs raised, as the symptoms are probably due to a transient, insufficient blood supply to the brain. Offer warm sweet drinks. The symptoms usually disappear after a short rest. In severe cases, first aid should be given and, when the patient is medically stable, the most appropriate of the following treatments may be applied:

Press Du-26 with the fingernail or puncture Du-26, P-9, Du-25, P-6 and St-36, or, apply moxibustion to Du-20, Ren-6 and Ren-4. The patient will usually respond, but if the symptoms persist, emergency medical assistance will be necessary.

Convulsions

All patients about to receive acupuncture should be asked if they have a history of convulsions. Patients who do have such a history should be carefully observed during treatment. If convulsions do occur, the practitioner should remove all needles and administer first aid. If the condition does not stabilise rapidly or if the convulsions continue, the patient should be transferred to a medical emergency centre.

Chapter 2
Manual Techniques Considerations

Introduction

There is a wide variety of manual techniques that can be applied specifically to the acu-points. They can be successfully combined with most types of bodywork. Furthermore, they are an excellent adjunct to many forms of medical and paramedical treatment.

The main types of bodywork that traditionally utilise the acu-points are *shiatsu, tuina, anma, and daoyin*. Other types of bodywork that can incorporate the use of acu-points include *any type of massage, reflexology, trigger point therapy, physiotherapy, chiropractic* and *osteopathy*.

Pressure Techniques

The simplest and most widely employed method is stationary perpendicular pressure. The main pressure techniques are:

- Perpendicular pressure
- Non-perpendicular (slanted) pressure
- Stationary pressure
- Moving pressure
- Sustained (continuous) pressure
- Intermittent (alternating) pressure
- Vibrational pressure
- Deep pressure
- Superficial pressure
- Strong pressure
- Gentle touch

Friction Techniques

A form of pressure. The main friction techniques are:

- Circular friction
- Cross-fibre friction
- Friction lengthways to the fibres
- Deep friction
- Superficial friction
- Fast friction
- Slow friction

Stretching and Opening Techniques

Stretching of muscles, tendons, fasciae and other soft tissues situated at or next to the acu-point:

- Stretching across the fibres (cross-fibre)
- Stretching along the length of the fibres
- Stretching and opening of channels
- Stretching of points around joints
- Opening of points and surrounding channel

Other Manual Techniques

There is a variety of other methods that can be used to access specific points:

- Pinching (a form of both pressure and stretching).
- Rolling (a form of both pressure and stretching).
- Hacking (a form of intermittent pressure).
- Rubbing (a form of superficial friction).
- Off the body qi projection (a form of Qigong).
- Muscular contractions (a form of exercise or Sotai).
- Mobilisation (used primarily around the joints to improve qi flow in all channels passing through the joint as well as the points situated around it).

Note
Cupping and guasha are also forms of 'massage'.

Manual Techniques Contraindications

General pressure contraindications

Pressure should not be applied on any area of inflammation or onto wounds or swellings such as cysts, lipomas and skin growths, eruptions such as moles and boils or areas of skin infection. Also, it should not be applied onto areas of distended vessels. Instead, other points are chosen either along the same channel, or adjacent to the problem area.

• Pressure and massage treatment is contraindicated during the first three months of pregnancy, unless otherwise specified by the primary health care practitioner.

• Pressure on abdominal points is contraindicated for the duration of the pregnancy.

• Pressure on the abdomen is contraindicated in any inflammatory condition affecting the abdomen such as gastric or intestinal inflammatory conditions, cysts anywhere in the abdomen including ovaries, fallopian tubes, etc.

• Pressure should not be applied to areas of neuralgia or lymphoedema.

Sensitive areas for pressure application

The application of correct pressure to many areas requires special skill, specifically:

• Pressure on, or next to, the spine

• Pressure on the abdomen

• Pressure on the neck

• Pressure on the throat

• Pressure on the face

• Pressure on the ribs and sternum

• Pressure or massage on areas superior to blood vessels and nerves

• Stretching of the back, neck and other joints

Points contraindicated for pressure and massage

In a normal bodywork situation, for practical reasons, Du-28, St-17, and Ren-1 are contraindicated for treatment.

Chapter 3
Moxibustion Considerations

Introduction

Moxibustion has been used by Classical Chinese Medicine for thousands of years to treat a wide range of disorders. It is often indicated where acupuncture and massage are not effective.

There is substantial variation in the use of moxibustion. The main method of *direct moxibustion* uses cones burnt directly on the skin. *Indirect moxibustion* is usually applied with a moxa pole, or with different types of burners including 'moxa boxes'. Indirect moxibustion can also be applied by placing cones on slices of ginger or garlic or using special ready made cones that stick to the skin. Moxa cones are also burnt on the navel on salt.

The times, quantities and types of moxibustion mentioned throughout the text are general guidelines only and should be carefully considered before application.

General Cautions

The size and number of cones or duration of indirect stimulation with sticks or other moxa burners depends on the constitution of the person receiving treatment, the underlying condition and the areas affected.

Therefore a strong patient with an acute disease and a thick fleshy area requires longer and stronger stimulation and more and larger cones.

Accordingly, a weak patient with a chronic disease and a thin, tendinous, bony or cartilaginous area requires less stimulation and fewer and smaller cones.

- Correct precautions must be taken to avoid burning. Therefore great care should be taken not to overstimulate areas of numbness, or when treating unconscious patients.

- Proper treatment should be applied to inadvertent burns (see page 18 for first aid for burn treatment).

- Moxibustion is contraindicated in febrile diseases.

- Moxibustion is contraindicated in cases of yin deficiency with marked heat signs.

- Moxibustion is contraindicated on the abdomen and lower back in pregnant women.

- Moxibustion is contraindicated close to sensory organs and mucous membranes, particularly the eyes and nose.

- Facial points, points of the throat and submandibular area are very sensitive and are rarely indicated for moxibustion. Overheating these areas can cause inflammation of the ears, eyes and local lymph glands, as well as causing possible damage to blood vessels and nerves.

- Direct moxibustion is contraindicated on all points of the head, face, throat, breast, axillary, pubic and perineal regions.

- Direct moxibustion should not be applied to the sites where tendons or major blood vessels are located close to the body surface. Also, it should not be applied on areas of inflammation, swelling and oedema, or if the patient's sensory awareness may be reduced.

- Special care should be taken with children and weak or elderly patients.

- Special care should be taken with thin or sensitive skin.

- Great care should be taken with diabetic patients and long-term steroid users as they burn much more easily.

- Areas of oedema and varicosities burn very easily.

- Care should also be taken with hairy patients.

Points Contraindicated for Moxibustion

The following points should not be treated with moxibustion:

GB-1, Bl-1, M-HN-8 Qiuhou, St-1, -2, -9, Ren-22, -23, Lu-8, -9, LI-19, -20, SJ-23, Du-26, -27, -28, Ren-1, Liv-12, and Sp-12.

Other points contraindicated for moxibustion, according to classical texts are:

St-8, Lu-3, -4, P-2, He-3, SI-18, Bl-2, GB-33, M-HN-8 Qiu Hou, Du-4 in persons less than 20 years old, Du-15, and -16.

! First Aid for Burns

Traditionally, a small burn from direct moxibustion is required for the treatment to be effective. Stronger burns that leave a scar have also been extensively used for therapeutic purposes. This method is called scarring moxibustion and should not be used in clinical practice.

Mild burns

Run the area under cold water for a few minutes, or apply a cold compress until the burning sensation stops. Apply aloe vera or lavender and a moisturising skin lotion. Also, hydrocortisone cream can be used.

Severe burns

Do not dress the wound or put anything over the area of the burn. Take the patient to hospital.

A 12 ch or 30 ch belladonna homeopathic remedy is effective for burns and can help if the area is very red and hot, particularly if there is throbbing. A 12 ch or 30 ch cantharis remedy can also be used for painful, blistering or peeling burns.

Hydrocortisone cream is the most effective medication for burns and if applied immediately, effectively limits tissue damage.

Chapter 4
Cupping Considerations

Introduction

Cupping is a very effective form of treatment in which a special cup is attached to the body surface. The cup sticks to the skin by means of suction, usually produced by introducing a flaming object into it. The flame burns up the oxygen and produces negative pressure within the cup, thus pulling the skin and subcutaneous tissue upward into it. As a result, qi and blood is activated and drawn to the area.

With *light suction*, the cutaneous and subcutaneous tissues are affected. However, *strong cupping* influences deeper tissues and structures (e.g. deep muscles and internal organs such as the lungs, kidneys and intestines).

Many different types of 'cups' have been employed to apply suction. These include animal horns, hollow pieces of bamboo, earthenware and glass or plastic jars or cups. There are also specially designed pump cups that create the suction without the need to use an ignited object.

Suction cups come in a variety of sizes and some even vary in shape. They are usually shaped like a rounded vase with a narrower rim.

Cupping has been widely used in many traditional Asian and European healing systems to treat a variety of disorders including respiratory diseases, coughing, fevers, intestinal disorders, arthritis and acute or chronic pain conditions.

Functions of Cupping

- Dissipates local stagnation of qi and Blood in both excess and deficiency conditions;
- Alleviates pain;
- Regulates the flow of qi and Blood;
- Causes vasodilation and improves blood circulation;
- Dispels exterior wind, particularly at initial onset;
- Dissipates heat, cold and dampness;
- Descends rising yang (applied down the back);
- Draws Qi to an area and tonifies (with empty cupping);
- Placed over internal organs, strong cupping of short duration can be of benefit (use cupping on the lower back for the kidneys, on the abdomen for the intestines, on the epigastrium for the stomach, etc.);
- Dispels phlegm from the lungs (applied to the thorax);
- Increases gaseous exchange in the lungs;
- Relaxes the body;
- Benefits the nervous system (applied next to the spine);
- Detoxifies the tissues;
- Improves elasticity of the connective tissues and fasciae;
- Reduces cellulite and water retention;
- Gentle cupping helps lubricate and moisten the skin and benefits scar tissue.

Guidelines and Precautions

- Warn the patient that the area may bruise;
- Apply a massage oil to lubricate the skin before placing the cups. If the area is hairy, use a larger quantity of lubricant, and apply vaseline, or similar, to the rim of the cup, so that it sticks to the skin more effectively;
- Begin gently. Use light or medium suction only for the first treatment to ascertain the patient's response and avoid the possibility of undesired reactions. Increase the strength as the treatments continue;
- Ensure the rim of the cup is not too cold, or too hot from excessive exposure to the flaming object, before positioning it.

If you are using a flaming object to create the suction, additionally ensure the following:

- Do not overheat the cup;
- Do not hold the ignited object directly over the patient;
- Use a small quantity of alcohol and ensure there is no excess before placing the flaming object in the cup.
  ! Drops of flaming alcohol can easily fall off;
- Always have an appropriate container close by, to place the flaming object into;
- Ensure there are no flammable materials in the vicinity (e.g. synthetic clothing, paper sheets and polyester pillows) and always have a fire extinguisher in the room;
- Leave the cup(s) in place for 20 minutes at the most. In many cases, 1 to 10 minutes is enough. Leaving the cups on for longer, particularly if the suction is strong, can damage the tissues and cause blistering, bleeding and even systemic symptoms including those of shock;
- When using strong suction and large cups, or if it is very hot, leave the cups in place for a shorter time;
- To remove the cup, press the skin down next to the rim with a finger or a cotton tip to release the vacuum.
  ! Never pull a cup to remove it.

Cupping Cautions

! Do not apply strong suction to the abdomen.

! Only use gentle suction of short duration if the skin is thin or sensitive, or if the person is taking anticoagulant medication.

! Only use gentle suction of short duration on children and weak or elderly patients.

! Only use gentle suction if the patient has hypertension and move downwards only.

Cupping Contraindications

Additional to the contraindications discussed in Chapter 9, cupping should not be applied in the following cases:

! Over broken or ulcerated skin;

! Over oedematous areas;

! Over enlarged blood vessels;

! Over areas where the muscle is thin;

! Over needles on the thorax (except next to the spine where the muscle is thicker);

! On the lower back or abdomen during pregnancy;

! On patients with high fever, convulsions, and cramps;

! On patients who are susceptible to bleeding profusely, or are on thrombolytic or anticoagulant medication.

After Cupping

• Massage the area gently to spread the qi and blood and reduce the congestion created by the suction;

• If strong cupping was used, or if there is any suspicion of inflamed skin, or burn, apply aloe vera gel, lavender water or lavender essential oil in a light plant oil base after the treatment. Also, arnica lotion helps reduce bruising;

• An arnica homeopathic remedy of 12 ch or 30 ch (sometimes a higher potency is given) helps reduce bruising, and also treats systemic symptoms of shock;

• Wash and sterilise the cups after use.

! **First aid for burns**, see page 18.

Methods of Cupping

1. Light suction cupping

The suction is just enough to hold the cup in place. The patient should not feel any pulling and there should be no bruising. The cup can be left on longer than other methods. Gentle or light suction is appropriate for debilitated patients and children.

2. Medium suction cupping

Suction is enough to lift the skin just a little in the cup. There will be very little bruising even if the cup is left on for a long time. There will be a slight pulling sensation.

Medium suction is used in the first treatment before moving onto a stronger method. It is also appropriate for children aged 7–14, and for adults on the abdomen.

3. Strong suction cupping

Suction is strong enough to pull the skin and subcutaneous tissue into the cup. It causes bruising rapidly. Leave the cup in place for no longer than 3 to 5 minutes. Massage the area afterwards to relax the patient.

This method is only appropriate for the back, shoulders and knees on strong adults who are used to medium cupping. It strongly dissipates stasis and draws out pathogenic factors, particularly heat. This is observed in the redness and bruising that occurs. With further treatments, this reaction decreases, indicating that the heat and/or stagnation has been reduced.

! Do not use strong suction on debilitated patients, children or the elderly because it drains Qi.

4. Moving cupping

The cup is moved around with medium suction while it is attached to the skin. The redness and bruising indicates the treatment is working. This reaction decreases with further treatments.

This is a very effective method to draw out pathogenic heat rapidly, descend rising yang (applied down the back), regulate the flow of qi and blood, dissipate stasis and alleviate pain.

5. Alternating cupping

This method uses several cups by removing and re-applying them in sequence. This method draws out cold and dissipates stasis without draining qi.

6. Empty cupping

This is strong suction of up to one minute duration. It immediately draws qi to the area and is used to tonify. It is appropriate for weak adults and children.

7. Moxa cupping

The cup can be positioned without any suction over a medium or large sized moxa cone that has been placed either directly on the skin, or a slice of ginger or garlic. The smouldering moxa will burn up the oxygen to create the suction and then will go out by itself. Alternatively, place the cup with medium or light suction over a half burnt cone (the burning will soon stop).

Furthermore, a large cup can be placed over a warm needle (burn the moxa on the needle).

8. Needle cupping

A large or medium sized cup is applied over an inserted needle after deqi has been achieved. If the suction is strong, blood may be sucked into the cup. This method is used for acute painful conditions such as inflamed, swollen and painful knees, spine or shoulders.

Chapter 5
Deqi

The Importance of Deqi

In Chinese, *'De Qi'* literally means *'to find the qi'*. The term is used to describe the situation where the qi of the point and channel is being mobilised for therapeutic purposes.

In order to explain deqi, we must first describe an acu-point, called *Xue* in Chinese and *Tsubo* in Japanese, as a specific place where the energy from the channels and body tissues gathers and converges. Acu-points are likened to vessels whose function is to hold and contain the qi, but also to offer an opening or doorway that allows the qi to flow harmoniously from the inside of the body to the outside and vice-versa. They are the entrances connecting the outside with the inside thus allowing the practitioner to achieve therapeutic results by activating the qi and Blood of the channels via the body's surface.

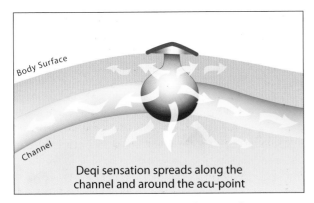

Deqi sensation spreads along the channel and around the acu-point

Figure 5.1: Modified acu-point character depicting the point like a vase.

Because the qi fills up the acu-point, it inevitably flows outward to the body's surface through the 'opening' of the 'vase' (see figure 5.1). In this sense, acu-points are the 'gates' or 'windows' of the person's physical and energy body. It is for this reason that there is an inherent connection between the external and internal environment and a continuous ebb and flow of qi.

When an acu-point is stimulated for therapeutic purposes, its 'door' must first be 'opened' to access the channel passing through it. When correct stimulation is applied, the qi is activated in the desired channels and areas of the body, offering appropriate therapeutic results. It is thus inevitable that when the channels and areas are being properly activated, a 'qi sensation' is felt, indicating that

the qi is being mobilised. This can be likened to opening the door or window into the passageway of a building: when it has been opened, the 'breeze' can be felt clearly.

Deqi sensation has been described in many ways by millions of people throughout the centuries. Some of the most widely used descriptions include 'a relieving ache or pain', 'a spreading feeling', 'numbness', 'tingling', 'distension', 'pulling', 'dullness', 'heaviness', 'warmth', 'dull spreading pain', and 'soreness'. Strong deqi can also produce a sensation of electricity or intense pain extending around the point and along the channel pathway.

Other indications of deqi include changes in the depth and rate of the breathing, pulse rate and rhythm and body temperature. Furthermore, deqi often brings about other manifestations such as abdominal rumbling, sighing, coughing, sweating, itching or lacrimation. It may also induce emotional changes such as sadness, crying or laughing.

Furthermore, deqi can be seen by visible flushing or other colour changes of the skin surrounding the point.

Deqi sensation varies from person to person and is different from one channel or point to another. Moreover, it depends on the state of the person's underlying condition and constitution, the nature and location of the disease as well as other physical, environmental or psychological factors (such as medications used now and in the past, the environmental temperature and weather, time of day, food intake, stress levels, etc.).

Each point is connected to different energetic and neural pathways and consequently produces different sensations. Some produce strong sensations, whereas others do not. Moreover, apart from the intensity of the sensation achievable at a point, there are many variations in the *'quality'* of the sensation. The latter is attributable to the different *intrinsic energetic characteristics* ascribed to the channels and points by the numerous classical Eastern medical practitioners of the past four millennia or more.

Additionally, current research suggests that deqi is apparent on many levels, which we are normally unaware of, thus boosting our understanding of more subtle biological functions. This helps to confirm many traditional theories regarding the movement of qi in the body, thus aiding the modern therapist achieve a deeper understanding of the nature of the channels and of qi.

Specific Therapeutic Deqi

It becomes apparent that because an acu-point may have *a number of different functions, it must also have a similar amount of distinguishable deqi manifestations.* This means that the *specific deqi sensation achieved must be for the specific therapeutic purpose for which the acu-point was chosen.* Thus the sensation varies depending on the desired result. Three different aspects of deqi are briefly analysed:

1. The specific area(s) it reaches;

2. The direction the sensation travels in;

3. The particular quality of the sensation.

1. Areas affected by deqi

When treating disorders of specific body areas, *it is important that the deqi sensation reaches the affected sites* because treatment will not be so effective if this does not occur.

This becomes even more apparent when treating painful conditions. One could go so far as to say that if the sensation does not reach and extend over the entire area of pain, the treatment has little or no result at all.

2. Direction of sensation

The direction the sensation travels in varies greatly from one case to another. However, in general, the qi sensation travels in the following directions, often simultaneously (see also figure 5.1, page 21):

- Extending (radiating) out around the point. *Considered more tonifying.*

- Travelling distally toward the fingers and toes along the course of the channel (applicable mainly to points on the limbs, but may also be induced from treatment applied to spinal and paraspinal points). *Considered more dispersing.*

- Travelling proximally up the limb toward the chest, abdomen or back (applicable only to points on the limbs). *For specific internal disorders. Can tonify and harmonise.*

- Extending inward into the thoracic cavity or abdomen (applicable only to points on the chest, abdomen, back and neck). *For specific internal disorders. Can tonify and harmonise.*

- Extending outward across the back, chest or abdomen (applicable only to points on the back, chest and abdomen). *For specific disorders.*

- Extending from the back to the chest and abdomen (applicable only to spinal and paraspinal points). *For spinal nerve disorders and internal complaints.*

Furthermore, it is common that a sensation is perceived in a completely unrelated area of the body that doesn't seem to have any relationship with the channels, areas or conditions being treated, or with the patient's history. Although there is no general explanation for this phenomenon, it may be simply interpreted as a re-adjustment in the flow of qi within the energy system, brought about by the organism's innate tendency to preserve homeostasis.

When treating systemic disorders with points on the limbs, it is most effective to achieve the sensation travelling proximally toward the target organs and areas. Proximally achieved deqi seems to have better therapeutic results, particularly when treating disorders with manifestations of deficiency.

When treating local channel disorders and pain using proximal and distal points, the sensation should traverse through the diseased area and beyond, distally toward the fingers and toes.

3. Quality of sensation

The quality of the deqi sensation varies from person to person and from location to location. Deqi may be difficult to achieve and varies greatly in patients who are on analgesic, anti-spasmodic, anti-inflammatory, anti-depressant or other forms of medication. Also, persons who are under [a lot of] stress or who have psychological disturbances may react unexpectedly to deqi. They may be hypersensitive to any method of acu-point therapy, reacting in an extreme manner. However, the opposite may also occur, making it impossible to obtain deqi.

Also, there seems to be a certain [small] percentage of the population who do not seem to be able to feel deqi. Another [small] percentage of the population seems to achieve an extremely strong sensation with the slightest stimulation, thus requiring that treatment be applied extremely lightly and superficially (no deep pressure or needling required).

If there is no sensation at all, one of the following may have occurred:

- The pressure or needle was not applied at the right location (the point was mis-located);

- The pressure or needle was not applied correctly (the pressure or needle was applied either too superficially or at the wrong angle, or in some cases the needle tip went too deep through the acu-point);

- The pressure or needle manipulation was applied without qi projection (the practitioner's qi is weaker than the recipient's);

- The patient was extremely deficient in qi and Blood;

- The patient had neurological damage, cerebral transient ischaemic attack or had taken drugs that alter sensation, such as sedatives, analgesics or anti-depressants;

- The needle was too thin or short.

If none of the above applied, the wrong point was chosen for treatment. Choose a point from an area or channel that is more reactive or full of qi and Blood.

If there is 'pain'
When the term 'pain' is used by your client, two questions should be asked:

(1) Does the pain feel sharp, like something is being bruised or injured by pressure, or pricked by a needle, like an injection? *This type of pain may be considered bad pain and indicates wrongly applied treatment.*

! It is often unavoidable to feel a small prick when a needle is being inserted. Although this indicates minor tissue damage, it is not dangerous, except when major blood vessels are punctured. Unfortunately, puncturing of small vessels is sometimes unavoidable, particularly if there is a lot of subcutaneous fat or weakened vascular walls.

(2) Is there also a sensation of 'relief', 'release', 'warmth', 'pulling', 'stretch' or something 'opening up' at the same time? *This type of pain, as long as it is not too excessive, may be considered a good pain and indicates that the qi is being mobilised.*

Terms such as 'dull spreading pain or aching', 'tingling' and 'heaviness' indicate deqi and should be distinguished from the other presentations of pain (such as those caused by wrong pressure or clumsy needling).

Some people are more sensitive to pain than others, thus in general:

- Men are more sensitive to pain than women;

- Children and elderly people are more sensitive than the middle aged;

- Those suffering from stress are usually more sensitive;

- Women during the premenstrual phase tend to be more sensitive;

- Athletes tend to be more sensitive;

- People with a sedentary lifestyle tend to be more sensitive to pain;

- Diabetics and those on long-term corticosteroid use have more sensitive skin;

- In the morning the skin may be more sensitive than toward the end of the day;

- In cold temperatures, the skin and muscles tend to tighten up, causing both acupuncture and acupressure to be more painful;

- Pain sensitivity can also vary significantly between different races.

Additionally, a certain small percentage of the population is extremely sensitive to pain for reasons that are not clear, and are thus put down to constitution or psycho-emotional factors.

In any case, where there may be heightened sensitivity to pain, the practitioner should apply all forms of treatment lightly and gently. Use the thinnest needles applicable and apply all other techniques gently and lightly.

Sharp pain during pressure
The pressure was applied too strong or too hard, too deep, at the wrong angle and/or too suddenly, or the pressure was applied to an inappropriate area; usually a blood vessel being pressed at the wrong angle and too deeply [this can cause bruising].

Electric pain during pressure (or sudden shooting pain)
The pressure was [wrongly] applied directly to a nerve that is either inflamed or located at a very superficial level [usually in thin bony areas]. Excessive and wrongly applied pressure may cause inflammation of the nerve.

! Pressure is contraindicated on areas of neuralgia.

Sharp pain or pricking during needle insertion
Unskilful needling, particularly inserting the needle tip too slowly or at the wrong angle to the skin, causes a strong pricking sensation. Use of a blunt, bent or excessively thick needle can also do the same. In addition, using too thin a needle can cause a strong prick because the shaft is too flexible and thus more difficult to insert, particularly if the skin is thick or tight.

Inserting the needle too quickly below the subcutaneous layer into the deeper tissues is dangerous and can result in damage to nerves, blood vessels and even internal organs. The needle should always be inserted slowly to the correct depth, so that if pain or a strong sensation occurs, deeper insertion is avoided.

! It is generally normal for a small prick to be felt when a needle is inserted, although a competent acupuncturist should generally be able to needle without causing any pain. Using a guide tube helps to minimise the risk of causing a prick, because the needle tip can be inserted more quickly and easily. It is recommended to use a guide tube on very sensitive patients and very thin needles (0.14 to 0.22 mm).

Pain when the needle is inserted deeply

This can be due to hitting pain receptor nerve fibres, in which case the needle should be lifted until the tip is in the subcutaneous layer and carefully re-inserted in a different direction. Also this could indicate blood vessel injury, particularly if accompanied by a burning sensation.

Pain during needle manipulation

This usually occurs when the needle is rotated with too wide an amplitude, or during lifting and thrusting manipulation, and is normally due to it becoming entwined with fibrous tissue or muscle fibres. To relieve the pain, gently rotate the needle back and forth until the fibre is released.

Burning pain during needle retention

This means a vessel has been punctured. The burning pain sensation is from the bleeding in the tissues. Remove the needle and apply pressure to the point. Additionally a cold compress can be applied.

Sharp or electric pain during needle retention

Sharp pain occurring while the needle is in place is commonly caused by it changing position or bending due to the patient moving, and is relieved by resuming the original position.

If this is not the case, it means needling was done too suddenly, too deeply, at the wrong angle or the wrong location. Consequently, the needle could have pricked a blood vessel or be close to a nerve.

In an extreme situation, this could mean the needle has damaged the nerve. In such a case, the patient may feel the pain for several weeks after the needling. As far as thoracic points are concerned, remove the needles immediately if there is pain associated with breathing.

Excessively strong sensation, electric or spreading pain during needle retention

This could mean a strong deqi, or the needle tip is close to a nerve sheath. (Compare the anatomy of local channel and nerve pathways, to ensure deqi manifests along the channel, not the nerve pathway.)

Pain after withdrawal of the needle

This is usually due to unskilled or excessive manipulation and is either caused by bruising or nerve damage. In the former, the pain will subside after a few days. However, if a nerve has been damaged, the pain may continue for several weeks.

There are also many cases where pain is perceived after the withdrawal of the needle but subsides very quickly in minutes or a few hours. This generally indicates a continuation of the qi sensation.

To relieve pain, apply stationary pressure to the affected area. Moxibustion can also be helpful. Also, apply arnica lotion if bruising is suspected. In the case of nerve damage, apply lavender, geranium or chamomile essential oil in an appropriate base, daily until the pain has disappeared.

Chapter 6
Classification of Points

All the body's points may be divided into two broad categories: those whose location and functions have been precisely charted and described, known as *Fixed points* or *Classified points*, and those that have not been charted, known as *Transient points*.

The first broad category includes all the channel and non-channel points. The channel points have been grouped into various categories according to their energetic quality and the areas, substances and types of conditions they treat. The main categories of the points are discussed in the following pages.

The *Non-channel points* (also known as *Extra*, or *Miscellaneous points*) include both the traditional extra points, mapped out thousands of years ago, and other more recently discovered ones, called *New points*. They are used in the treatment of specific conditions or body areas.

The second broad category, the *Transient points*, are points whose locations vary, as they are an immediate reflection of the particular disharmony and its relationship to the person. They are therefore inherently unchartable.

Transient points are found either as reactive points along the channel pathways and other specific areas treated, or anywhere else on the body. In this case they are known as *Ashi points* (meaning 'that's it'). Ashi points are found anywhere there is pain, tenderness or other abnormal sensations, manifesting either on palpation or spontaneously. They are usually used to treat pain conditions and their local area, but are also effective in other cases. Pain should be diminished after treatment. Additionally we will emphasise another two, albeit nonclassical, broad point categories based on worldwide popularity and frequency of use in acupuncture and bodywork.

The Top Most Commonly Used Points

This category includes those points that seem to be used most often: **LI-4, -11, St-36, Kd-3, Sp-6, P-6, GB-34, Liv-3, Lu-5, -7, -9, SJ-5, He-7, Ren-4, -6, -12, -17, St-25**, Back Transporting Shu points (particularly **Bl-23, -20, -18, -17, -15, -13), Du-4, -14, -20, Ren-3, -17, St-40, -44.**

The most commonly used points are important for a variety of reasons, including:

- They have a wider range of indications and therefore are used in more cases.

- They are very dynamic and powerful points having stronger therapeutic results than other points of the same channel or category. For example, Liv-3 is the most commonly used liver point.

- They are also chosen in many cases where the treatment principle and diagnosis are not clarified in detail so that choosing such a point, even without a diagnosis, is more likely to be of benefit.

Special Point Categories (Classifications)

The Back-Shu and Front-Mu Points

Both the *Front Collecting Mu* and the *Back Transporting Shu* points have an immediate and powerful effect on their pertaining organs. They may be tender, either spontaneously or on palpation, and are therefore also useful in diagnosis. Employing Mu and Shu points together offers a particularly powerful treatment.

The *Front Collecting Mu points*, also known as *Alarm points*, or *Bo points* in Japanese, are located on the chest and the abdomen, directly above their pertaining organs (see figure 6.1, page 27). It is here that the qi of each internal organ converges and gathers. The Mu points have an immediate and direct effect on the internal organs and are therefore used more often in acute conditions to treat the Yang Organs. They are:

Lung	**Lu-1**	Bladder	**Ren-3**
Large Intestine	**St-25**	Kidney	**GB-25**
Stomach	**Ren-12**	Pericardium	**Ren-17**
Spleen	**Liv-13**	San Jiao	**Ren-5**
Heart	**Ren-14**	Gallbladder	**GB-24**
Small Intestine	**Ren-4**	Liver	**Liv-14**

The *Back Transporting Shu points*, also known as *Associated points*, or *Yu points* in Japanese, are located on the back, directly above their pertaining organs to which they send, or 'transport', qi directly (see figure 6.1, page 27). They have a direct tonifying influence on the internal organs and are used in both acute and chronic conditions, particularly when there is depletion of the vital substances. The Shu points also treat the orifices that pertain to their associated organ, and are:

Lung	**Bl-13**	Bladder	**Bl-28**
Large Intestine	**Bl-25**	Kidney	**Bl-23**
Stomach	**Bl-21**	Pericardium	**Bl-14**
Spleen	**Bl-20**	San Jiao	**Bl-22**
Heart	**Bl-15**	Gallbladder	**Bl-19**
Small Intestine	**Bl-27**	Liver	**Bl-18**

Additional Back Shu points

These points, although not directly related to the Zangfu organs, could be considered extra Back Shu points because they have a special effect on their associated areas, body functions and psycho-emotional aspects:

Du Mai Shu point	**Bl-16**
Diaphragm Shu point	**Bl-17**
Sea of Qi Shu point	**Bl-24**
Original Qi Gate Shu point	**Bl-26**
Backbone (lower spine)	**Bl-29**
White ring (anus) Shu point	**Bl-30**
Uterus	**Bl-32**
Vital Region Shu point	**Bl-43**
Upper Arm Shu point	**SI-10**
Outer Shoulder point	**SI-14**
Middle Shoulder point	**SI-15**

Psycho-emotional Back Shu points:

Corporeal Soul Door	**Bl-42**
Gate of the Ethereal Soul	**Bl-47**
Willpower Room	**Bl-52**
Spirit Hall	**Bl-44**
Abode of Thought	**Bl-49**

The Source-Yuan Points

The *Source-Yuan points* for each of the Twelve Regular Channels are located at the wrists and ankles. They have a profound tonifying effect on the underlying energy of the organs and are very important in the treatment of any chronic condition, particularly when there is depletion of the vital substances. In general, they are of increased significance on the Yin channels.

The Source-Yuan points are: **Lu-9, LI-4, St-42, Sp-3, He-7, SI-4, Bl-64, Kd-3, P-7, SJ-4, GB-40,** and **Liv-3.**

The Accumulation Cleft-Xi Points

The *Accumulation Cleft-Xi points* are where the qi of the channels accumulates, just as water gathers in a crevice or cleft. They are therefore used to treat acute, excess conditions either of the organ itself or the channel, particularly when there is pain. On the Yin channels, they also treat disorders of the Blood (including heat and stasis of Blood).

There is one accumulation point on each of the Twelve Regular Channels: **Lu-6, LI-7, St-34, Sp-8, He-6, SI-6, Bl-63, Kd-5, P-4, SJ-7, GB-36,** and **Liv-6.**

Additionally, there are four accumulation points for the Eight Extraordinary Vessels:

Yang Qiao Mai	**Bl-59**
Yang Wei Mai	**GB-35**
Yin Qiao Mai	**Kid-8**
Yin Wei Mai	**Kd-9**

The Connecting-Luo Points

The *Connecting-Luo points* are employed to harmonise the qi between the yin and yang paired channels via opening their Connecting channel. For this reason, they are often used to transfer pathogenic factors from one channel to another (usually from the Yin channel to its Yang pair). They are also employed in the treatment of signs and symptoms of disharmony of the fifteen Connecting Luo channels, disorders of the five emotions and the five openings (sensory organs).

The Connecting points of the Twelve Regular channels are: **Lu-7, LI-6, St-40, Sp-4, He-5, SI-7, Bl-58, Kd-4, P-6, SJ-5, GB-37** and **Liv-5**.

There are also three additional Connecting Luo points:

Great Luo of the Spleen	**Sp-21**
Du Mai	**Du-1**
Ren Mai	**Ren-15**

The Four and Six Command Points

These points are very important and commonly used because they treat any disorder of these areas:

Face and Mouth	**LI-4**
Neck and Head	**Lu-7**
Abdomen	**St-36**
Back	**Bl-40**
Chest (thorax)	**P-6**
Mind (resuscitation)	**Du-26**

The Eight Gathering Hui Points

The *Eight Gathering Hui points*, also called *Influential* or *Meeting points*, are points where the energy of the organs, certain tissues and vital substances, gathers and accumulates. The Gathering points have a direct influence on these and are used to treat various conditions affecting them.

Qi	**Ren-17**
Blood	**Bl-17**
Vessels	**Lu-9**
Marrow	**GB-39**

Bone	**Bl-11**
Sinews	**GB-34**
Yin organs (zang)	**Liv-13**
Yang organs (fu)	**Ren-12**

The Five Transporting Shu Points

The *Five Transporting Shu points* are five points on each channel located distal to the elbows and knees, whose quality of qi can be likened to the flow of water along its course, starting at a well and reaching a distant ocean. Each of these points has an individual energetic character that distinguishes the nature of the qi flowing through it. This is irrespective of the other categories they may be grouped into. The Five Transporting Shu points can also be classified in relation to the Five Phases and are employed in the treatment of imbalances among the Elements (see figure 6.2).

The *Well-Jing points* are located at the distal ends of the Twelve Regular channels, at the tips of the fingers and toes. At these points, the qi of the channels is at its most superficial, flowing rapidly in an outward direction. It is here that the polarity of Yin/Yang changes as the paired channels flow into one another. The Well-Jing Points have a powerful effect on the mind and are used for insomnia, anxiety, irritability and to restore consciousness. They also activate the channel pathways in cases of pain and other channel disorders. On the Yin channels they are allocated to the Wood Element, and on the Yang, to the Metal Element.

The *Spring-Ying points*, the second points along the channels, are located at the base of the fingers and toes. The qi here is likened to a swirling spring where the water gushes outward. Their function is similar to that of the Well-Jing points insofar as the qi here is dynamic and moves rapidly. Thus they are used to clear pathogenic factors, particularly Heat and Fire. On the Yin channels they are allocated to Fire, and on the Yang, to Water.

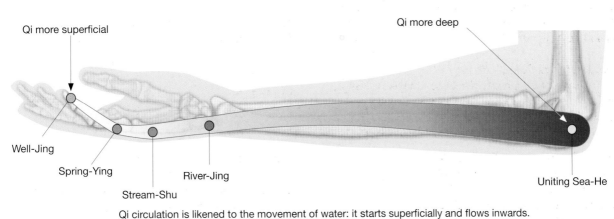

Qi circulation is likened to the movement of water: it starts superficially and flows inwards.

Figure 6.1: Schematic representation of the Five Transporting Shu points.

5 Transporting Points	Well-Jing	Spring-Ying	Stream-Shu	River-Jing	Sea-He
Lungs	11	10	9	8	5
Large Intestine	1	2	3	5	11
Stomach	45	44	43	41	36
Spleen	1	2	3	5	9
Heart	9	8	7	4	3
Small Intestine	1	2	3	5	8
Bladder	67	66	65	60	40
Kidney	1	2	3	7	10
Pericardium	9	8	7	5	3
San Jiao	1	2	3	6	10
Gallbladder	44	43	41	38	34
Liver	1	2	3	4	8

Figure 6.2: The Five Transporting Shu and Five Phase points.

The *Stream-Shu points*, the third points along the channels, are located on the wrists and ankles on the Yin channels, and on the dorsal aspect of the hands and feet on the Yang channels. The qi here, although still moving quickly, begins to enter a little deeper into the circulation and broadens out. It is at these points that pathogens penetrate deeper into the channels and the Defensive qi (Wei qi) gathers here to protect the interior of the body. On the Yin channels they are primarily used to tonify and nourish the organs, and on the Yang, to expel pathogenic factors. On the Yin channels they are also source points (see page 26) and are allocated to the Earth Element. On the Yang channels they belong to Wood.

The *River-Jing points* are located on the forearm and leg on the Yin channels and are allocated to Metal, whereas on the Yang channels they are found at the wrists and ankles and pertain to Fire. The qi at the River-Jing points flows like a strong current after coming a long way from its source. The qi at these points is much bigger, wider and deeper, and it is here that pathogens enter into the joints, tendons and bones. River-Jing points are commonly used in the treatment of painful obstruction syndrome and arthritis.

The *Uniting Sea-He points*, located at the elbows and knees, are where the qi of the channel becomes deep and joins the systemic circulation of the body, like a river flowing into the sea. The qi at these points moves slowly inwards towards the pertaining organ. The Uniting Sea-He points have a deeper but less immediate effect. They are used to harmonise the qi of the internal organs in both acute and chronic conditions by clearing interior pathogenic factors and regulating the flow of qi. Some are also important to tonify the vital substances. On the Yin channels they are allocated to the Water Element, and on the Yang channels, to the Earth Element.

There are three additional *Uniting Sea-He points*, known as the *Lower Sea points*, one each for the Large Intestine, Small Intestine and San Jiao, respectively. They are: **St-37, -39**, and **Bl-39**.

The Five Phase points correspond to the Five Transporting Shu points:

Point	Well-Jing		Spring-Ying		Stream-Shu		River-Jing		Sea-He
Yin channel	Wood	→	Fire	→	Earth	→	Metal	→	Water
Yang channel	Metal	→	Water	→	Wood	→	Fire	→	Earth

Figure 6.3: Schematic representation of the Five Phase points.

Five Phase Point Selection

There are a variety of different applications for the Five Phase points. These depend on the specific emphasis the practitioner wants to give. Some examples are given below:

In cases of deficiency of an Element, the point pertaining to the *Mother Element* may be chosen to tonify it. In the case of deficiency of the Liver and Wood Element, for example, the point Liv-8 can be chosen (Liver pertains to Wood and Liv-8 is a Water point: Water generates Wood).

These points are known as *Tonification points* and are: **Lu-9, LI-11, St-41, Sp-2, He-9, SI-3, Bl-67, Kd-7, P-9, SJ-3, GB-43,** and **Liv-8.**

In the case of excess, the *Child Element* point is dispersed (sedated). For example, Liver fire may be treated using the point Liv-2 (Liv-2 is a fire point: Fire is the child of Wood and therefore sedates it).

The *Sedation points* are: **Lu-5, LI-2, St-45, Sp-5, He-7, SI-18, Bl-65, Kd-1, P-7, SJ-10, GB-38,** and **Liv-2.**

Another use of the Five Phase points is the reinforcing of a particular element using the *Horary points*. These points belong to the same Element as the one we want to affect. For example we could use Lu-8 to reinforce the Lung Qi (Lu-8 is a Metal point).

The *Horary points* are: **Lu-8, LI-1, St-36, Sp-3, He-8, SI-5, Bl-66, Kd-10, P-8, SJ-6, GB-41,** and **Liv-1.**

The Five Phase points are also employed in the treatment of associated psychosomatic and emotional disorders ascertained by the Five Phase diagnosis.

Additionally, conditions caused by the related pathogenic factors are commonly treated via these points: Water points treat cold, dampness and phlegm conditions; Wood points treat wind; Fire points treat heat and fire; Earth points treat dampness and phlegm; whereas Metal points treat dryness.

Reinforcing of particular qualities associated with the Five Phases is also employed in order to tonify and harmonise the vital substances. For example, the Earth points are used to tonify and nourish qi and Blood while Water points are used to cool and moisten fluids and yin. Accordingly, Fire points can tonify yang.

The Five Phase method of point selection is generally combined with an understanding of the other actions a point may have. He-9, for example, is the Tonification point for the Heart, but is not as commonly used to treat deficiency of the Heart as He-7, because Well-Jing points are mostly used in the treatment of acute conditions.

5 Phase Points	Wood	Fire	Earth	Metal	Water
Lungs	11	10	9	8	5
Large Intestine	3	5	11	1	2
Stomach	43	11	36	45	44
Spleen	1	2	3	5	9
Heart	9	8	7	4	3
Small Intestine	3	5	8	1	2
Bladder	65	60	40	67	66
Kidney	1	2	3	7	10
Pericardium	9	8	7	5	3
San Jiao	3	6	10	1	2
Gallbladder	41	38	34	44	43
Liver	1	2	3	4	8

Figure 6.4: The Five Phase points.

The Window of Heaven Points

The *Window of Heaven points*, also known as *Window of the Sky points*, were traditionally considered to treat the 'Five Regions of the Window of Heaven', i.e. the five sense organs or orifices.

These points are often used for treating psychological disturbances and disorders of the sense organs and neck area. Also, many of these points are indicated for rebellious qi and disorders of sudden onset.

Indications include headache, dizziness, aphasia, epilepsy, fainting, mental confusion, excessive dreaming, insomnia, diminished memory and concentration, deafness, tinnitus, diminished hearing or vision, eye pain, inability to open the eyes, excessive lacrimation, epistaxis, loss of sense of smell, redness and swelling of the face, aphasia, coughing, dyspnoea, spitting blood, vomiting, goitre, and lymphadenopathy.

Originally there were five points listed. Subsequently the other five were added to this list. However, there is a great deal of discrepancy as to their functions. Also, various sources differ in their opinion on which points are included in this category. For example, according to some sources, SI-17 should in fact be GB-9.

The original Window of Heaven points are: **Lu-3, St-9, LI-18, SJ-16,** and **Bl-10.** The additional five points are: **Ren-22, SI-16, SI-17, Du-16,** and **P-1.**

The Nine Points for Returning Yang

According to classical texts, these nine points are most important for treating yang collapse. Symptoms include cyanosis, profuse sweating, tachycardia, aversion to cold, shivering and loss of consciousness. They are: **LI-4, St-36, Sp-6, Kd-1, -3, P-8, GB-30, Du-15,** and **Ren-12.**

The Thirteen Ghost Points

The use of these points to treat psychiatric disorders and epileptic conditions was established in the Tang dynasty (8th century). They are: **Du-26, Lu-11, Sp-1, P-7, Bl-62, Du-16, St-6, Ren-24, M-HN-37 (Haiquan), Du-23, Ren-1, LI-11,** and **P-8.**

The Twelve Heavenly Star Points

These points were considered the most useful by the renowned physician Ma Dan Yang in the Song Dynasty (10th/11th century). They are: **St-36, St-44, LI-11, LI-4, Bl-40, Bl-57, Liv-3, Bl-60, GB-30, GB-34, He-5,** and **Lu-7.**

The Points of the Four Seas

According to the Yellow Emperor's inner medical classic, there are four 'Seas' in the human body. These are: the Sea of Qi, the Sea of Blood, the Sea of Nourishment (or Sea of Water and Grain), and the Sea of Marrow.

The Sea of Qi points
These points are traditionally indicated for both excess and deficiency disorders of qi. Symptoms include fullness of the chest, dyspnoea, weak breathing and exhaustion. They are: **St-9, Ren-17, Du-14,** and **Du-15.**

The Sea of Blood points
These points are traditionally indicated for both excess and deficiency disorders of the Blood, and are: **Bl-11, St-37,** and **St-39.**

The Sea of Nourishment points
These points, also known as the *Sea of Water and Grain,* are traditionally indicated for both excess and deficiency disorders of the abdomen. Indications include fullness and pain of the abdomen, hunger and inability to eat. They are: **St-30,** and **St-36.**

The Sea of Marrow points
They are traditionally indicated for both excess and deficiency disorders of the Marrow. Indications include dizziness, tinnitus, poor vision, and on a psychological level, they are recommended for laziness. They are: **Du-16,** and **Du-20.**

The Eight Extraordinary Vessels

The Eight Extraordinary Vessels, unlike the Twelve Regular Channels, are not directly related to individual Zangfu organs, although they do have a close relationship to the Kidneys, Uterus and Brain. They aid the flow of qi and Blood in the regular channels by acting as reservoirs (the Twelve Regular Channels are more like rivers). When there is a surplus of qi and Blood in the regular channels, it overflows into the Extraordinary Vessels. Conversely the qi and Blood from the Extraordinary Vessels is transferred to the Regular Channels as needed. The latter may occur in times of greater demand, such as during a chronic illness, shock or pregnancy.

'*The Eight Extraordinary Vessels are so named because they do not conform to the norm. Qi and Blood constantly flow through the twelve regular channels and, when abundant, overflow into the Extraordinary Vessels*'.

The filling and emptying of the Extraordinary Vessels ensures a constant and uninterrupted flow of qi and Blood in the Regular Channels, so that homeostasis is maintained. Thus, the Extraordinary Vessels do not have their own continuous pattern of circulation but rather respond to the fluctuations of the Twelve Regular Channels. According to the Yellow Emperor's classic of internal medicine (*Nei Jing*), '*When there are heavy rains, canals and ditches are full to the brim...similarly, the extraordinary vessels are left out of the channel system so that they can take the overflow from the main channels*'.

The Extraordinary Vessels regulate the circulation of Essence, acting as a link between the Pre-heaven Qi (Xian Tian Qi) and Post-heaven Qi (Hou Tian Qi) They are mostly used for treating problems of the Essence and constitution. The Chong and Ren Mai (Penetrating and Conception Vessels) particularly influence the cycles of the Essence that control growth, development, reproduction and the ageing process. Each cycle lasts seven years in women and eight years in men.

The Chong, Ren and Du Mai also circulate the Defensive qi over the thorax, abdomen and back thus aiding in the protection of the body from exterior pathogenic factors.

The Eight Opening and Coupled Points

With the exception of the Ren Mai and Du Mai, the Extraordinary Vessels do not have their own points, but rather share the points of the Twelve Regular Channels. Their qi is accessed via a special point that opens them, known as the *Opening point* (also called the *Master point* or *Confluent point*) and a *Paired point*, known as the *Coupled point*. The Eight Opening points are those where the Extraordinary Vessels connect to the Twelve Regular Channels. They are listed below.

The Extraordinary Vessels are grouped into pairs according to their Yin-Yang polarity. Each pair shares the Opening and Coupled point. Thus, the Opening point on the upper limb is combined with the one on the lower limb.

	Opening point	Coupled point
Du Mai	SI-3	Bl-62
Ren Mai	Lu-7	Kd-6
Chong Mai	Sp-4	P-6
Dai Mai	GB-41	SJ-5
Yang Qiao Mai	Bl-62	SI-3
Yin Qiao Mai	Kd-6	Lu-7
Yin Wei Mai	P-6	Sp-4
Yang Wei Mai	SJ-5	GB-41

The *Du Mai*, also known as the *Governing Vessel*, traverses the entire spine up the posterior midline, ascending to the head and face, and joining all the yang channels at Du-14. It is considered to be the most yang of all the channels and is known as the *Sea of Yang*.

The *Ren Mai*, also known as the *Conception Vessel* or *Directing Vessel*, ascends across the abdomen and chest, up the posterior midline to reach the face. It connects all the Yin meridians and is also called the *Sea of Yin*.

The *Chong Mai*, known as the *Penetrating Vessel*, runs parallel to the Kidney channel up the legs, through the abdomen and chest, reaching the face. It connects the Twelve Regular Channels and acts as a reservoir for their Qi and Blood. Thus, it is also called the *Sea of Blood*.

The *Yin Wei Mai*, known as the *Yin Linking Vessel*, connects and regulates the flow of Qi in all the Yin channels and dominates the interior of the body.

The *Yin Qiao Mai*, known as the *Yin Heel Vessel* or *Yin Motility Vessel*, starts at the medial aspect of the heel and travels up the inside of the body, following the Kidney channel, reaching the face where it joins the Yang Heel Vessel at the inner canthus of the eye. It regulates the ascending and descending of Yin Qi.

The *Yang Qiao Mai*, known as the *Yang Heel Vessel* or *Yang Motility Vessel*, starts at the lateral aspect of the heel and travels up the lateral side of the body to join the Yin Qiao Mai at the eyes. It regulates the ascending and descending of Yang Qi and the movement of the lower limbs.

The *Yang Wei Mai*, known as the *Yang Linking Vessel*, connects and regulates the flow of Qi in all the Yang channels and dominates the exterior of the body.

The *Dai Mai*, also known as the *Girdle Vessel* or *Belt Meridian*, originates at the hypochondrium, encircles the waist, and binds all the other channels.

In practice, however, the Eight Opening points are also used independently for their specific functions.

- Sp-4 is combined with P-6 to treat diseases of the Heart, chest, or Stomach.

- Lu-7 is combined with Kd-6 to treat diseases of the Lung, chest, throat, or diaphragm.

- SJ-5 is combined with GB-41 to treat diseases of the outer canthus, ear, shoulder, neck, or cheek.

- SI-3 is combined with Bl-62 to specifically treat diseases of the inner canthus, neck, or shoulder.

The Six Divisions

There are Twelve Regular Channels, divided into *six Yin* and *six Yang*. These channels are grouped into two sets of six pairs. The first set is known as the *interiorly-exteriorly related channels*, or the *yin-yang paired channels*. The yin-yang paired channels meet at the tips of the fingers and toes, where the polarity of yin-yang changes.

The Twelve Regular Channels are further subdivided into *three pairs of Yin* and *three pairs of Yang channels* known as the *Six Divisions*. The three pairs of Yang channels meet at the face whereas the Yin meets on the chest.

The channels running along the anteromedial surface of the limbs are the *Greater Yin channels*. Those traversing the anterolateral surface of the limbs are the *Bright Yang channels*. Those traversing the middle of the medial surface of the limbs are the *Absolute Yin channels*. Those traversing the middle of the lateral surface of the limbs are the *Lesser Yang channels*. The channels running along the posteromedial surface of the limbs are the *Lesser Yin channels* and finally those running along the posterolateral surface of the limbs are the *Greater Yang*.

Thus, the Six Divisions reflect the similarity of the energy flowing in the upper and lower limbs.

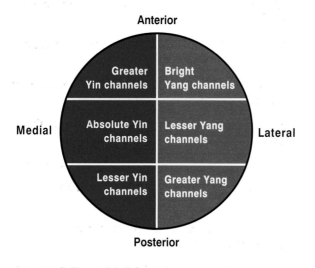

Figure 6.5: Schematic representation of the channel distribution on the four limbs.

The Chinese Clock

As the rhythms of nature fluctuate from day to night, winter to summer and so on, so the qi in the channels waxes and wanes. During the daily 24-hour cycle, the qi surges through each of the twelve channels for two hours. It does this following the Six Divisions schema. Starting at 3 a.m. the qi enters the Lung channel and every two hours flows to the next, ending in the Liver.

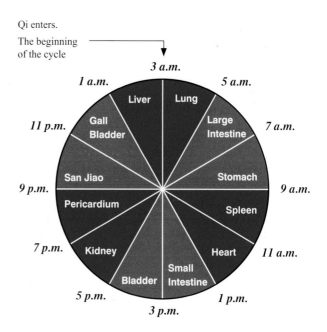

Figure 6.6: The Chinese Clock.

Thus each channel has a particular time during which it is fullest of qi and an opposite one, during which its qi is at its lowest. A symptom occurring daily at the same time may be related to the channel that is at its peak, or the one that is at its lowest. A problem occurring around 5 a.m. may therefore be related to either the Large Intestine or the Kidney, or to both. Treatment effects can be maximised by applying the treatment at certain times of day.

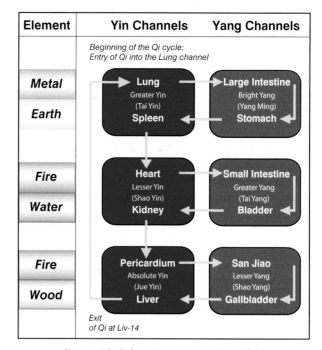

Figure 6.7: Schematic representation of the flow of qi throughout the 12 channels.

Chapter 7
Principles of Point Selection

How to Choose Points

Choosing a set of points that work together harmoniously to treat the whole person plus the specific complaint is accomplished according to the principles laid out over thousands of years of clinical experience by the practitioners of Traditional Chinese Medicine. In order to make the most effective choice, all the energetic qualities of a point must be studied in detail, in addition to the patient's case history and current symptoms plus those environmental, psycho-emotional and physical factors that may play a role in the outcome of the treatment.

It is most important to remember that an effective choice of points cannot be achieved without an accurate diagnosis. It is therefore of great importance to ensure that the diagnosis is concise and clear. The selection of points is based on the treatment principle and should thus include:

- Points that treat the *cause*, or '*Roots*' (*Ben* in Chinese) of the disease;
- Points that treat the *manifestation*, or '*Branches*' (*Biao* in Chinese) of the disease.

In general, if the disorder is primarily due to deficiency of the Vital substances, treat the cause (root), whereas if it is due to excess, treat the manifestations (branches).

Furthermore, if the problems manifest primarily with signs of *deficiency* and *emptiness*, points and techniques that bring the energy inwards close to the centre of the body, toward the affected area(s) are chosen. In these cases, points on the affected area, or close to it, are of most significance. Such points are known as *Local points*, and can be further divided into:

- **Local points**: Exactly on the affected area.
- **Adjacent points**: Close to the affected area.

Conversely, if there are many manifestations or symptoms of excess and blockage in the form of pathogenic factors or stagnation of qi and Blood, points and techniques that dissipate, expel and move the qi outwards are chosen (generally, the qi moves toward the surface of the body and the extremities). Therefore, points located away from the problem area toward the extremity are of most importance. These are known as *Distal points*, as many of the most important points are located on the limbs.

The selection of Distal points can be further divided as follows:

- Selecting points on the extremities to treat the centre of the body and vice-versa.
- Selecting proximal and distal points on the limbs.
- Selecting points on the upper body to treat the lower part.
- Selecting points on the lower body to treat the upper part.
- Selecting points contralaterally (on the left of the body to treat the right and vice-versa).
- Selecting points on the front of the body to treat the back and the opposite.
- Selecting points on the yin and yang related channels.
- Selecting points on the Six Divisions' related channels.
- Selecting points according to specific channel connections and intersections.
- Selecting special Distal points that are beyond the scope of this text, such as ear, Sujok or reflexology points.

Chart A
Selecting Points According to Area
(Local and Distal Points)

Further to the differentiation of syndromes, a skilled practitioner will observe the channels, points and areas of the entire body as well as those directly related to the specific complaint, in order to ascertain the best points' prescription. Assessing the channels and points is a very important facet of diagnosis.

Selection of points according to the diseased area is especially important when dealing with disorders of the channel pathways and pain conditions. A temporal headache, for example, may be treated according to the affected channels: the Gallbladder in this case.

Points are also selected to treat their Yin/Yang paired channel and organ, as well as the channel related along the Six Divisions.

Liv-3 may for example, be selected to treat the Gallbladder channel, whereas SJ-5 may also be chosen in the same case, because the San Jiao channel is related to the Gallbladder along the Six Divisions. Additionally, other channels may also be affected at the intersection points. A selection of local, adjacent and distal points should be combined.

Chart B
Selecting Points According to Syndromes

As mentioned, the areas of the problem are located and the main points that treat it are selected. Then, points that also treat the underlying disharmony are chosen. A thorough evaluation of all the signs and symptoms and aspects of the person (physical, energetic, emotional, psychological, etc.) is necessary to reach an accurate diagnosis. This is achieved through the information obtained from the Four Methods of Diagnosis *(Si Zhen)*.

First, a *principle of treatment* is determined. Second, points and techniques that tonify and nourish or disperse excess are chosen from the Eight Principles of Diagnosis. Points and techniques that influence the *Qi, Blood, Body Fluids, Jing* and *Shen* are chosen from the Vital Substances Diagnosis, whereas points and techniques that eliminate exterior or interior dampness, heat, fire, cold, phlegm, wind and dryness are chosen from the Pathogenic Factors (Six Evils) Diagnosis. Points of the affected channels are chosen according to their energetic quality and its relationship to the disharmony determined by the Internal Organ Diagnosis.

The Six Divisions differentiation offers a way to ensure that the chosen points have a direct influence on the affected channels and stage of development of the condition.

An analysis of the patient's disharmony according to the Five Phases also offers a clear and precise method for selecting points.

Chart C
Selecting Points According to Diseases and
Conditions from Empirical Knowledge and
Clinical Practice

These are symptomatic treatments based on the thousands of years of clinical experience gained by the practitioners of Traditional Chinese Medicine.

These selections of points are commonly employed for the conditions and symptoms mentioned and are intended to help the practitioner make an effective prescription. However, they *are not prescriptions in themselves*. Many of these points can also be used, separately or in combinations, for *symptomatic treatments*.

Important note on the points lists
The points are generally listed in order of importance so that the first point(s) are more important than the ones at the end of each list.

Chart A: Selecting Points According to Area (Local and Distal Points)

DISEASED AREA	LOCAL POINTS	DISTAL POINTS
HEAD		
Whole head	Du-20 G✓	Liv-3, Kd-1, -6, Sp-6, He-7
Vertex	Du-20, -23	Liv-3, Kd-1
Temple	Taiyang, GB-8, -20	SJ-5, GB-41
Forehead	Yintang, Du-23, St-8, GB-14, -15	LI-4, St-44, -41
Occiput and neck	Bl-9, -10, Du-14, -15, -16, -17, Bailao	SI-3, Lu-7, GB-39, Bl-60, -63, SI-6
FACE	varying	LI-4, St-44, Lu-7, SJ-5
Eyes	Bl-1, -2, GB-1	Liv-3, GB-37, GB-20
	St-1, -2, SJ-23, Taiyang, St-3	LI-4, Kd-6, Liv-2, -3
Nose	LI-19, -20, Du-23, Yintang, Bitong	Lu-7, LI-4
Teeth	St-6, -4, Ren-24	LI-4, St-44, Lu-7
Ears	SJ-21, SI-19, GB-2, -20, SJ-16, -17	SJ-3, -5, GB-41, -43, -39, Kd-3, -6
Tongue	Ren-23 C✓	He-5, Du-15, Kd-6
Throat	St-9, LI-18, SI-17, Ren-23	Lu-10, -11, LI-4, -1, Lu-7, Kd-6, Liv-2
Neck	Du-14, -15, -16, Bailao, Bl-10, -11	SI-3, Lu-7, GB-39, P-6
	Huatuojiaji (C1–T2), SI-13, -14, -15	Luozhen
TRUNK		
Chest	Ren-17, Lu-1, Liv-14, Kd-25, St-12–18,	P-6, Lu-5, LI-4, St-40, Sp-4
	Bl-12–18, Sp-20, -21	
Breasts	Ren-17, St-18, Liv-14, P-1	P-6, GB-41, Sp-4, SI-1
ABDOMEN	Ren-4, -6, -12	St-36, Sp-4, -6
Epigastrium	Ren-12, St-21, Liv-14, Bl-21	St-36, Sp-4, P-6
Middle of abdomen	St-25, Sp-15, Ren-6, -8, Bl-20–22	St-36, -37, -39
Lower abdomen	Ren-3–6, Bl-23–26	Sp-6, -8, -9, St-36, Bl-40
Bladder	Ren-3, St-28, Bl-28	Sp-6, -9
Genitals	Ren-2–4, St-28–30, Zigong	Sp-6, -9, Liv-5, GB-41, Kd-5, Bl-67
Sides of abdomen	Liv-13, -14, GB-24, -27, -28, Bl-18, -19	SJ-6, GB-34, -41, Liv-3
LUMBAR REGION	Bl-22–26, Bl-52, Du-4, Shiqizhui,	Bl-40, -60, Kd-3, GB-30, Du-26,
	Huatuojiaji (T10–L5)	Yintang, Yaotong, LI-4, He-7
Rectum	Bl-30, -35, Du-1	Bl-57
UPPER LIMB	varying, LI-10	Huatuojiaji (C3–T2)
Shoulder	SJ-14, LI-15, GB-21	St-38, SJ-5, LI-4, -11
Elbow	LI-10, -11, -12, SI-8, SJ-10, Lu-5	LI-4, SJ-5, SI-6, GB-34
Wrist	SJ-4, -5, LI-5, SI-4, -5, P-7, Lu-9	GB-40
LOWER LIMB	varying, St-36	Huatuojiaji (L3–S1)
Hip	GB-29, -30, St-31	GB-34, -41
Knee	St-35, -36, Sp-9, Bl-39, -40	Bl-23
Ankle	Bl-60, -62, Kd-6, St-41, GB-40	SJ-4

Chart B: Selecting Points According to Syndromes

SYNDROMES	POINTS
QI	
Qi deficiency	St-36, Ren-6, Sp-3, Ren-12, -17, Kd-3, Bl-20, -21, Lu-9, He-5, LI-4
Qi stagnation	GB-34, Liv-3, -14, SJ-5
Sinking Qi	Du-20, St-36
Qi and Blood deficiency	St-36, Sp-6, Ren-4, Bl-20, -23
BLOOD	
Blood deficiency	Sp-6, Ren-4, St-36, Liv-8, Bl-15, -17, -20, -21, -23, Liv-3, He-7, Sp-10
Blood Heat	He-8, P-8, Liv-2, -3, Sp-10, Bl-40, LI-11
Blood stasis	Liv-3, Sp-4, -6, -8, -10, P-6, Ren-17, Bl-17, -18
Blood loss	Sp-1, -10, Bl-17, Liv-1, -14
BODY FLUIDS	
Dampness	Sp-3, -9, -6, Bl-20, -22, -23, Ren-4, -6, Liv-13
Phlegm	St-40, Sp-3, Lu-5, Bl-20, -13
Oedema	Kd-3, -7, Sp-6, -9, Lu-7, LI-4, Bl-22, -23, Ren-9
Dryness	Ren-12, St-36, Kd-6, Lu-7, Sp-6, Kd-7
ESSENCE	
Decline of the Kidney Essence	Du-4, Bl-23, -52, Kd-3, Sp-6, GB-39, Du-16, Bl-11, Ren-4
SHEN	
Restlessness of the mind	He-7, -5, SI-3, P-6, -7, Sp-6, Kd-1, -6, Bl-15, -43, -44, LI-4, Liv-3
Mental agitation	St-40, He-8, P-8
Poor concentration	He-7, -9, St-40, Du-20, Bl-15, -20, -45
Loss of consciousness	Du-26, He-9, the twelve Well-Jing points
EMOTIONAL	
Anger	Liv-2, -3, -5, LI-4
Sadness	Lu-7, Ren-17, Bl-13, -42
Worry	Sp-3, -4, ST-40, Bl-20, -21, -49, Sp-6
Fear	Bl-23, -52, Kd-4
Overexcitement	He-7, P-6, Bl-15, LI-4, Sp-6
YIN YANG	
Yin deficiency	Kd-6, Sp-6, Lu-7, Ren-4, -12, Bl-23, Kd-3, St-36
Yang deficiency	St-36, Ren-6, Kd-3, Du-4, Bl-23, Kd-7
Yin collapse	Kd-3, Kd-7, Ren-6, Ren-4
Yang collapse	Ren-8, St-36, Kd-3, Du-20, Ren-6, Ren-12

PATHOGENIC FACTORS

SYNDROMES	POINTS
HEAT	
Exterior wind heat	SJ-5, LI-4, Du-14, Bl-13, LI-11
Interior full heat and fire	Liv-2, St-44, Lu-10, He-8, P-8, LI-4, -11, Liv-3, Kd-1, Du-14
Empty heat	see *Yin deficiency* (page 36)
COLD	
Exterior wind cold	Lu-7, LI-4, Bl-12, -13
Interior cold	St-36, Sp-6, Kd-3, Ren-4, -6, -8, -12, Du-4
Empty cold	see *Yang deficiency* (page 36)
WIND	
Exterior wind	Lu-7, LI-4, SJ-5, Bl-12, -13, Du-14, -15, Bl-10
Interior wind	Liv-1, Liv-3, Bl-18, Du-16, GB-20, Du-20 and the other Well points.
DAMPNESS	see *Body Fluids* (page 36)
DRYNESS	see *Body Fluids* (page 36)

Chart B: Selecting Points According to Diseases and Conditions from Empirical Knowledge and Clinical Practice

SYMPTOMS	POINTS
Abdominal distension	St-36, Sp-6, -3, -9, Sp-15, -25, Ren-6, -9, -12
Abdominal distension and pain	St-36, Sp-4 , -6, -3, St-25, Sp-15, Ren-4, -6, -12, LI-4, -11, Liv-3
Amenorrhoea	Sp-6, -4, -10, Liv-3, Kd-3, Liv-8, Bl-18, -20, -23, St-29, -30, LI-4
Asthma	Lu-9, -7, -1, LI-4, Bl-12, -13, Ren-22, -17, Dingchuan, Chuanxi
Breast swelling and pain	Liv-14, St-18, Liv-3, GB-41, -34, P-1, -6, St-36, -40
Chest pain	Ren-17, P-4, -6, LI-4, Bl-13–17, Huatuojiaji (C3–T9)
Cough	Lu-1, -7, Bl-12, -13, LI-4
Cough with profuse phlegm	Lu-1, -5, St-40, Sp-3
Cough, unproductive, dry	Lu-9, -7, Kd-6, St-36
Coma or fainting	Du-26, the twelve Well-Jing points, especially Kd-1 and He-9
Constipation	Sp-15, St-25, -36, -37, Bl-25, Ren-6, -4, Sp-6, LI-4, SJ-6, Huatuojiaji (T10–L5)
Cystitis	Ren-3, St-28, Bl-23, -28, Sp-6, -9, Liv-5, -8
Diarrhoea	St-25, Sp-9, -6, -3, St-36, -37, Ren-6, -8 (moxa), Bl-25, Huatuojiaji (T10–L5)
Dreaming, excessive	He-7, Bl-15, Liv-3, GB-44, LI-4
Dysphagia	Ren-22, P-6, Liv-3, LI-4, St-9, LI-18
Dysmenorrhoea	Sp-4, -6, -10, Liv-3, Ren-4, St-25, GB-27, -28, Bl-23, -32, Shiqizhui
Epigastric pain	Ren-12, P-6, St-34, -36, Bl-21
Fainting, loss of consciousness	Du-26, -20, Ren-4, St-36, LI-4, P-9, Kd-1
Fullness of the chest	P-6, LI-4, Ren-17, Lu-1, -7
Fever	Du-14, LI-4, -11, Lu-10, Liv-3
Gastrocnemius muscle spasm	Bl-56, -57, -60, GB-34
Genital pain or itching	Liv-5, Sp-6, St-30, Bl-32
Haemorrhage	Sp-1 (moxa), Sp-10, Liv-1 (moxa)
Haemorrhoids	Du-1, -20, Bl-57, Sp-6, Bl-30
Hiccup (spasm of the diaphragm)	P-6, Bl-17, St-12, -13, GB-24, Liv-14, St-36
Hot flushes	St-9, Kd-6, -3, He-6, Sp-6, Ren-4, Liv-3, Du-15
Hypertension	St-9, Liv-2, -3, LI-11, -4, Sp-6, Kd-6, GB-20, -21, SJ-5, SI-3, Du-14
Hypochondrial pain	GB-34, Liv-14, SJ-5, -6, P-6, GB-41, -24, Bl-17, -18, -19, -20
Hysteria	P-6, He-7, SI-3, Du-26, LI-4, Liv-3, the twelve Well-Jing points
Indigestion	St-36, Sp-4, Ren-12, St-25, P-6
Infertility	Bl-23, -52, -32, Sp-4, -6, -10, Kd-3, -6, Ren-4, -6, St-29, -30, -36, P-6
Impotence, premature ejaculation	Ren-4, -6, Sp-6, Kd-3, Bl-23, -52, St-29, -30, Kd-3, -6

SYMPTOMS	POINTS
Insomnia	He-7, Sp-6, Kd-6, GB-13, Anmian, GB-20, -21
Insufficient lactation	St-18, Ren-17, St-36, SI-1, Liv-14, Sp-3
Itching	Sp-10, Baichongwo, LI-11, Sp-6, Lu-7
Labour (delayed or prolonged)	Bl-31, -32, Sp-6, Liv-3, -5, LI-4, GB-21, Bl-60, -67
Loss of sense of smell	LI-20, Lu-7, LI-4
Loss of voice	St-9, LI-18, -4, P-5, He-5, Du-15, Ren-23
Malposition of the fetus	Bl-67 (moxa)
Mastitis	Liv-14, St-18, Ren-17, Liv-2, SI-1, P-6
Miscarriage, threatened	Sp-1, St-36, Du-20
Morning sickness in pregnancy	Ren-12, P-6, St-36, -30, Bl-20, -21
Nausea and vomiting	P-6, St-21, -36
Pain, anywhere	LI-4, Liv-3, Sp-21, Bl-17, SJ-5, P-6, GB-34, Du-26
Palpitations	H-7, P-4, -6, Ren-17, Bl-15, -14, Huatuojiaji (T2–T6)
Poor appetite	St-36, Sp-6, -3, Ren-12, Bl-20, -21
Prolapse of the uterus or rectum	Du-20, St-36, -30, Du-1, Bl-30, -32
Salivation, excessive	Ren-24, Du-26, St-4, -6, LI-4, Sp-3, LI-4
Sciatica	Bl-23, -30, GB-30, -34, -31, Bl-36, Bl-39, 40, -57, -60
Sore throat	LI-4, Lu-10, -11, LI-1, -18, St-9, Lu-1
Sweating, excessive	LI-4, Kd-7, Du-14, Liv-3, LI-11, He-6
Sweating, spontaneous	LI-4, Kd-7, St-36, Lu-9, -7, Du-14, Bailao
Sweating, night	He-6, Kd-7, SI-3, LI-4, Bl-43, Du-14
Sweating, absence	LI-4, Bl-13, Kd-7, Lu-7, SI-3
Temporomandibular syndrome	St-6, -7, LI-4, GB-34, SJ-5
Vaginal discharge (leucorrhoea)	Sp-6, -9, -3, Ren-6, GB-26, St-36, -28, Kd-3, GB-41
Weakness, general	St-36, Ren-4, -6, Du-4, Bl-23, Liv-13
Weakness of the limbs	St-36, Liv-13, Sp-3, LI-10

Chapter 8
Cun Measurements

Introduction

The traditional method of locating the points includes a comprehensive measurement system that uses *Body Inches,* or *Proportional Anatomical Measurement Units.* These units are relative to the size of the area being measured, and they are called *Cun* in Chinese.

For example, 1 cun on the abdomen may be a slightly different size to 1 cun on the forearm, or face. Furthermore, 1 cun on the adult differs greatly from one cun on a child.

General Guidelines

- 1 cun is approximately the length of the middle phalanx of the middle finger.

- 1 cun is approximately the width of the interphalangeal joint of the thumb.

- 3 cun is approximately the width of the four fingers at the level of the first interphalangeal joint of the index finger.

- 2 cun is approximately the length of the middle and distal phalanges of the index finger.

- 1.5 cun is approximately the width of the index and middle finger at the level of the first interphalangeal joint.

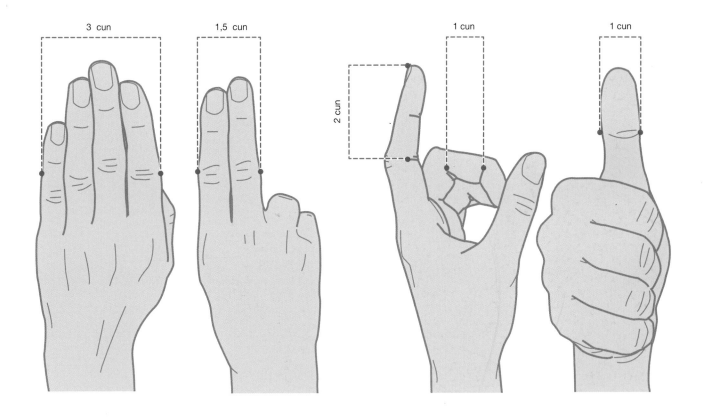

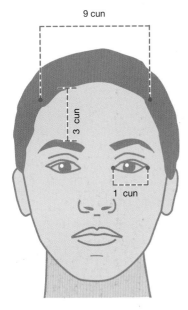

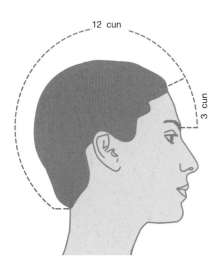

Cun Measurements According to Body Area

Head and Face
- Anterior to posterior hairline   12 cun
- Glabella (between the eyebrows) to anterior hairline   3 cun
- Glabella (between the eyebrows) to posterior hairline   15 cun
- Left to right St-8 (at the corner of the forehead)   9 cun
- Left to right mastoid processes   9 cun
- Eye, inner to outer canthus   1 cun

Chest
- Anterior midline to tip of acromion   8 cun
- Anterior midline to midmamillary line   4 cun
- Distance between the nipples   8 cun
- Distance between the midpoint of the clavicles   8 cun
- Centre of axilla to inferior border of eleventh rib   12 cun

Back and Neck
- Posterior midline to medial border of scapula   3 cun
- Medial border of PSIS to posterior midline   1.5 cun
- Lower border of C7 (Du-14) to posterior hairline   3 cun

Abdomen
- Umbilicus to xiphisternal junction (sternocostal angle)   8 cun
- Umbilicus to upper border of pubic symphysis   5 cun
- Anterior midline to lateral border of the rectus   4 cun
  abdominis muscle or medial aspect of ASIS

Upper Limb
- Upper arm, anterior axillary fold to cubital crease   9 cun
- Forearm, cubital to wrist crease (or LI-5 to LI-11)   12 cun

Lower Limb
- Upper border of greater trochanter to knee crease   19 cun
- Protuberance of greater trochanter to knee crease   18 cun
- Gluteal crease to popliteal crease   14 cun
- Patella: superior to inferior borders   2 cun
- Medial malleolus to knee crease   15 cun
  (or inner eye of the knee)
- Lateral malleolus to knee crease   16 cun
  (or outer eye of the knee, or St-35)

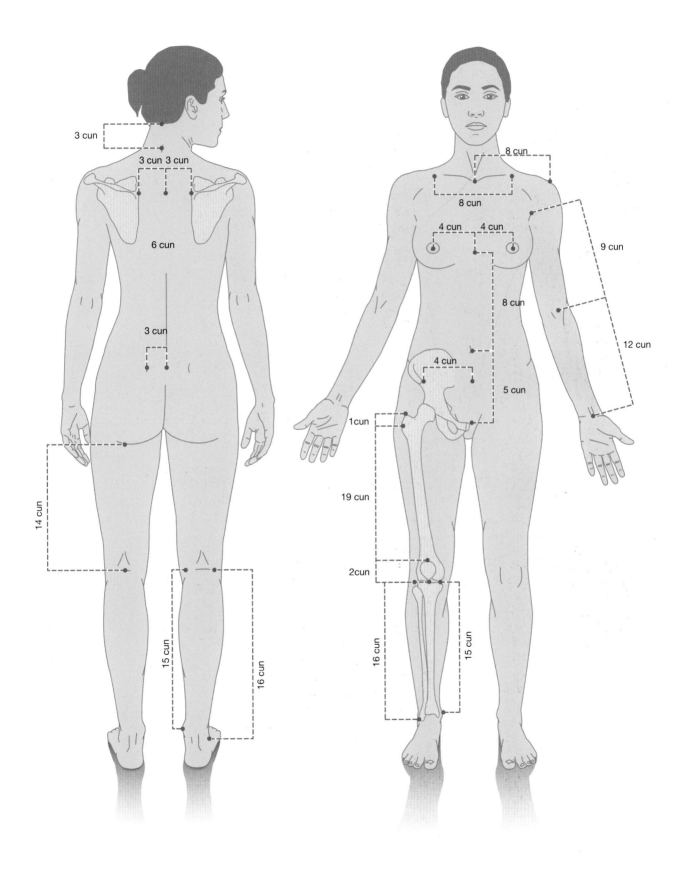

Chapter 9
Considerations, Cautions and Contraindications

Before applying any of the relevant therapeutic methods, one should conscientiously take into account all factors that could play a role in the outcome of the treatment.

Thus, after careful analysis of the case history, the clinical signs and symptoms, and the patient's physical and psychological state at the time, one can form the treatment principle and prescription.

A useful prescription includes those points that will be *most reactive in each case and bring about the best therapeutic results*. Bear in mind that using a purely theoretical approach to point selection will not take into account important factors such as the condition of the tissues surrounding the point and along the channel pathway, or the patient's localised sensitivity or pain levels. Therefore, before applying any form of treatment, one should always examine the location by looking, palpating and asking about that point.

The length of time and strength of the treatment to be applied varies from one case to another. The person's underlying energy, constitution and psycho-emotional state, as well as the particular disorder and inherent or acquired characteristics of the specific site to be treated, are all important factors requiring consideration.

General Contraindications

In view of the unregulated nature of acupuncture and many bodywork methods, it is difficult to specify absolute contraindications for these forms of therapy. However, for reasons of safety, all methods of treatment should be used with caution or avoided in the following conditions.

Pregnancy
Both acupuncture and massage techniques should be applied with great caution during pregnancy because they may induce labour. Stimulation of certain acupoints may cause strong uterine contractions and induce abortion. Therefore, it is generally best to avoid any form of treatment in the first three to four months of pregnancy. Needling points on the lower abdomen and lumbosacral region during the first trimester is contraindicated. After the third month, points on the upper abdomen and points that cause strong sensations should also be avoided.

Moxibustion should not be used on the abdomen or lower back at any time during pregnancy.

Cupping is not often recommended during pregnancy. However, gently applied cupping can be employed in certain cases (not on the abdomen). Furthermore, cupping can be useful during labour.

Medical emergencies and surgical conditions
Acupuncture, moxibustion, cupping and acupressure are contraindicated in medical emergencies. In such cases, first aid should be applied and transport to a medical emergency centre arranged.

These methods should not be used to replace necessary surgical intervention.

Malignancy
Acupuncture, moxibustion, cupping or any form of acupressure should not be used for the primary treatment of malignant tumours*. In particular, needling at the tumour site should be prohibited. However, these methods can be used as a complementary measure to support medical treatment, in combination with other therapies, for the relief of pain or other symptoms, to alleviate side-effects of chemotherapy and radiotherapy, and thus to improve the quality of life.

Bleeding disorders
Needling, moxibustion, guasha and cupping should be prohibited in patients with bleeding and clotting disorders. Manual pressure should also be avoided in clotting disorders and is contraindicated if there is any suspicion of thrombosis. However, gentle acupressure and qi projection techniques, applied by skilled practitioners, can be beneficial in certain cases.

* It is interesting to note, however, that acupuncture and qigong therapy have been successfully employed in a wide variety of cases involving both benign and malignant tumours.

Considering Sensitive, Dangerous and Contraindicated Points

The previous chapters mention important information regarding the correct use of points. However, this information should be taken as a guideline only and each case should be studied individually before applying any form of treatment.

Sensitive and dangerous points

Sensitive and dangerous points include most points of the face, abdomen, back, chest, neck and throat, but also points on the limbs located superior to major blood vessels and nerves. All these points are surrounded by fragile anatomical structures and can be tender or painful during the application of treatment.

Some of these points require special skill in needling; however, inappropriately applied manual techniques and moxibustion can also be dangerous.

For more details, see the relevant chapters on needling (page 11), manual techniques and shiatsu (page 15), cupping (page 19) and moxibustion (page 17).

Contraindicated points

Throughout the text, the classical contraindications are specified as well as those based on contemporary medical practice. The dangerous and contraindicated points mentioned, apply to specific modes of treatment and particular cases. For example, moxibustion is contraindicated on St-2, but acupuncture and manual pressure techniques are not.

Contraindications relating to specific cases may be general or specific. For example, moxa is contraindicated on Du-4 in persons under the 20th year of age, according to classical texts; needling any abdominal point during pregnancy is contraindicated, according to any standard medical advice.

Chapter 10

Points of the

Arm Tai Yin
Lung Channel

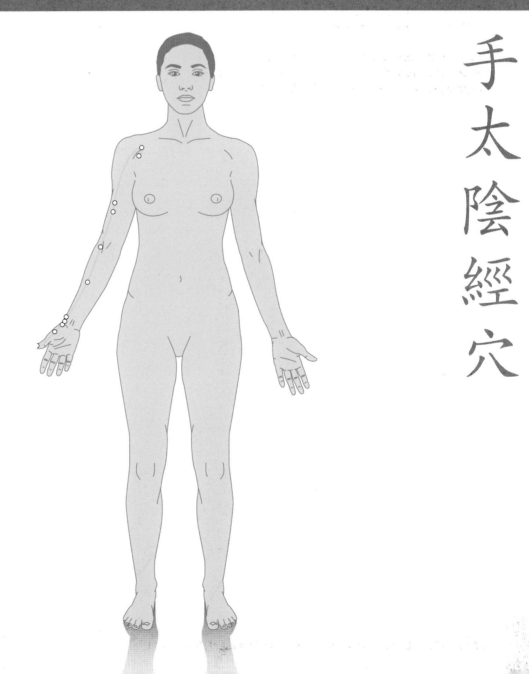

手太陰經穴

Lu-1   Zhongfu

中府

Central Mansion

Alarm *Mu* point of the Lungs
Intersection of the Spleen on the Lung channel

On the anterior lateral aspect of the chest, approximately 1 cun inferior and slightly lateral to Lu-2, just medial to the coracoid process of scapula. In the pectoralis major muscle, and more deeply, at the insertion of the pectoralis minor.

Also, medially in its deep position, the muscles of the second intercostal space (ICS), or the body of the rib, depending on the individual structure of the rib cage and the shoulder girdle.

To aid location, ask the patient to stretch the arm out forward (flexion of the shoulder). First, locate Lu-2 at the centre of the depression of the deltopectoral triangle, and then, following the contour of the rib cage, move the tip of the finger inferiorly approximately 1 cun to locate Lu-1.

Most acupuncture texts locate Lu-1 in the first intercostal space, which is misleading for a number of reasons.

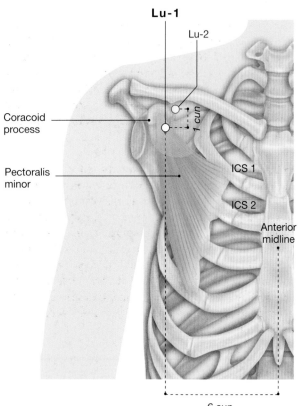

Lu-1

Lu-2

Coracoid process

1 cun
1 cun

Pectoralis minor

ICS 1

ICS 2

Anterior midline

6 cun

Firstly, Lu-1 is located lateral to the rib cage; therefore the intercostal spaces are not found at this site at all.

Secondly, if manual pressure* is applied deeply in a medial direction, it can reach the second intercostal space or the body of the second rib (depending on the individual structure of the surrounding tissues and the specific angle of pressure employed). However, it will definitely *not access the first intercostal space*, which is situated much closer to the anterior midline.

A possible reason for this discrepancy is that if the intercostal spaces are counted next to the sternum, Lu-1 can be described as being *at the same level as the medial end of the first intercostal space* (approximately).

To clarify, place the tip of the finger at the medial end of the first intercostal space and then draw a line extending laterally, following the contour of the rib cage. The finger will naturally stop at the depression of Lu-1, between the coracoid process and the rib cage.

This also infers that other points located in relation to Lu-1, including Sp-20 and Sp-17, should in fact be placed one intercostal space below their usual descriptions.

Best treatment positions
Lu-1 is generally best treated with the patient lying down in a supine position, with the arm lying by their side at an angle of approximately 45 degrees to the body.

In cases of severe coughing and dyspnoea, massage, cupping and moxibustion are more appropriate in a sitting position. However, needling is not recommended whilst the patient is sitting up.

For (unilateral) shoulder joint problems, Lu-1 and Lu-2 can be effectively treated in a side-lying position. These points can be opened by extending the shoulder girdle posteriorly.

! Excessive stimulation of Lu-1 can deplete the qi in deficient patients. In predisposed patients it can aggravate the respiratory system, possibly triggering an asthma attack.

! Do not overactivate the Lungs' descending functions during pregnancy, heavy menstrual flow and generally in weak patients.

* Although in theory the same would apply to needling, do not insert the needle at a medial angle because this holds a substantial risk of puncturing the lung.

Another consideration is that it can be easier to effectively stimulate Lu-1 by manual techniques because needling it correctly requires a great deal of competence and is potentially dangerous.

Needling
- 0.3 to 0.6 cun lateral oblique insertion.
- 0.5 to 1 cun transverse oblique insertion inferiorly and laterally, following the contour of the rib cage.
- 0.5 to 1 cun transverse oblique insertion upward toward Lu-2.

!! Do not needle in a medial direction because this holds a considerable risk of puncturing the lung and causing a pneumothorax.

Additionally, needling deeply in a lateral direction can puncture any of the numerous axillary vessels: superficially, the cephalic vein; deeper, the thoracoacromial artery and vein; inferiorly, the lateral thoracic artery and vein; in its deep position, the long thoracic nerve, the axillary artery and vein and nerves of the brachial plexus.

Manual techniques and shiatsu
Perpendicular pressure and friction techniques are applicable to the intercostal space with the tips of the fingers or thumbs. Dispersing type stimulation, such as rubbing or friction, is best applied superficially to the surrounding area to treat exterior conditions, whereas a deeper pressure, usually applied at right angles to the rib cage, is used to dissipate interior stagnation and tonify the Lung qi.

Lu-1 can be effectively opened by stretching the shoulder girdle posteriorly while extending and laterally rotating the arm.

Deep friction and stretching of the pectoralis major and minor and coracobrachialis muscles is also very effective for problems of the shoulder and chest.

! This area can be quite sensitive or tender. Do not apply strong pressure to the rib cage.

Moxibustion
Cones: 3–5. Pole: 5–15 minutes. Light or medium stimulation.

Cupping
Medium, light or empty cupping with small or medium cups is applicable. Do not exceed 10 minutes.

Guasha
Guasha is applicable across the pectoralis major and the pectoralis minor insertion on the coracoid process.

Magnets
The application of magnets is also very effective, particularly for chronic breathing complaints. For acute dyspnoea, apply north poles on Lu-1 and south poles on Ren-17 and Bl-12 or Bl-13 (depending on which is most reactive during pressure palpation). Also, the following combination is very effective: south on left LI-4, north on left Lu-1, south on left Bl-13, north on right Bl-13, south on right Lu-1 and north on right LI-4 (or vice-versa).

Stimulation sensation
Deqi may be perceived radiating down into the chest (through the lobes of the lungs to the diaphragm and even reaching the epigastrium and abdomen) or extending around the region, across the front of the chest and shoulder to the upper arm, reaching the upper back, neck, throat or face depending on the treatment required.

Also, the breathing rhythm and depth may change or the person may cough or sigh.

Actions and indications
Lu-1 is a *very important and extensively used point* for *many types of breathing disorders*, especially *coughing* and *dyspnoea.*

Its primary actions are to *improve the flow of Qi in the chest and benefit respiration* by promoting the *Lung dispersing and descending functions,* thus *clearing, relaxing and dissipating fullness from the chest.* It effectively *clears interior heat, stagnation and phlegm from the chest* as well as *releasing exterior wind, cold and heat.* Furthermore, Lu-1 *strengthens the upper Jiao and tonifies Lung qi.*

Indications include fullness, oppression and pain of the chest, shortness of breath, most types of coughing and wheezing (particularly if symptoms are worse when lying down), asthma, bronchitis, respiratory tract infections, chronic weak breathing, haemoptysis, pain and swelling of the throat, neck or axilla, tonsillitis, laryngitis, pharyngitis, lymphadenopathy, goitre, difficulty swallowing, nausea, retching and vomiting (particularly in relation to coughing), gastric flu, fever, aversion to cold, sweating, swelling of the face, rhinitis and nasal obstruction.

Lu-1 has also been employed in a variety of other cases including respiratory and skin allergies, painful or itchy skin rashes, excessive perspiration, intercostal neuralgia, palpitations, chronic exhaustion, abdominal distension, hypochondrial pain and disorders of the gallbladder.

As *a local point*, it is effective in the treatment of *channel disorders* including pain of the shoulder, difficulty in abducting and extending the arm, frozen shoulder, pain of the upper arm and upper back, periarthritis of the shoulder and spasm or shortening of the pectoralis major and minor and the coracobrachialis muscle.

Lu-1 is also one of the *Eight Points to Clear Heat from the Chest* (together with St-12, Bl-11 and Bl-12).

> **Main Areas:** Chest. Lungs. Nose. Shoulder.
> **Main Functions:** Benefits respiration.
> Regulates chest qi. Dispels stagnation and heat.
> Releases the exterior. Tonifies Lung qi.

Lu-2   Yunmen   雲門

Cloud Gate

At the centre of the deltopectoral triangle. This sizeable depression is formed by the clavicle (above), the superior border of the pectoralis major (below) and the anterior border of the deltoid muscle on the lateral side.

To aid location, ask the patient to stretch the arm forward (flexion of the shoulder) to emphasize the pectoralis and anterior deltoid muscle.

Best treatment positions
Similar to Lu-1.

Needling
• 0.5 to 1 cun transverse oblique insertion inferiorly toward Lu-1.

!! Do not needle in a medial direction. Do not needle deeply. This holds a considerable risk of puncturing the lung and causing a pneumothorax.

Actions and indications
Lu-2 has *similar functions to Lu-1*. However, it is not considered as effective for interior Lung disorders and is *preferred for channel complaints*, particularly *pain and stiffness of the shoulder*.

Furthermore, Lu-2 is considered to be the point where the qi enters the diurnal cycle, and may be used to engender the flow of qi throughout the entire body as well as to ease stagnation.

Lu-2 is also employed to *clear heat*, and is mentioned as one of the *Seven Points for Draining Heat from the Extremities*. The others are LI-15, Bl-40 and Du-2.

> **Main Areas:** Shoulder. Arm. Chest. Lungs.
> **Main Functions:** Regulates qi. Alleviates pain.

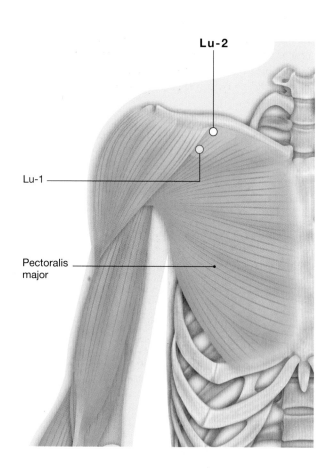

Lu-5   Chize

尺澤

Cubit Marsh

Uniting Sea-*He*, Water (Sedation) point

On the cubital crease, in the depression on the radial side of the tendon of the biceps brachii and medial to the brachioradialis muscle.

To aid location, ask the patient to flex the elbow to emphasize the biceps brachii tendon.

Best treatment positions

Lu-5 is usually treated with the patient lying supine and the arm by the side at an angle of approximately 45 degrees to the body. The forearm should be supinated and the elbow slightly flexed (use cushion support under the forearm). However, it can also be effectively stimulated with the elbow in extension. The former seems to be more effective for situations where there is excessive tightness or fullness of this area and the latter in cases of flaccidity or weakness.

Needling

- 0.3 to 1 cun perpendicular insertion, between the tendon of the biceps brachii muscle and the brachioradialis muscle.
- Oblique lateral insertion toward LI-11, or vice-versa.

! Do not puncture the cephalic vein or the lateral antebrachial cutaneous nerve; more deeply, the radial nerve and the radial recurrent artery.

Manual techniques and shiatsu

Pressure is best applied perpendicularly to the cubital fossa. A useful technique is to mobilise the elbow joint in a circular motion, whilst applying the pressure.

Friction can be applied laterally to the brachioradialis muscle and medially to the biceps brachii tendon. Additionally, opening and stretching of the region can be achieved by extending the elbow and supinating the forearm.

Moxibustion

Cones: 3–5. Pole: 5–10 minutes. Light or medium stimulation.

Stimulation sensation

Regional aching and distension is usually perceived. Also, electricity giving way to numbness may extend down the forearm toward the wrist and palm. Furthermore, deqi often travels proximally up the arm toward the shoulder and chest.

Actions and indications

Lu-5 *is a major point, used for many disorders of the Lungs*. Its primary functions are to *resolve chronic or acute lung phlegm conditions, clear heat, nourish yin and moisten the Lungs*. It is particularly indicated for *Lung phlegm heat*. Furthermore, Lu-5 can also be employed to *dissipate cold and tonify Lungs qi*.

Indications include acute or chronic productive cough, thick yellow, dark, green, brown turbid or blood stained sputum, chronic dry cough with expectoration of small quantities of dry, sticky, dark or blood stained sputum, chronic weak cough, dry throat, profuse white or colourless sputum, dyspnoea, asthma, bronchitis, pneumonia, pain, fullness and heaviness of the chest, shortness of breath, gurgling sound in the chest, painful or swollen throat, tonsillitis, epistaxis and fevers.

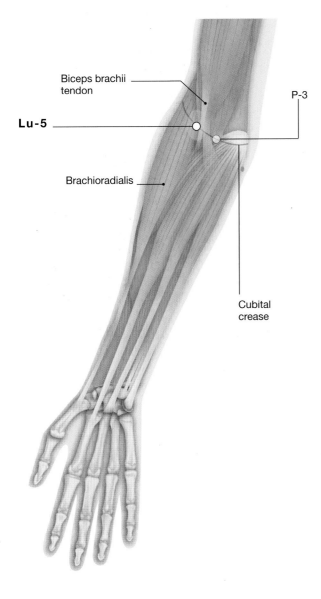

Biceps brachii tendon

P-3

Lu-5

Brachioradialis

Cubital crease

Lu-5 has also been employed to *open the water passages* and treat cases such as frequent urination, enuresis, urinary retention, oedema, diarrhoea and swelling of the four limbs.

Furthermore, it has been used to treat a variety of other disorders including nausea, vomiting, diarrhoea, abdominal distension, hypochondrial pain, epilepsy and lower back ache.

As *a local point*, Lu-5 is important to relax the sinews and alleviate pain at the lateral and anterior aspect of the elbow and arm. Indications include pain and stiffness of the elbow and arm, lateral epicondylitis, tendinitis and frozen shoulder.

> **Main Areas:** Lungs. Chest. Elbow. Upper jiao.
>
> **Main Functions:** Dispels phlegm. Opens the water passages. Alleviates cough. Clears the Lungs.

Lu-6 Kongzui

Collection Hole

孔最

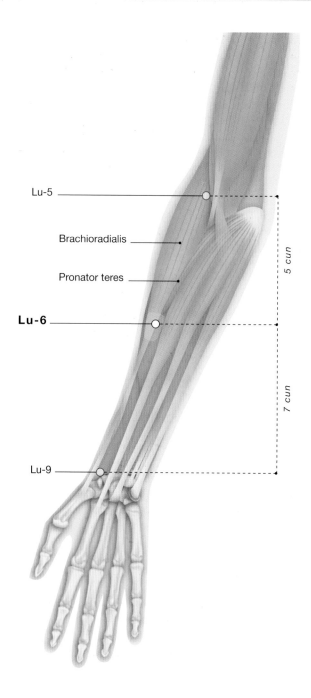

Accumulation Cleft-*Xi* point

On the anterior aspect of the forearm, 7 cun above Lu-9, on the line joining Lu-5 and Lu-9. Situated superficially in the brachioradialis muscle, more deeply, in the pronator teres and deeper still, in the flexor pollicis longus.

To aid location, Lu-6 is 1 cun above the midpoint of the line connecting Lu-5 with Lu-9.

Best treatment positions
Lu-6 is best treated in a supine position, with the patient's arm lying by their side at an angle of approximately 45 degrees to the body, and the forearm in a relaxed position (if necessary use cushions).

Needling
- 0.3 to 1 cun perpendicular or oblique insertion (insert needle on lateral margin of brachioradialis).
- 0.5 to 1.5 cun oblique insertion proximally or distally along the channel.

! Do not puncture the cephalic vein, the superficial branch of the radial nerve, the lateral antebrachial cutaneous nerve and the radial artery and vein; more deeply, in a medial direction, the median nerve.

Manual techniques and shiatsu
Stationary pressure and friction techniques are applied with light or medium pressure because this location can be quite sensitive.

Moxibustion
Cones: 3–7. Pole: 5–15 minutes. Light or medium stimulation only (do not overheat this location).

Stimulation sensation
Local distension and soreness is easily achieved because this is a sensitive point. Sometimes electricity extending up or down the channel is also perceived.

Actions and indications

Lu-6 is mainly used for *acute, excess conditions of the Lung channel and organ*, of both *interior and exterior origin*. It has been widely employed to treat absence of sweating in febrile diseases because it *augments the Lung function of dispersing qi and controlling the opening and closing of the pores*. Indications include epistaxis, haemoptysis, loss of voice, fever without sweating, acute cough and sore throat, dry throat, asthma, and chest pain.

As a local point, Lu-6 effectively treats pain and stiffness of the arm, elbow and forearm and difficulty flexing the elbow and fingers.

> **Main Areas:** Nose. Lungs. Skin. Forearm.
>
> **Main Functions:** Releases the exterior. Diaphoretic. Clears heat from the upper jiao. Arrests bleeding.

Lu-7　Lieque　　列缺

Interrupted Sequence
Thunder and Lightning

Connecting *Luo* point
Opening (Master) point of the Ren Mai
Command point of the head and neck
Heavenly Star point

On the most lateral aspect of the radius, at the base of the styloid process, 1.5 cun proximal to the transverse wrist crease. In the narrow 'V' shaped crevice, between the tendons of brachioradialis and abductor pollicis longus.

To aid location, slide the tip of the index finger proximally up from LI-5, to slip into the shallow crevice.

Best treatment positions

Treatment is usually applied with the patient in a supine or sitting position. The best needling position is with the forearm in a semi-supinated position.

! Lu-7 can release emotional states such as sadness, depression or worry in predisposed patients.

Needling

- 0.3 to 1.5 cun transverse insertion into the crevice, distally or proximally, along the channel pathway. The former may be more effective to release the exterior, whereas the latter can be considered more tonifying.

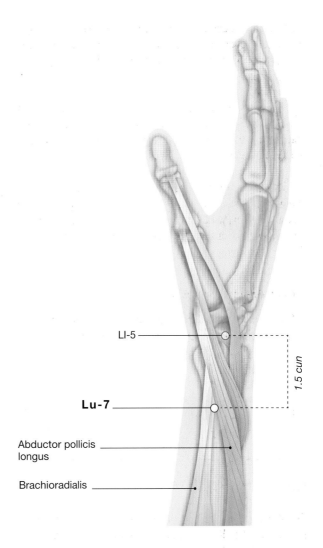

LI-5

Lu-7

1.5 cun

Abductor pollicis longus

Brachioradialis

Note: it is often helpful to lift up (pinch) the skin and subcutaneous tissue to insert the needle.
- 0.2 to 0.3 cun perpendicular insertion into the crevice.

! Do not puncture the superficial branches of the radial artery, vein or nerve, the cephalic vein or the lateral cutaneous antebrachial nerve.

Manual techniques and shiatsu

Pressure must be applied carefully to ensure reaching the epicentre of the point inside the crevice. Cross-fibre friction can be applied to the tendons. Additionally opening of this point can be achieved by stretching the anterolateral aspect of the wrist and pulling the thumb slightly medially.

Treatment is applied regularly until symptoms subside, particularly if there is acute difficulty breathing.

Moxibustion

Cones: 2–5. Pole: 5–15 minutes. Also, rice-grain moxibustion can be effective.

Stimulation sensation

Deqi can be difficult to achieve and is generally not very strong. This is partly because this is a very superficial location and the surrounding vasculature causes it to be painful and sensitive. Deqi is commonly experienced as regional aching or dull heaviness possibly extending proximally up the channel, or distally toward the thenar eminence. In some cases it produces an electric or tingling sensation due to branches of the lateral antebrachial cutaneous nerve or the superficial branch of the radial nerve being stimulated.

Actions and indications

Lu-7 is a *very important and widely used point*, because it is effective in *a large variety of exterior and interior Lung conditions*. It *releases the exterior, promotes sweating, circulates defensive qi, stimulates the descending and dispersing of Lung qi and opens the nose*. Also, it effectively *moistens the Lungs, nourishes fluids and yin and tonifies Lung qi*.

Indications include sneezing, dry, tickly, itchy or sore throat due to exterior wind, dryness, heat or yin deficiency, tonsillitis, chronic or acute pharyngitis, itchy nose, nasal discharge or obstruction, rhinitis, loss of smell, chills and fever, upper respiratory tract infections, acute or chronic asthma and cough due to excess or deficiency, shallow breathing, chronic weak breathing, dyspnoea, constriction and fullness of the chest.

Lu-7 also *opens the Ren Mai* and *nourishes fluids and yin throughout the body*. It treats general symptoms of *Yin deficiency*, particularly in relation to the Lungs and Kidneys. They include heat in the five hearts, night sweating, insomnia, malar flush, sensitive skin, scant urination and weakened sexual or reproductive functions.

Furthermore, it helps *open the water passages and benefits the urinary system*. Indications include oedema and swelling of the face, urinary incontinence (particularly if related to coughing), dysuria and urinary retention.

Lu-7 is the *Command point for the back of the head and neck* and is useful in such cases as stiffness of the neck, headache, facial pain or paralysis and toothache.

Additionally, it has a *strong emotional effect* and can be helpful following bereavement. It helps release excessive emotional states, and is especially indicated for excessive weeping, grief, depression and melancholy. It is commonly used in *smoking cessation* treatments and is also helpful in other types of addictions.

As a *local point*, Lu-7 can be beneficial to treat pain or impaired movement of the forearm, wrist, thumb or index finger.

Main Areas: Head. Face. Back of neck. Nose. Throat. Lungs. Chest. Bladder. Forearm.

Main Functions: Descends and disperses Lung qi. Releases the exterior. Opens the Ren Mai. Nourishes yin and moistens fluids. Benefits the neck.

Lu-8   Jingqu   經渠
Channel's Ditch

River-*Jing*, Metal (Horary) point

On the medial margin of the radius, in the depression approximately 1 cun above the transverse wrist crease, level with the high point of the radial styloid process, on the radial side of the radial artery.

Best treatment positions

Similar to Lu-9.

Needling

• 0.1 to 0.3 cun perpendicular insertion.

!! Do not puncture the radial artery. Lu-8 and Lu-9 are listed as potentially dangerous points for needling (see page 13) and require special skill and experience.

Moxibustion

Contraindicated.

Actions and indications

Lu-8 is not a commonly used point, because its effects are not as strong as other Lung channel points. It can however be effective to *tonify the Lung qi* and *harmonise the Metal Element*.

Main Areas: Lungs. Upper jiao.

Main Function: Tonifies Lung qi.

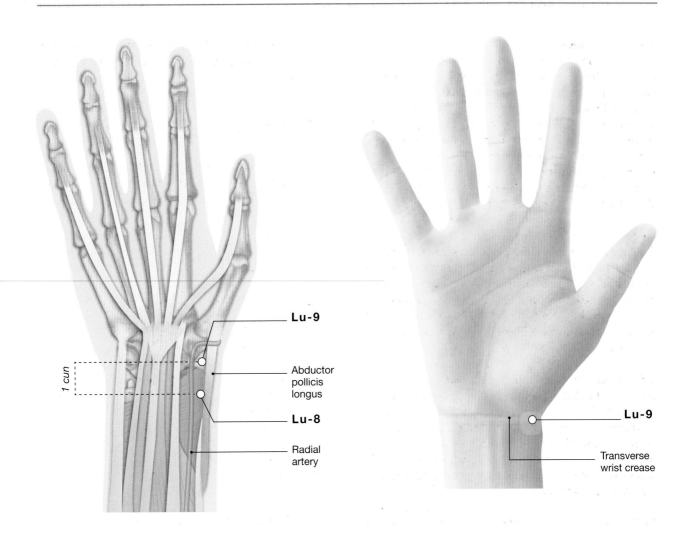

Lu-9

Abductor
pollicis
longus

Lu-8

Radial
artery

Lu-9

Transverse
wrist crease

Lu-9   Taiyuan

太淵

Great Source

Source-*Yuan* point
Stream-*Shu*, Earth (Tonification) point
Gathering *Hui* point for the Vessels

On the transverse wrist crease, in the depression on the radial (lateral) side of the radial artery. Lateral to the tendon of flexor carpi radialis and medial to the tendon of abductor pollicis longus.

To aid location, the sizeable depression of Lu-9 is emphasized when the patient abducts the thumb.

Best treatment positions
Lu-9 can be treated easily with the patient lying or sitting.

! This is a very sensitive point and should be stimulated carefully, particularly in deficient patients, for whom it is often a point of choice.

Needling
- 0.2 to 0.5 cun perpendicular insertion between the radius and scaphoid bones into the wrist joint space.
- 0.2 to 0.5 cun insertion angled under abductor pollicis longus tendon toward LI-5.

!! Do not puncture the radial artery. Lu-9 and Lu-8 are listed as two of the most potentially dangerous points for needling, requiring special skill and experience in their use (see page 13).

Moxibustion
Contraindicated.

Magnets

Magnets applied directly over the radial artery may be helpful in circulation and blood vessel disorders due to the magnets' anticoagulant effect on the blood passing through the radial artery. Use opposite poles on each side or alternate poles between Lu-9 and Lu-8.

Manual techniques and shiatsu

Sustained perpendicular pressure is most effective, including gentle pressure of the artery.

Note: In many cases it is not possible to apply finger pressure to the acupuncture point on the radial side of the artery because the point is too small, unless the practitioner has small enough fingers in relation to the recipient.

Lu-9 can be opened, and thus accessed more deeply, by extending the thumb simultaneously to apply pressure. However, if the point is very tight and full, it may be best to apply the pressure with the wrist in a flexed position.

Additionally, pressure can be applied simultaneously to mobilising the thumb and wrist gently in various directions.

Furthermore, carefully applied gentle friction can be applied to the abductor pollicis longus tendons.

! Do not rub or apply friction to the artery; press perpendicularly only. Avoid strong pressure of the artery, particularly in the elderly, those suffering from weak vessels and very deficient patients.

Stimulation sensation

Generally, Lu-9 produces a gentle sensation extending around the location and into the wrist. Deqi may also extend up the arm toward the chest, or distally toward the thumb.

Actions and indications

Lu-9 is a major and *extensively used point to tonify the Lung and chest qi, benefit respiration, alleviate coughing and strengthen the voice*. At the same time, it *resolves phlegm, clears heat, nourishes yin and moistens the Lungs*. It is primarily used in *chronic and deficient conditions to boost Lung qi and strengthen the chest*.

Indications include shortness of breath, weak or shallow breathing, dyspnoea, weak or hoarse voice, inability to talk, chronic weak cough, productive cough, dry cough, asthma, chronic bronchitis, emphysema, chronic sore throat, pharyngitis, chronic tiredness, exhaustion, depression and spontaneous or night sweating.

Additionally, it is effective to *moisten and improve the voice* and is of benefit to professionals such as singers and actors. Lu-9 is also used in *smoking cessation* prescriptions.

Furthermore, Lu-9 is the *Gathering Hui point for the vessels and pulses* and has been extensively used for *weakness of the circulation and blood vessels*. Indications include weak, irregular or absent pulse, arrhythmia, palpitations, sluggish circulation, cold extremities, tendency to thread veins, varicose veins and other vessel disorders, including chilblains and Raynaud's syndrome, anaemia, haemoptysis and chest pain.

As a *local point*, Lu-9 can help in the treatment of chronic pain in the wrist, stiffness or inability to move the thumb and weakness of the forearm.

Furthermore, Lu-9 is located on the distal pulse point (inch point) which is used to determine the condition of the Lungs, Heart and upper jiao functions.

Main Areas: Chest. Lungs. Blood vessels.

Main Functions: Tonifies chest qi. Strengthens the breath and the voice. Nourishes Lung yin. Transforms phlegm. Benefits the vessels and improves circulation.

Lu-10 Yuji

Fish Border
(Thenar Eminence)

Spring-*Ying*, Fire point

On the thenar surface, halfway along the first metacarpal bone, at the junction of the skin or the palmar and dorsal surfaces.

To aid location, palpate gently with the fingertip for the depression between the flesh and bone.

The best needling site is in the small space between the opponens pollicis and abductor pollicis brevis muscle.

Best treatment positions
Lu-10 is best treated with the palm in a semi-supine position so that the thenar surface faces upwards.

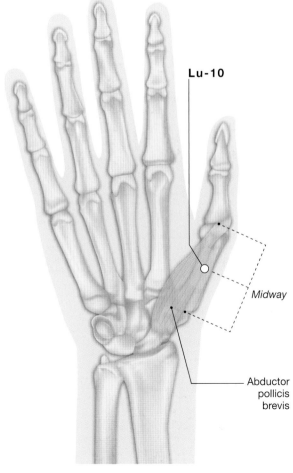

Lu-10

Midway

Abductor
pollicis
brevis

Palmar view

Needling
- 0.3 to 0.8 cun perpendicular insertion.
- Bleeding Lu-10 is effective in cases of severe interior heat or exterior wind-heat affecting the throat.

Manual techniques and shiatsu
Strong stimulation with perpendicular pressure or friction is most effective applied regularly until symptoms subside. Additionally, opening of this point can be achieved by stretching the thumb and rolling the thenar muscles medially toward the palm.

Hold the recipient's thumb with your fingers in order to press perpendicularly with your thumb into the space between the muscle belly and bone.

Moxibustion
Cones: 1–3. Pole: 1–5 minutes. Moxibustion is not commonly used at Lu-10, because it is mostly employed in the treatment of heat conditions. However, rice-grain moxibustion can be effective.

Guasha
Carefully applied guasha can be helpful in cases of acute sore throat.

Magnets
Stick-on magnets can also be beneficial.

Stimulation sensation
Regional aching and numbness possibly extending proximally toward the wrist and forearm.

Actions and indications
Lu-10 is an important point for *acute symptoms caused by excessive exterior or interior heat or phlegm-fire in the Lungs*. It is widely used to *soothe and moisten the throat*.

Indications include acute inflammation of the throat, hoarse voice, tonsillitis, pharyngitis, bronchitis, pneumonia, fever, thirst, cough with chest pain, thick yellow sticky, dry or blood stained sputum, epistaxis, toothache and headache.

Furthermore, Lu-10 has been employed for a variety of other disorders including vomiting, abdominal pain, genital itching and psycho-emotional disturbances such as anger, sadness, fright and restlessness.

Main Areas: Lungs. Throat. Thumb.

Main Functions: Clears exterior heat and phlegm and fire toxins. Benefits the throat.

Lu-11   Shaoshang

少 商

Lesser Metal

Well-*Jing*, Wood point
Second Ghost point

On the radial (lateral) side of the thumb, approximately 0.1 cun proximal to the corner of the nail. At the intersection of two lines following the radial border of the nail and the base of the nail.

Best treatment positions

Lu-11 can be treated easily with the patient sitting or lying. A strong stimulation is most effective if applied regularly until symptoms subside.

Needling

- 0.1 to 0.2 cun perpendicular insertion.
- Bleeding Lu-11 with a three-edged needle is effective in cases of severe interior heat or exterior wind-heat causing acute swelling and inflammation of the throat.

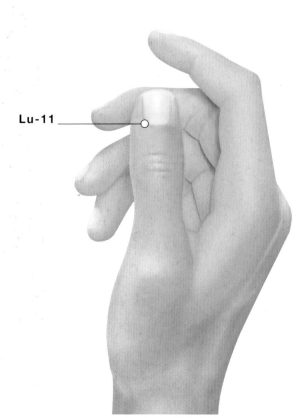

Lu-11

Manual techniques and shiatsu

Friction or stationary pressure may be applied quite strongly with the thumb or fingertip.

Rubbing the Well-Jing points at the ends of the fingers and toes is also an effective technique.

Self-acupressure or even 'biting' this point oneself is a useful first aid method for sore throat.

Moxibustion

Cones: 1–3. Pole: 5 minutes. Rice-grain moxibustion is also effectively employed.

Stimulation sensation

Regional aching or numbness. In common with the other Well-Jing points, Lu-11 may be quite painful locally and strong stimulation can engender a very powerful sensation reaching the chest.

When deqi is perceived, the breathing rhythm and depth may change, or the person may sigh.

Actions and indications

Lu-11 is primarily employed in cases of *inflammation of the throat due to exterior heat*. Indications include sore, swollen and painful throat, acute tonsillitis, laryngitis or pharyngitis, goitre and inflammation of the eyes due to wind-heat.

Furthermore, *in common with to the other Well-Jing points*, Lu-11 helps *pacify the Heart, calm the mind and restore consciousness* in cases of fainting or coma due to wind-stroke.

It also *activates the Lung sinew channel* and can treat pain and paralysis or spasticity of the arm following cerebrovascular accident.

Main Areas: Throat. Lung channel. Mind.

Main Functions: Dispels exterior heat and wind. Restores consciousness.

Chapter 11

Points of the

Arm Yang Ming
Large Intestine Channel

手陽明大腸經穴

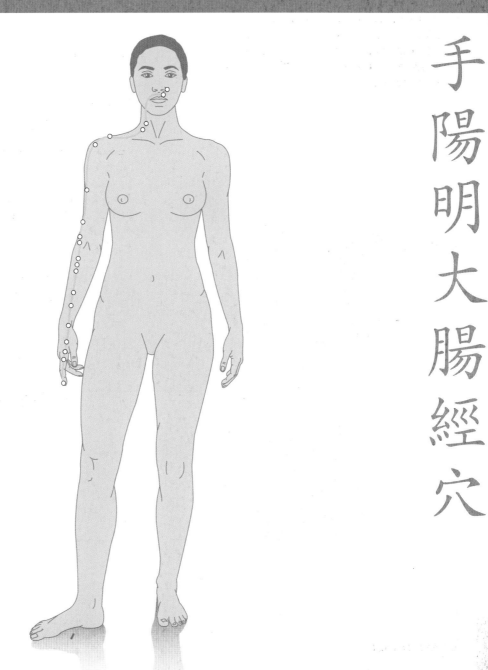

LI-1 Shangyang
Metal Yang

商陽

Well-*Jing*, Metal (Horary) point

On the radial (lateral) side of the index finger, approximately 0.1 cun proximal to the corner of the nail. At the intersection of two lines following the radial border of the nail and the base of the nail.

Best treatment positions
Similar to Lu-11 and the other Well-Jing points.

Needling
• 0.1 cun perpendicular insertion.
• Prick to bleed.

Stimulation sensation
Local ache or distension, maybe extending along the channel. Similar, but not as powerful, as Lu-11.

Actions and indications
LI-1 *clears both interior and exterior heat and wind* and is mainly used to treat *acute pain, swelling and inflammation of the throat*.

In common with the other Well-Jing points, LI-1 will *help restore consciousness* in cases of coma or fainting.

Additionally, it opens the Large Intestine sinew channel and *treats pain along the channel pathway*.

Main Areas: Throat. Large Intestine channel. Mind.

Main Functions: Restores consciousness. Benefits the throat.

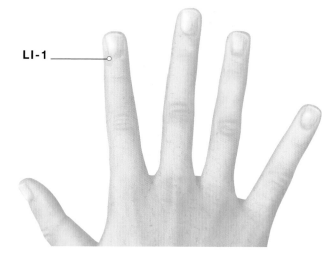

LI-1

LI-3 Sanjian
Third Space

三間

Stream-*Shu* point, Wood point

On the radial border of the index finger, just proximal to the head of the second metacarpal bone. In the depression dorsal to the insertion of the first dorsal interosseous muscle. To aid location, make a loose fist.

Best treatment positions
LI-3 can be treated with the patient sitting or lying.

Needling
• 0.3 to 1 cun perpendicular insertion.

Manual techniques and shiatsu
Perpendicular pressure is best applied between the muscle and bone. Friction is also effective.

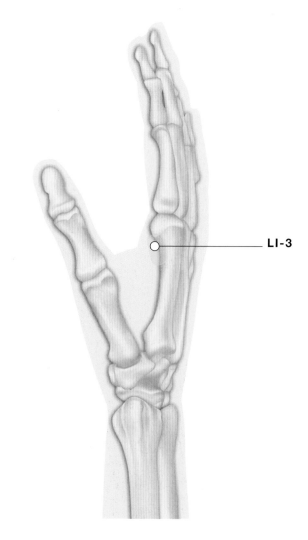

LI-3

Moxibustion
Cones: 3–5. Pole: 5–10 minutes.

Stimulation sensation
Local ache or distension possibly extending proximally or distally along channel.

Actions and indications
LI-3 is primarily indicated to *dispel wind and clear heat* and *benefit the face and throat*. Symptoms include painful, inflamed and swollen throat or eyes, toothache, chills and fever, stiffness of the neck and epistaxis.

Furthermore, it *dispels fullness from the Large Intestine* and can be used to treat such cases as diarrhoea, and abdominal distension and pain.

As *a local point* it can be used to treat pain and stiffness of the index finger or second metacarpophalangeal joint.

> **Main Areas:** Throat. Teeth. Finger. Intestines.
>
> **Main Functions:** Dispels wind and clears heat. Benefits the face and throat. Alleviates regional pain.

LI-4   Hegu
Junction Valley

合谷

Source-*Yuan* point
Command point for the Face and Mouth
One of the nine points for Returning Yang

There are a number of variations to the location of Hegu (it is a 'large point', as its Chinese name suggests). It is therefore recommended to palpate the entire area for the most reactive points. Furthermore, LI-4 may be treated at more than one location in the same session.

Standard location
At the centre of the flesh between the first and second metacarpal bones, at the highest point of the bulge of the dorsal interosseous muscle when the thumb is adducted, level with the midpoint of the second metacarpal bone.

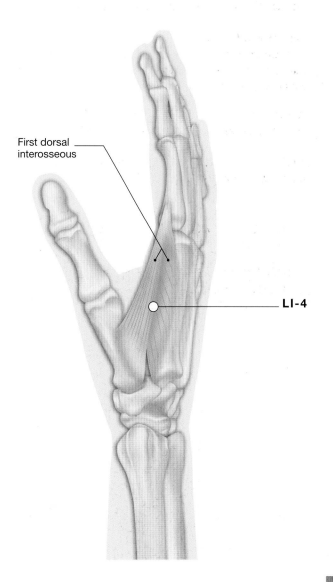

First dorsal interosseous

LI-4

LI-4

Midway

In the dorsal interosseous muscle attaching to the second metacarpal bone, or between the two bellies of the interosseous muscles attaching to the first and second metacarpal bone. In its deep position, situated in the adductor pollicis muscle.

If deqi cannot be achieved at this position, locate LI-4 a little more proximally toward the base of the metacarpal bone, or use one of the alternative locations.

Alternative locations
At the end of the crease formed between the index finger and thumb when the thumb is adducted.

At a number of points, level with the end of the crease, and closer to the second metacarpal bone than the previous location.

At variable sites in the interosseous muscles, distal to the junction of the bases of the first and second metacarpal, located with the thumb and index finger separated. These points can also be found more proximal to the previous locations.

! The radial artery is situated just distal to the junction of the base of the first and second metacarpal.

Contraindications
! LI-4 induces menstruation and labour so treating it is therefore contraindicated during pregnancy and heavy menstrual bleeding.

!! LI-4 is an extremely powerful point, and strong stimulation should be avoided in patients with deficiency conditions. In certain cases, even light stimulation can cause sudden sinking of the qi.

Best treatment positions
LI-4 can be treated with the patient sitting or lying. Try supporting the hand in a semi-supinated position.

Needling
- 0.3 to 1 cun perpendicular insertion, directed under the midpoint of the second metacarpal bone. The needle should aim to insert into the fascia joining the two bellies of the interosseous muscle. Palpate gently while adducting the thumb to ascertain the small gap.
- 1.5 to 3 cun insertion on the palmar surface (under the metacarpals) to join with P-8 and/or SI-3.
- 0.5 to 1.5 cun oblique insertion, directed distally toward LI-3 or proximally upward along the channel toward the base of the second metacarpal bone.

! Do not puncture the cutaneous branches of the radial nerve and the dorsal metacarpal artery and vein; and more deeply, the perforating branch of the radial artery; and proximally, the radial artery.

!! LI-4 is one of the most common points to cause needle shock.

Manual techniques and shiatsu
Pressure can be applied in a variety of different ways depending on the desired results and the underlying condition. The strongest method is to apply the pressure perpendicularly onto the second metacarpal bone palpating along its lateral and palmar border for the most reactive sites.

In cases where there is a lot of tension, apply friction (with careful small movements) alternating with sustained perpendicular pressure into the tight fibres, spasms and nodules in the muscle and surrounding soft tissues.

Press the point opposite LI-4 on the palmar surface simultaneously with the thumb on the dorsal surface and the index finger on the palmar. Pinch and press the muscle belly in order to access the adductor pollicis and flexor pollicis brevis muscles.

Also, apply friction to the dorsal surface with the thumb whilst holding stationary pressure on the palmar surface.

Self-treatment is highly recommended at LI-4, especially because acupressure should be applied regularly until symptoms subside. This may be done hourly.

Moxibustion
Cones: 3–10. Pole: 5–15 minutes, light or medium stimulation only. Rice-grain moxa is also effective.

! Do not overheat this area, due to underlying vessels.

Guasha
Guasha is most effective applied distally toward LI-3 or across the fibres of the interosseous muscle.

! Do not injure the dorsal metacarpal vein.

Magnets
Magnets are also effectively employed at this location.

Stimulation sensation

Stimulation of LI-4 by pressure or needling can engender extremely strong sensations of soreness, tingling, numbness, aching or electric sensation spreading out around the point and distally toward the fingers or upward toward the wrist, arm, elbow, chest and abdomen.

These sensations normally give way to numbness. The patient often sighs or breathes deeply when deqi is achieved.

Furthermore, deqi may release stuck emotions and the person may cry or start talking excessively. Additionally, because LI-4 strongly descends qi, it may induce a feeling of dizziness or tiredness. In certain cases it may also lead to symptoms of shock, including pallor, weak pulse, sweating, dizziness and nausea.

For best results, a strong sensation should be achieved. Pain and other acute symptoms should be reduced after treatment.

Actions and indications

Due to its *extremely powerful effect on the body and mind, LI-4 is possibly the most commonly used acu-point of the entire body and has been employed in the treatment of most diseases and symptoms.*

LI-4 *strongly moves stuck qi and descends excessive yang, thus alleviating pain and calming the mind.* Due to the powerful effect it has on moving qi and dispelling stasis, LI-4 is known as the *analgesia point* and is often combined with Liv-3 to relax the patient and *alleviate pain of any cause or location.* LI-4 and Liv-3 are known as the *Four Gates*, and combined, have an extremely strong pain relieving effect.

They are also considered the most important body points in acupuncture anaesthesia (combined with ear points). These two points have similarly powerful qi moving qualities (a possible reason for this is that they share the equivalent anatomical location in the largest and strongest muscular areas of the dorsal aspects of the hand and foot).

LI-4 has been extensively used to treat various *acute and chronic pain conditions*, including pain anywhere in the body, pain following injury, pain of the upper limbs, acute pain or cramping of the abdomen, painful defecation, epigastric pain, tightness, heaviness and pain of the chest, back or neck pain, headaches, pain of the eyes, ears, nose and throat.

On the *psycho-emotional* level it is effective in cases of anxiety, physical or emotional stress, frequent sighing, constriction of the throat, mental restlessness or agitation, insomnia, irritability, depression, grief, mood swings, psychological shock, extremely introverted or extroverted behaviour, aphasia and panic attacks.

Furthermore, it is helpful in the *treatment of substance abuse*, bulimia, smoking and addiction related disorders (see also Liv-3) and can help boost the metabolism and detoxify the body in weight loss or other health programmes.

LI-4 strongly *descends qi and rising yang, sedates interior wind and treats symptoms of windstroke.* Indications include convulsions, loss of consciousness, fainting, dizziness, epilepsy, numbness of the limbs and body, transient ischaemic attack, paralysis or spasticity of the arm following cerebrovascular accident, hemiplegia, hypertension, palpitations, goitre and fever.

It is a *very important point to dispel exterior wind, cold and heat, induce sweating and regulate the defensive qi* (wei qi). It *clears interior heat and Yang Ming heat, transforms phlegm, clears the Lungs, descends rebellious qi and stops coughing.* It is extensively employed to treat *febrile diseases* and most *exterior and interior Lung disorders.*

It is commonly employed to treat upper and lower respiratory tract infections, chills and fever, aversion to cold, tidal fever, excessive or absent sweating, sneezing, nasal obstruction, runny nose, pain of the nose, sore, swollen or itchy throat, tonsillitis, pharyngitis, cough, dyspnoea, shortness of breath, asthmatic wheeze and tightness, pain, heaviness and fullness of the chest.

Additionally, LI-4 helps in cases of *allergies and skin disorders due to wind, heat or toxin accumulation.* Indications include itchy or red skin rash, acne, boils, eczema, urticaria, nettle rash, insect stings, hay fever and allergic asthma. Acupuncture at LI-4 may also be employed as a medical adjunct in cases of serious allergies or anaphylaxis.

LI-4 is probably the most powerful distal point to treat *disorders of the face, mouth and sense organs.* Indications include facial paralysis, facial pain, trigeminal neuralgia, stiffness and pain of the jaw, tinnitus, inflammation of the ears, painful or bleeding gums, mouth abscesses, toothache, swelling of the face, throat or submandibular area, lymphadenopathy, goitre, itchy, painful, red, swollen and inflamed eyes, conjunctivitis, excessive lacrimation, frontal headache, migraine, pain of the whole head, redness of the face, acne, pain or swelling of the nose, epistaxis, allergic rhinitis and sinusitis.

LI-4 is the Source-Yuan point of the Large Intestine channel and can be employed to *benefit the intestine* and treat constipation, acute or chronic diarrhoea, gastroenteritis, prolapse of the large intestine and haemorrhoids.

LI-4 is also very important in the treatment of *gynaecological disorders* because it *descends qi and clears the lower jiao*, inducing menstruation, abortion or labour. Indications include dysmenorrhoea, amenorrhoea, delayed or irregular menstruation, premenstrual syndrome, delayed or prolonged labour, inadequate cervical dilation and difficulty in expulsion of the placenta.

Additionally, with the application of moxibustion, LI-4 can help *tonify yang and restore yang collapse*.

Furthermore, it is also very important in the treatment of *channel disorders* to alleviate pain and treat atrophy or paralysis. Indications include pain and stiffness along the course of the channel, particularly of the forearm, elbow and shoulder, tendinitis, frozen shoulder, cramp or spasm, spasticity, atrophy and paralysis of the arms.

Main Areas: Hand. Face. Sense organs. Mouth. Teeth. Eyes. Nose. Chest. Throat. Mind. Lungs. Abdomen. Intestine.

Main Functions: Moves stuck qi and dissipates fullness. Releases the exterior. Alleviates cough. Analgesia point.

LI-5 Yangxi
Yang Stream

River-*Jing*, Fire point

On the lateral aspect of the wrist, at the centre of the sizeable depression of the anatomical snuffbox formed by the tendons of the extensor pollicis longus and brevis muscles, between the scaphoid and radius. To aid location, extend the thumb to define the anatomical snuffbox.

Best treatment positions
LI-5 can be treated with the patient sitting or lying.

Needling
• 0.3 to 1 cun perpendicular insertion, directed into the wrist joint space between the scaphoid and radius.

! Do not puncture the cephalic vein or the cutaneous branch of the radial nerve; more deeply, the radial artery.

Manual techniques and shiatsu
Sustained perpendicular pressure is effectively applied with the thumb or fingertips. Friction of the extensor pollicis longus and brevis and abductor pollicis longus is effective for wrist and thumb mobility problems.

Another technique is to grasp the tendons of extensor pollicis brevis and abductor pollicis longus at the lateral aspect of the wrist so that the thumb presses LI-5 and the index finger Lu-9.

An effective technique is to apply the pressure into the joint space with the thumb extended, simultaneously to mobilising the wrist joint (grasp the patient's thumb with the fingers of your right hand, so that the thumb presses into LI-5. Hold the patient's wrist in a stable position with your left hand to effectively mobilise the wrist).

Moxibustion
Cones: 3. Pole: 5–15 minutes. Light or medium stimulation only. Rice-grain moxa is also effective.

! Do not overheat this area.

Stimulation sensation
Localised ache, tingling or numbness spreading into the wrist joint or up and/or down the channel.

Actions and indications
LI-5 is a very *important point for disorders of the wrist* and thumb including pain, swelling, stiffness and inflammation, soft tissue injuries, fracture, arthritis and tendinitis.

Although it is rarely used for interior complaints, it has traditionally been employed to *clear yang ming heat and calm the mind*.

Main Areas: Wrist. Hand.

Main Function: Alleviates pain and swelling.

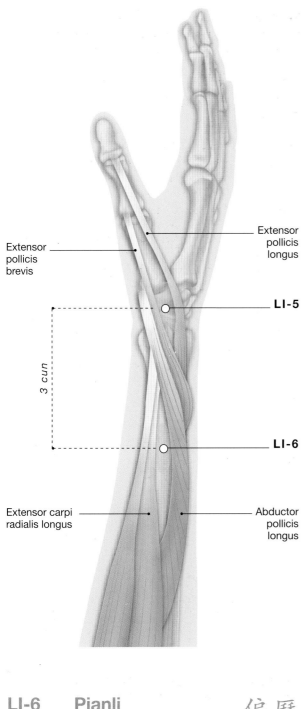

Extensor pollicis brevis

Extensor pollicis longus

Extensor carpi radialis longus

Abductor pollicis longus

LI-5

LI-6

3 cun

LI-6   Pianli

偏歷

Diverging Passage

Connecting *Luo* point

On the most lateral (radial) aspect of the forearm, in the shallow depression 3 cun proximal to LI-5, one quarter of the way along the line connecting LI-5 with LI-11.

To aid location, a visible depression appears at LI-6 when the forearm is pronated and the wrist extended.

Best treatment positions
This location can be treated with the patient lying down or sitting up. The forearm should be pronated and the elbow slightly flexed.

Needling
• 0.3 to 1 cun perpendicular insertion.
• 0.5 to 1.5 cun oblique insertion upward or downward along the channel pathway.

! Do not puncture the cephalic vein or the branches of the posterior antebrachial cutaneous nerve.

Moxibustion
Cones: 3–5. Pole: 5–10 minutes.

Guasha
Guasha is effectively applied down the channel or across the fibres of extensor carpi radialis longus and brevis, and the brachioradialis muscle.

! Do not injure the cephalic vein.

Manual techniques and shiatsu
Friction and sustained perpendicular pressure may be applied with the thumbs or fingertips.

Friction is effective across the fibres of extensor carpi radialis longus and brevis (and brachioradialis).

! Do not injure the cephalic vein or the lateral antebrachial cutaneous nerve.

Stimulation sensation
Localised ache, distension, tingling or numbness spreading up and/or down the channel.

Actions and indications
Although it is a connecting *Luo* point, LI-6 is rarely used for interior complaints. It is *mainly employed in the treatment of channel disorders and pain* of the forearm, although even for this, it is not as commonly used as other points.

It has, however, been *traditionally employed to treat a variety of disorders* including sneezing, runny nose, nasal congestion, epistaxis, sore throat, inflammation of the eyes, facial paralysis, deafness, tinnitus, earache, toothache, oedema, swelling of the face and upper body, urine retention and even madness.

Main Areas: Forearm. Wrist.

Main Function: Alleviates pain.

LI-7 Wenliu
Warm Flow

溫溜

Accumulation Cleft-*Xi* point

On the most lateral (radial) aspect of the forearm, in the shallow depression 2 cun proximal to LI-6 (5 cun proximal to LI-5), on the line connecting LI-5 with LI-11.

Best treatment positions
Similar to LI-6.

Needling
• 0.3 to 1 cun perpendicular insertion.
• 0.5 to 1.5 cun oblique insertion proximally or distally.

! Do not injure the accessory cephalic vein and the lateral antebrachial cutaneous nerve; more deeply, the radial nerve.

Actions and indications
LI-7 is primarily used in *excess conditions to alleviate pain*, particularly acute pain of the arm. It also *expels exterior pathogenic factors* causing symptoms such as sore, swollen throat, ulceration of the mouth, epistaxis, headache and paralysis, or pain of the face.

Furthermore, it *clears yang ming heat and calms the mind*, but is rarely used for these purposes.

Main Area: Forearm.

Main Function: Alleviates pain.

LI-10 Shousanli
Arm Three Miles

手三里

In the depression 2 cun distal to LI-11 on the line joining LI-11 and LI-5.

Lateral to border of the brachioradialis muscle, situated in the extensor carpi radialis longus and more deeply, in the extensor carpi radialis brevis. In its deep position lies the supinator muscle.

To aid location, define the lateral border of the brachioradialis by asking the patient to flex the elbow against resistance given to the lower part of the forearm, which should be in a semi-supine position.

Best treatment positions
LI-10 can be treated with the patient sitting or lying. It can be located and treated more easily with the elbow flexed and the forearm in a semi-supine position.

! LI-10 is often sensitive or tender.

Needling
• 0.5 to 1.5 cun perpendicular insertion into the extensor carpi radialis longus and brevis, and more deeply, the supinator muscle.

! Do not puncture the branches of the posterior or lateral antebrachial cutaneous nerve, and more deeply, the radial collateral artery and the branches of the radial nerve.

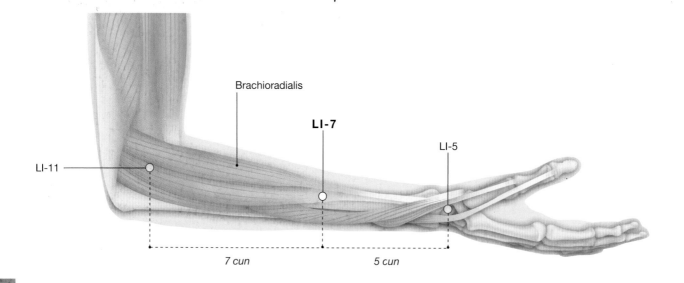

LI-11 — Brachioradialis — **LI-7** — LI-5

7 cun — 5 cun

Manual techniques and shiatsu

Friction or sustained perpendicular pressure is best applied with the thumbs or fingertips. Pressure should be strong enough for a warmth or distending soreness to extend up and down the arm.

Moxibustion

Cones: 3–7. Pole: 5–15 minutes. Light-medium stimulation only.

Cupping

Light or medium cupping with a small cup can be effective.

Guasha

Gentle guasha is effective applied across the muscle fibres or along the channel pathway.

Stimulation sensation

Warmth or a distending ache should extend around the location and up and down the forearm.

Actions and indications

LI-10 is an *important point to treat pain, stiffness, weakness, motor impairment, atrophy or paralysis of the upper limb* and shoulder.

LI-10, called *Arm Three Miles,* is the equivalent upper limb point to St-36 *Leg Three Miles,* and has similar functions such as *tonifying Qi and Blood* and *harmonising the yang ming,* albeit not as powerfully.

Arm and Leg Three Miles are commonly combined in order to *strengthen the four limbs.*

> **Main Areas:** Forearm. Arm. Shoulder. Stomach. Intestines.
>
> **Main Functions:** Strengthens the arms. Alleviates pain. Harmonises the Yang Ming.

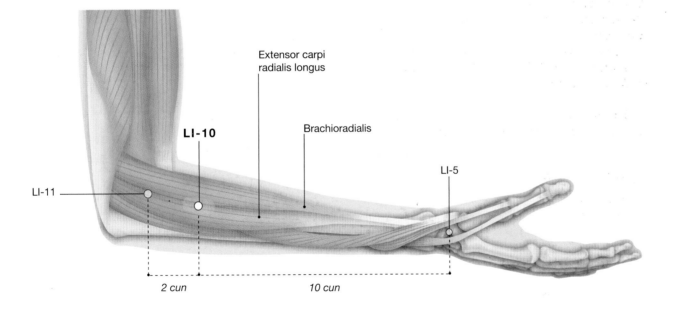

Extensor carpi radialis longus

Brachioradialis

LI-10

LI-11

LI-5

2 cun

10 cun

LI-11   Quchi

曲池

Pond at the Bend

**Uniting Sea-*He*, Earth (Tonification) point
Twelfth Ghost point**

At the lateral end of the transverse cubital crease when the elbow is flexed. Approximately midway between Lu-5 and the lateral epicondyle of the humerus.

Situated lateral to the border of the brachioradialis muscle near the origin of the extensor carpi radialis longus muscle.

To aid location, apply pressure palpation to determine the most reactive site. If there is no deqi reaction during pressure palpation try locating and treating it with the elbow extended (this helps bring the qi closer to the surface and subsequently increases deqi).

Best treatment positions
LI-11 can be treated with the patient sitting or lying. It is most often treated with the elbow flexed and the forearm lying across the abdomen. However, it can also be treated with the elbow extended and the forearm pronated.

Needling
• 0.5 to 1.5 cun perpendicular insertion (elbow flexed).
• 1 to 3 cun perpendicular insertion angled to connect with Lu-5 or He-3 (elbow flexed).
• 1 to 2 cun oblique insertion into the extensor carpi radialis longus and extensor carpi radialis brevis directed distally down the channel (elbow extended).
• 0.5 to 1 cun insertion directed slightly laterally into the joint space between the humerus and radial head (elbow flexed).

! Do not puncture the branches of the posterior antebrachial cutaneous nerve; more deeply, the radial collateral artery and the branches of the radial nerve; deeper still, the brachial artery and median nerve.

Manual techniques and shiatsu
Friction or sustained perpendicular pressure can be applied quite strongly to this location with the thumbs or fingertips. Friction techniques are effective applied across the muscle fibres inserting at the lateral epicondyle, including the common extensor tendon and the extensor radialis longus. These techniques are stronger if applied with the elbow extended and the forearm pronated.

Additionally, mobilise the elbow joint simultaneously to pressure application.

Another effective technique for elbow and arm disorders is to apply the pressure simultaneously to LI-11 and Lu-5. An efficient way to achieve this is to apply the thumb to Lu-5, and middle finger to LI-11 while grasping and pressing the muscles between the two points.

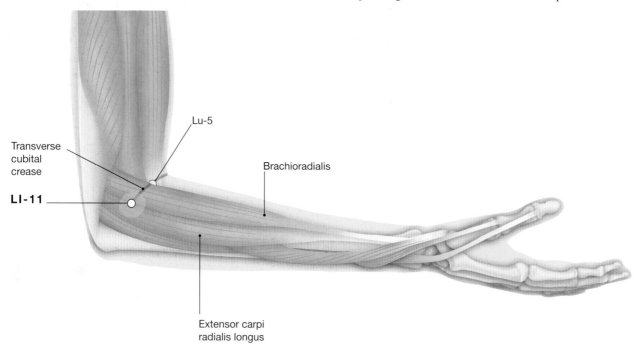

Transverse cubital crease

Lu-5

Brachioradialis

LI-11

Extensor carpi radialis longus

Moxibustion

Cones: 3–10. Pole: 5–20 minutes. Rice-grain moxa is also effectively employed.

Cupping

Medium or strong cupping with small cups can be very effective for chronic inflammation of the extensor tendons.

Guasha

Apply guasha across the muscle fibres or distally along the channel pathway.

Magnets

Stick-on magnets can be very beneficial for a variety of complaints. Use alternating poles on LI-11, LI-12, Lu-5, LI-4, LI-15 and GB-21.

Stimulation sensation

A strong aching or electric sensation should extend around the location and down the anterior and lateral aspects of the forearm (Lung and Large Intestine channels) toward the wrist and hand. The sensation may also be perceived travelling proximally toward the shoulder and chest. Deqi at this location can be quite intense and often gives way to numbness. It varies considerably depending on the exact location and style of treatment applied. See note on locating LI-11.

Actions and indications

LI-11 is one of the *most important and commonly used points for a wide variety of disorders*. Its primary functions are to *dispel wind and release the exterior, clear heat, dampness and damp-heat, descend excessive yang, cool the Blood and alleviate itching*. Furthermore, it *regulates qi and blood, dispels stasis, sedates interior wind and harmonises the yang ming*.

Indications include low or high fever with or without chills and sweating, aching body, headache, red, inflamed or itchy eyes, nasal obstruction, pain and swelling of the throat, earache, toothache, headache, goitre, phlegm nodules, lymphadenopathy, cough, asthma, dyspnoea, expectoration of yellow sticky phlegm, fullness and heaviness of the chest, upper respiratory tract infections or allergies, abdominal distension and pain, nausea, vomiting, hypochondrial pain and distension, jaundice, hepatitis, liver diseases, diarrhoea, dysentery, gastroenteritis, urinary tract infections, cystitis, dry scaly skin, itchy red skin rash, itching in general, acute or chronic skin diseases such as acne, eczema, urticaria, systemic or local inflammatory or allergic conditions, swelling and oedema, hypertension, windstroke, facial paralysis, hemiplegia and dizziness.

Psychologically, LI-11 helps in cases of depression, restlessness and irritability.

LI-11 *activates the channel, dispels stasis and alleviates pain* and is one of the most important points for *disorders of the elbow and forearm*. Indications include impaired movement or atrophy of the elbow, arm and forearm, pain and stiffness of the shoulder, periarthritis, lateral epicondylitis and ankylosis of the elbow.

> **Main Areas:** Elbow. Forearm. Throat. Face (nose, eyes, mouth, ears). Lungs. Abdomen. Intestines.
>
> **Main Functions:** Clears heat and damp heat. Descends rising yang. Regulates qi. Dispels stasis.

LI-12　Zhouliao

肘髎

Elbow Bone Hole

In the depression just above the lateral epicondyle of the humerus, approximately 1 cun supralateral to LI-11 when the elbow is flexed at 90 degrees. On the lateral aspect of the triceps brachii muscle at the origin of the anconeus muscle.

Best treatment positions
This location can be treated with the patient lying down or sitting up in a chair. It should be treated with the elbow flexed at approximately 90 degrees.

! This location can be extremely painful to the slightest touch, particularly if there is inflammation or stiffness of the elbow.

Needling
• 0.5 to 1 cun perpendicular insertion (elbow flexed).

!　Do not puncture the posterior cutaneous antebrachial nerve, and more deeply, branches of the radial collateral artery and radial nerve.

Manual techniques and shiatsu
Friction or sustained perpendicular pressure can be applied with the thumbs or fingertips. Friction techniques are effective applied across the triceps brachii and anconeus muscle fibres.

!　This location is often painful.

Moxibustion
Cones: 3. Pole: 5–10 minutes.

Guasha
Effective.

Actions and indications
LI-12 is an *important local point* for disorders of the elbow including difficulty in flexing and extending the elbow, pain, atrophy or paralysis of the arm.

Main Area: Elbow.

Main Functions: Regulates qi and Blood. Alleviates pain.

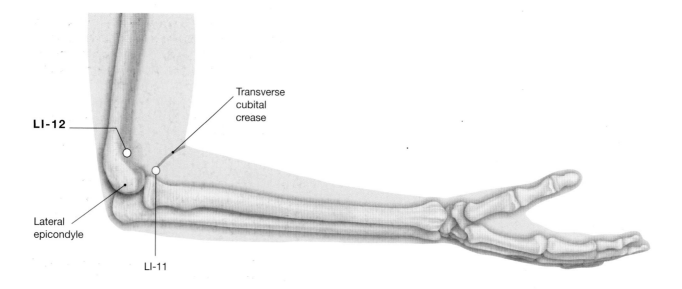

LI-12

Transverse
cubital
crease

Lateral
epicondyle

LI-11

LI-14 Binao

臂臑

Upper Arm Prominence

Intersection of the Small Intestine, Bladder and Yang Wei Mai on the Large Intestine

On the lateral aspect of the humerus along the line joining LI-11 to LI-15, in the depression slightly anterior and superior to the insertion of the deltoid muscle when the arm is hanging down by the side.

Ask the patient to lift (abduct) the arm against resistance to contract the deltoid and define its insertion.

Alternative locations
(1) In a depression between the deltoid muscle fibres just superior to its insertion.
(2) In the depression posterior to the deltoid insertion.

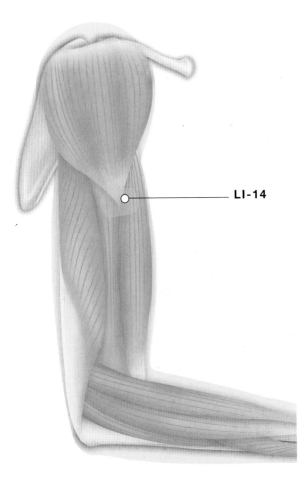

LI-14

Best treatment positions
This location can be treated with the patient lying supine or sideways, or sitting up.

Needling
• 0.3 to 0.7 cun perpendicular insertion.
• 0.5 to 1.5 cun oblique upward insertion into the muscle.
• 1 to 1.5 cun horizontal insertion under the deltoid insertion posteriorly or anteriorly. Insert the needle at the main location to needle posteriorly. To needle anteriorly, use the second alternative location, just posterior to the deltoid insertion.

! Do not puncture the posterior brachial cutaneous nerve, and more deeply, branches of the deep brachial artery and vein.

Moxibustion
Cones: 3–5. Pole: 5–10 minutes.

Guasha
Guasha is effectively applied across the deltoid insertion and upwards between the deltoid muscle fibres.

! This location can be painful.

Manual techniques and shiatsu
Friction or sustained perpendicular pressure may be applied with the thumbs or fingertips. Friction of the deltoid insertion and up the channel between the anterior and middle fibres of the deltoid is also extremely effective.

Shiatsu pressure is best applied in a side-lying or sitting position.

Actions and indications
LI-14 is mainly used to *treat pain, stiffness, atrophy, paralysis or impaired mobility of the arm and shoulder*. It is particularly indicated for frozen shoulder and difficulty in lifting the arm.

Other symptoms it has been traditionally used for include pain and inflammation of the eyes, phlegm nodules in the neck and arm, goitre and chest pain.

> **Main Areas:** Arm. Shoulder.
>
> **Main Functions:** Regulates qi and Blood. Alleviates pain.

LI-15 Jianyu

Shoulder and Clavicle

肩髃

Intersection of the Small Intestine and Yang Qiao Mai on the Large Intestine channel

On the anterolateral aspect of the shoulder, in the anterior of the two distinct depressions between the anterior and middle belly of the deltoid muscle. Between the acromion and the greater tubercle of the humerus.

To define the depressions, ask the patient to lift (abduct) the arm. Use resistance if necessary.

Locate LI-15 directly anterior to SJ-I4.

Best treatment positions
LI-15 is usually treated with the arm down by the sides of the body, although it can also be needled with the arm abducted (raised).

Needling
• With the arm down by the side, 0.5 to 1 cun perpendicular insertion. The needle should enter the space between the subacromial bursa inferiorly and the acromion process superiorly.

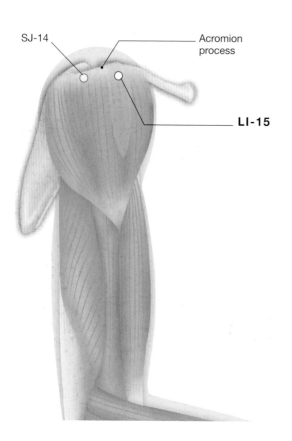

SJ-14

Acromion process

LI-15

• With the arm down by the side, 0.5 to 2 cun oblique or transverse insertion down the channel between the anterior and medial fibres of the deltoid.
• With the arm abducted (raised), 1 to 3 cun perpendicular insertion directed toward He-1.
• With the arm abducted, 0.5 to 2 cun transverse-oblique distal insertion into the deltoid fibres.
• Posterior transverse insertion to join with SJ-14.

Moxibustion
Cones: 3–5. Pole: 10–20 minutes. Indirect moxibustion is most effective applied for 15–30 minutes at LI-14 and other major points surrounding the shoulder (including LI-15, SJ-14, LI-16, GB-21, LI-14, Lu-2 and M-UE-48 Jianqian).

Cupping
Small or medium cups may be used. Curved rim cups are best. Medium to strong suction is effective over needles or separately.

Guasha
Guasha is very effective around the entire shoulder joint, particularly in cases of stiffness and pain.

Magnets
Use opposite poles on LI-15 and SJ-14.

Manual techniques and shiatsu
Sustained perpendicular pressure or friction techniques may be applied into the space between the acromion process and head of humerus with the thumbs or fingertips. Friction down the channel between the anterior and middle fibres of the deltoid is also extremely effective. Shiatsu pressure can also be applied to the surrounding area with the forearms or elbows (carefully) in a side-lying or sitting position.

Stimulation sensation
Distension, aching, soreness or electricity extending to the areas being treated (commonly into the shoulder joint, up toward the neck and down the arm toward the elbow, forearm, hand and fingers).

Actions and indications
LI-15 is very useful in *many disorders of the shoulder*. It effectively treats pain and stiffness of the shoulder particularly if there is *difficulty in lifting the arm* and moving it forward (abduction and flexion of the shoulder). It is particularly indicated for supraspinatus tendinitis, periarthritis of the shoulder, heat in the shoulder (inflammation), frozen shoulder and atrophy or paralysis of the upper limb.

LI-15 is also mentioned as one of the Seven Points alongside Lu-2, Du-2 and Bl-40.

Other traditional indications include skin rashes due to exterior wind-heat, goitre, toothache and hypertension.

> **Main Area:** Shoulder.
>
> **Main Functions:** Regulates qi and Blood. Dispels stasis. Alleviates pain.

LI-16 Jugu

Great Bone

巨骨

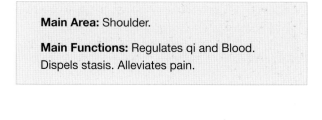

Intersection of the Yang Qiao Mai on the Large Intestine channel

On the superior aspect of the shoulder, at the centre of the large depression medial to the acromion process. In the trapezius and supraspinatus muscles.

To aid location, slide the tip of the finger over the acromion. It should fall into the depression of LI-16.

Best treatment positions
This location can be treated with the patient in a supine, side-lying or sitting position.

! This is a sensitive point and both pressure or acupuncture treatment can be dangerous if incorrectly applied.

Needling
• 0.5 to 1.5 cun perpendicular insertion, directed laterally.

! Do not puncture the branches of the lateral (middle) supraclavicular nerve.
!! Do not needle deeply medially because the lung apex may be punctured.

Moxibustion
Pole: 5–10 minutes. Direct moxibustion is not recommended at this location. Rice-grain moxa can be used.

Guasha
Guasha is applicable across the trapezius fibres and upwards toward GB-21 or posteriorly toward SI-12.

Manual techniques and shiatsu
Deep, sustained perpendicular pressure is most effectively applied with the person sitting up or lying sideways. Friction techniques are not so easily applicable, particularly if the gap between the bones is quite small. Self-acupressure is also applicable.

Stimulation sensation
A distending, aching or tingling sensation should radiate into the shoulder and down toward the lungs and chest. Also the sensation can extend upwards toward the throat and submandibular area, or distally down the arm.

Actions and indications
LI-16 is a powerful point to *regulate qi and Blood, dispel stasis* and *alleviate pain.* It is primarily used to treat pain and impaired mobility of the shoulder and arm.

Furthermore, it relaxes, opens and clears the chest, aiding the Lung function of dispersing and descending, and helps clear phlegm accumulation from the upper jiao. Indications include pain and swelling of the neck and supraclavicular area, lymphadenopathy, goitre, thyroid disease, heaviness of the chest, dyspnoea and cough.

LI-16 has also been traditionally employed to treat blood stasis in the chest causing coughing or vomiting blood and epilepsy.

> **Main Areas:** Shoulder. Chest.
>
> **Main Functions:** Regulates qi and Blood. Dispels stasis. Alleviates pain. Opens the chest.

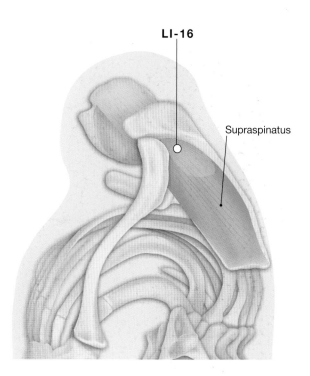

LI-16

Supraspinatus

LI-18 Futu

扶突

Beside the Prominence

Window of Heaven point

On the anterolateral aspect of the neck, in the depression between the two heads of the sternocleidomastoid muscle, directly lateral to St-9 Renying, approximately 3 cun lateral to the tip of the laryngeal prominence (Adam's apple).

To emphasize the sternocleidomastoid border, ask the patient to turn their head away from the side to be palpated whilst applying resistance.

Best treatment positions
Bilateral acupuncture treatment is best applied in a supine position without a pillow under the head so that the throat is in an open position. Unilateral treatment can be effective in a side-lying position. However, pressure techniques can also be applied sitting up. See also St-9.

! This is an extremely sensitive location and both massage or acupuncture treatment can be extremely dangerous if incorrectly applied.

Needling
• 0.3 to 0.5 cun perpendicular insertion.

! Do not needle deeply. Do not puncture branches of the greater auricular or transverse cervical nerve.

Moxibustion
Light indirect stimulation for 5–10 minutes. Direct moxibustion is contraindicated at this location.

Manual techniques and shiatsu
Light friction techniques and sustained perpendicular pressure are effectively applied carefully with the fingertips or thumbs. Stimulate regularly until symptoms subside.

! Do not apply strong pressure to this area.

Stimulation sensation
A distending, aching or tingling sensation spreading out around the point and extending toward the shoulder or into the throat upwards to the submandibular area and/or down toward the chest.

Actions and indications
LI-18 is primarily used for *disorders of the throat* including pain, swelling and acute inflammation of the throat and neck, loss of voice, cough and difficulty swallowing caused by exterior wind, phlegm or heat accumulation from febrile or thyroid disease. It can also be used for paralysis of the throat muscles.

Main Area: Throat.

Main Function: Alleviates swelling and pain.

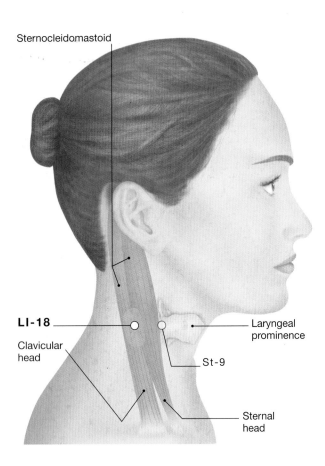

Sternocleidomastoid

LI-18

Clavicular head

St-9

Laryngeal prominence

Sternal head

LI-20 Yingxiang

Receiving Fragrance

Intersection of the Stomach on the Large Intestine channel
Window of Heaven point

In the nasolabial sulcus, level with the midpoint of the lateral border of the ala nasi.

Needling
- 0.3 to 1 cun transverse insertion directed upward and medially to join with Bitong (M-HN-14).
- 0.2 to 0.5 cun oblique or transverse insertion directed directly downward.
- 0.5 to 1.5 cun transverse insertion directed downward along nasolabial sulcus.

Manual techniques and shiatsu
Sustained perpendicular pressure or gentle friction in tiny circles is effective and may be applied with the thumb or fingertips. Also stretching the two points away from each other so that the nostril opens is effective.

Self-acupressure is most effective applied regularly throughout the day until symptoms subside. An effective self-shiatsu technique is employed in a sitting position. Place your thumb onto LI-20 so that your fingertips touch your forehead to offer support. Allow the weight of your head to fall onto the point (by leaning slightly forward) so that it is pressed against the tip of the thumb. This can be done unilaterally or bilaterally.

Stimulation sensation
Distension, ache or tingling is often perceived extending into the nasal cavity and back of the throat. It may also extend up the cheek toward the eye. Itching of the nose, runny nasal discharge and lacrimation often occur as a result of deqi here and indicate that the stimulation is working. In some cases sneezing or an itchy sensation in the throat can occur. The nose should start to open immediately when deqi is perceived.

Actions and indications
LI-20 is a *major point to open the nose and benefit the breathing*. It is extensively used to treat nasal obstruction, epistaxis, loss of sense of smell and facial pain caused by chronic or acute inflammatory conditions such as rhinitis, nasal polyps and sinusitis.

LI-20 can also treat facial paralysis, acne, swelling or itching of the face, mouth abscesses, toothache and redness and pain of the eye.

Breathing should be improved after treatment. If there is no difference, treat LI-20 again for longer, or with a different technique.

> **Main Area:** Nose.
>
> **Main Functions:** Improves breathing and smell. Clears heat and wind.

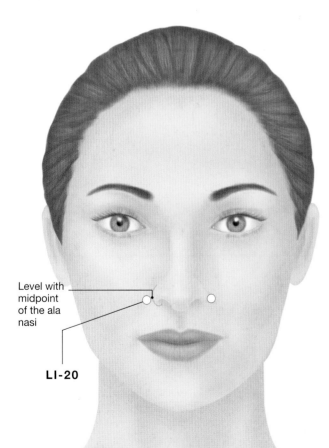

Level with midpoint of the ala nasi

LI-20

Chapter 12

Points of the

Leg Yang Ming
Stomach Channel

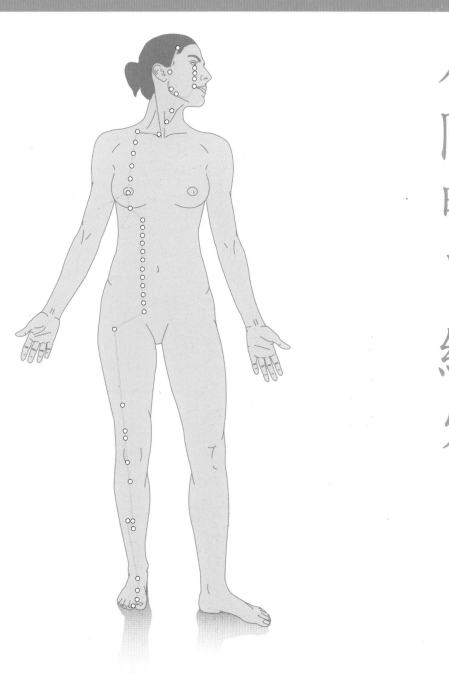

足
陽
明
胃
經
穴

St-1 Chengqi

承泣

Tear Container

Intersection of the Yang Qiao Mai and Ren Mai on the Stomach channel

Between the eyeball and the midpoint of the infraorbital ridge, level with the centre of the pupil when the eye is focussed straight ahead.

Situated in the orbicularis oculi muscle; in its deep position, in the inferior oblique and inferior rectus muscle.

!! This is one of the most sensitive and dangerous points and great care should be taken in all methods of treatment.

Best treatment positions
A supine position with head supported comfortably with pillows is best.

Needling
• 0.3 to 1 cun perpendicular insertion angled between the eyeball and inferior orbital ridge.
• 0.3 to 0.5 cun transverse insertion along the orbital ridge, toward the inner or outer canthus.

!! Needling St-1 is potentially dangerous and requires special skill and experience. Great care should be taken as wrongly angled insertion will damage the eye.

Use the thinnest needle possible (gauges: 36–40 mm: 0.18–0.14).

Support the eyeball with the tip of the finger and insert the needle slowly and carefully, whilst the patient looks upward. Angle the needle slightly downward and then perpendicularly along the inferior orbital wall under the eyeball. Do not manipulate the needle.

The patient should keep the eyes as relaxed and still as possible during needle retention and avoid unnecessary blinking. It is best that the eyes remain closed for the duration of the treatment, until after the needle is removed to avoid the skin being pulled.

Apply pressure with a cotton pad after removing the needle for up to one minute.

! St-1 can bruise easily. If any slight swelling is observed remove the needle immediately and apply pressure and a cold compress. If bruising occurs, apply a cold compress for 2 to 5 minutes. The patient can take an arnica homeopathic remedy of 30 ch or 200 ch, followed by 12 ch or 30 ch per day for a week (in some cases a higher potency may be given). The bruising should disappear within a week and will not affect the eyesight.

!! Do not puncture the infraorbital artery, vein and nerve, the oculomotor nerve, the opthalmic artery, and the optic nerve.

Manual techniques and shiatsu
Light, sustained pressure may be applied carefully onto the infraorbital ridge with the pad of the fingers (the illustration does not show a shaded pressure area).

! Pressure into the small space between eyeball and ridge is NOT applicable, although qigong therapy can be applied here. Do not friction or rub this location and avoid the use of oils or massage lubricants. Ensure hands are perfectly clean and void of dust, oil, etc.

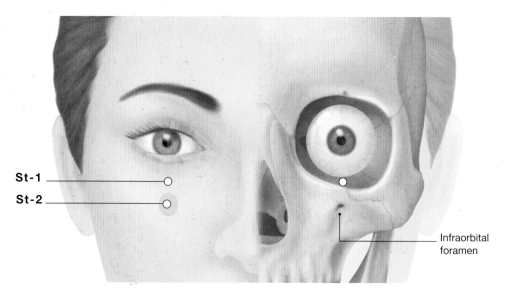

St-1
St-2
Infraorbital foramen

Moxibustion
Contraindicated.

Stimulation sensation
A distending or pulling sensation spreading out around the point and into the eye or down the cheek may be obtained. Lacrimation often occurs.

Actions and indications
St-1 is an important point, used in a *wide variety of eye disorders*. It *clears and brightens the eyes, dispels wind, clears heat and soothes inflammatory reactions* of the eye.

Indications include tired eyes, pain, swelling or redness of the eyes, excessive tearing, itching or dryness of the eyes, migraine, allergies, keratitis, squint, deviation of the eye, spasm or paralysis of the muscle under the eye.

It is also effectively employed to help *improve vision* in a variety of disorders including myopia, astigmatism, hypermetropia, retinitis, optic neuritis, glaucoma, night blindness, colour blindness and cataract.

St-1 is an *important beauty point to improve the appearance of the area under the eyes*. It treats dark circles, bags, puffiness and swelling.

> **Main Area:** Eyes and area below.
>
> **Main Functions:** Benefits the eyes and area below. Improves vision. Dispels wind and clears heat.

St-2   Sibai   四白
Four Direction Brightness

In the depression of the infraorbital foramen, in line with St-1 and St-3. To aid location, it is approximately 0.3 cun below St-1.

! This is a very sensitive point.

Best treatment positions
Similar to Chengqi St-1.

Needling
• 0.1 to 0.3 cun perpendicular insertion into the infraorbital foramen.

! Do not puncture the infraorbital neurovascular bundle.

• 0.3 to 0.5 cun transverse insertion upward and outward.
• 0.3 cun transverse insertion upward toward St-1.

!! Do not insert the needle too far to avoid damaging the eye ball.

• 0.5 to 1 cun transverse insertion outward toward SI-18 or other areas of the cheek.
• Transverse insertion downward toward St-3, Bitong M-HN-14, LI-20 or other areas of the cheek.

Manual techniques and shiatsu
Stationary pressure and light friction may be applied carefully and gently to the infraorbital foramen.

! This point is sensitive and can bruise if excessive or incorrectly angled pressure is applied.

Stimulation sensation
A distending sensation spreading out around the point, down the cheek toward the gums and nose or upward toward the eye should be achieved. Lacrimation often occurs.

Actions and indications
St-2 is an *important point employed in many eye disorders*. It has a general *brightening effect on the eyes and similar actions such as dissipating wind, clearing heat, stopping excessive lacrimation and helping to improve the vision*.

Additionally, it *regulates the qi and Blood circulation* helping to *alleviate pain of the front of the face, cheeks and eyes*. In comparison to St-1, St-2 is less effective for conditions of the eye but more effective for pain, paralysis or spasm of the under eye and cheek muscles. Also, it is easier to treat than St-1 and therefore more commonly used.

Indications include spasm or paralysis of the muscles under the eye, deviation of the eye or cheek, excessive lacrimation due to wind, any acute or chronic inflammatory eye condition, pain, swelling or redness of the eyes, rhinitis, sinusitis, facial pain or paralysis. St-2 is also used in the treatment of trigeminal neuralgia and migraine. It is also an *important beauty point for the under-eye area* as it treats puffiness, swelling, bags and dark circles.

> **Main Areas:** Eye. Area below eye. Cheek. Nose.
>
> **Main Functions:** Dispels wind and clears heat. Stops excessive lacrimation. Improves appearance.

St-3 Juliao
Great Bone Hole

巨髎

Intersection of the Yang Qiao Mai and Large Intestine on the Stomach channel

Below the zygomatic arch, directly below St-1 and St-2, approximately level with the lower border of the ala nasi. In the zygomaticus minor muscle and more deeply, the levator anguli oris.

Best treatment positions
St-3 is best treated with the patient lying down in a supine position. However, sitting can also be employed.

Needling
• 0.2 to 0.5 cun perpendicular insertion.
• Oblique insertion in various directions (e.g. toward Sibai St-2, Dicang St-4 or Yingxiang LI-20).

Manual techniques and shiatsu
Stationary perpendicular pressure and friction techniques are applicable with the fingertips or thumbs.

St-3

Moxibustion
Moxibustion is rarely recommended on facial points, except in cases of cold invasion and facial paralysis. It can however be very effectively employed with indirect, light stimulation for up to 5–10 minutes. Use smokeless moxa only.

Also, a moxa boat can be effectively employed over the front of the cheek.

! Avoid overstimulation.

Stimulation sensation
An aching, numb or tingling sensation is often achieved spreading out around the point, across the cheek, gums and nose and upward toward the eye. Also, lacrimation often occurs, indicating deqi.

Actions and indications
St-3 is a *primary point for the treatment of nasal obstruction*, sinusitis and pain of the cheek, as it *dispels wind and cold from the face, relieves swelling, promotes qi and Blood circulation and alleviates pain*. It also *effectively clears heat and benefits the eyes*.

Clinical manifestations include sinusitis, nasal obstruction, epistaxis, allergic rhinitis, allergic swelling of the lips and cheek, frontal headache, toothache, disorders of the upper gums and teeth, paralysis and pain of the face, deviation of the mouth, cheek or eye, spasm, tic or paralysis of the cheek, trigeminal neuralgia, twitching of the eyelids, excessive lacrimation, red, painful or swollen eyes, conjunctivitis, keratitis and deteriorating vision.

> **Main Areas:** Cheeks and centre of the face. Nose. Sinuses. Eyes. Gums and teeth.
>
> **Main Functions:** Dispels wind and clears heat. Opens the nose. Alleviates pain.

St-4   Dicang

Earth Granary

地倉

Intersection of the Large Intestine, Yang Qiao and Ren Mai on the Stomach channel

Directly below St-3, approximately 0.4 cun lateral to the corner of the mouth. In the risorius, zygomatic major and more deeply the buccinator muscle.

Best treatment positions
This point can be treated with the head facing upwards or slightly sideways, depending on the treatment to be applied, with the patient lying in a supine or side position.

Needling
- 0.5 to 2 cun transverse insertion outward toward St-5 or St-6.
- 0.5 to 1.5 cun transverse insertion upward toward St-3 or LI-20.
- 0.2 to 0.3 cun perpendicular insertion into the risorius (also the zygomaticus major) and buccinator muscles.

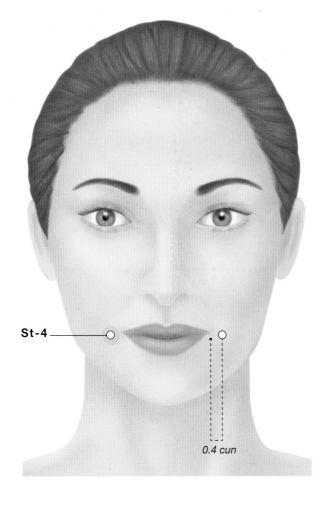

St-4

0.4 cun

!! Do not apply large or strong manipulation. Do not needle deeply. Do not puncture the buccal branch of the facial nerve (the facial artery and vein are situated laterally to St-4).

! This point can bruise easily. If any slight swelling is observed remove the needle immediately and apply pressure and a cold compress.

Manual techniques and shiatsu
Stationary pressure and friction can be applied taking care not to press the cheek too hard onto the underlying teeth. If stronger pressure must be applied, ask the patient to contract the risorius muscles (by pursing the lips slightly and smiling with the corners of the mouth).

An effective technique for tonifying and lifting the mouth and cheek area is to apply pressure into the risorius muscle with the fingertip whilst stretching the corners of the mouth in an upward and outward direction. At the same time the patient contracts the surrounding muscles in an opposite direction quite strongly by pursing the lips. This technique is most effective if applied regularly as a self-exercise.

Moxibustion
Not recommended. However, in some rare cases, light indirect stimulation for up to 5 minutes can be helpful. See also St-3 and St-5.

Stimulation sensation
Distension, ache or tingling is achieved locally or toward the nose, the eye or the cheek.

Actions and indications
St-4 is mainly used to treat *disorders of the mouth and cheek by clearing wind and cold, relaxing the channels and promoting circulation of qi and Blood.* Indications include facial paralysis and pain, trigeminal neuralgia, spasm or tic of the cheek, mouth or muscles under the eye, excessive salivation, drooling, aphasia, inability to eat, bulimia and excessive hunger.

St-4 is also commonly employed as a beauty point to release tension of the risorius muscle.

Treatment at St-4 is used to suppress the appetite during weight loss programmes. Self-acupressure can be applied regularly throughout the day or when food cravings are experienced.

> **Main Areas:** Mouth. Lips. Front of cheek.
>
> **Main Function:** Depresses appetite.

St-5 Daying

Great Reception

大迎

On the body of the mandible, in the groove-like depression anterior to the border of the masseter muscle.

To aid location, bulge the cheeks out (as if blowing into a wind instrument) or clench the jaw tightly to define the masseter muscle.

! This location can be painful or tender and all forms of treatment should be applied carefully.

Best treatment positions
St-5 can be treated with the head facing upwards or slightly sideways, depending on the treatment to be applied, with the patient in a supine or side-lying position.

Needling
• 0.3 to 0.5 cun perpendicular insertion.
• 0.3 to 1.3 cun transverse insertion towards St-6.
• 0.5 to 1.5 cun transverse insertion towards Ren-24 or St-4.

! Do not apply large or strong manipulation. Do not puncture the facial artery and vein or the branches of the facial nerve.

Moxibustion
Not recommended. However, in some rare cases, light indirect stimulation for up to 5 minutes can be helpful.

! Avoid overheating this location because of the underlying facial artery and vein.

Manual techniques and shiatsu
Stationary pressure and friction techniques with the fingertips are effectively applied perpendicularly and also in a posterior direction onto the anterior border of the masseter muscle. Friction of the border of the masseter is also very effective. Applying pressure simultaneously to St-5 and St-6 is also very helpful for disorders of the jaw.

Treat St-5 instead of St-6, in cases where the latter location is too painful or tight.

Stimulation sensation
A strong sensation spreading out around the point and across the jaw and cheek should be achieved for best results.

Actions and indications
St-5 is primarily employed to *clear the channel, circulate qi and Blood and alleviate pain*. Indications include pain or swelling of lower teeth or jaw, caries, periodonditis or other inflammatory conditions of teeth and gums, receding gums, deviation of the mouth, swelling of the cheek, inflammation of the parotid gland, facial paralysis and pain and clenched jaw.

St-5 is not as commonly used as St-6 for jaw problems, because the latter is usually more dynamic.

> **Main Areas:** Jaw. Cheek. Gums. Teeth.
>
> **Main Functions:** Regulates qi and Blood. Dispels stasis. Alleviates pain.

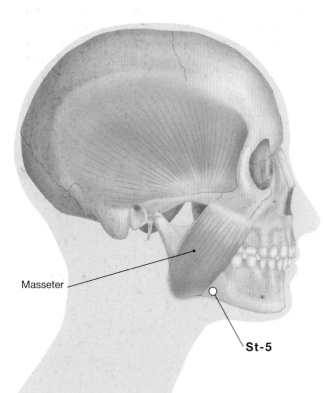

Masseter

St-5

St-6   Jiache

頰車

Jaw Bone

Seventh Ghost point

In the depression at the prominence of the masseter muscle, about one finger width anterosuperior to the tip of the angle of mandible. Locate with the jaw clenched.

Best treatment positions
This point can be treated with the head facing upwards or sideways, depending on the treatment to be applied, with the patient lying down supine or sideways. However, sitting can also be employed.

Needling
• 0.3 to 0.5 cun perpendicular insertion.
• 0.5 to 2 cun transverse insertion toward St-4.
• Upward transverse insertion into the masseter.

! Do not puncture the buccal branches of the facial nerve.

Moxibustion
Lightly applied indirect moxibustion can be applied in certain cases for up to 3 minutes.

Guasha
Light guasha can be effectively applied across or along the masseter fibres to treat pain and other disorders of the jaw.

Manual techniques and shiatsu
Perpendicular pressure and friction can be applied with the fingertips or thumbs simultaneously to both sides in a supine or sitting position. Additionally unilateral pressure can be applied with the patient lying sideways or supine with the head rotated slightly. If this location is very tight and painful apply gentle circular and cross-fibre friction with a lubricant applied to the fingertips.

! This location can be extremely tender or painful to the slightest touch.

!! Wrongly applied or excessive unilateral pressure may damage the temporomandibular joint.

Stimulation sensation
A strong sensation is easily achieved because in most people there is much tension in this area. The sensation should spread out around the point toward the jaw, cheek, ear and/or sides of the face.

Actions and indications
St-6 is *very powerful and commonly used in the treatment of disorders of the jaw and temporomandibular joint (TMJ)*. Its primary functions are to *clear the channel, remove obstructions, relax the sinews and alleviate pain*. Indications include tightness and pain of the jaw, temporomandibular joint syndrome, clenching or grinding of the teeth, tension headache, migraine, toothache, swelling of cheeks, parotitis, swelling and inflammation of the gums, deviation of the mouth, facial paralysis and pain, and trigeminal neuralgia.

St-6 can also be used to *calm the mind and relax the head and neck* in cases of mental restlessness causing symptoms such as stress, tension headaches, stiffness and pain of the neck, and insomnia. It has also been traditionally employed to treat excessive salivation.

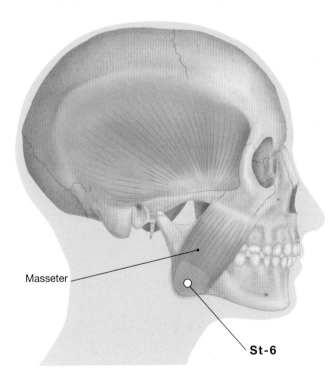

Masseter

St-6

> **Main Areas:** Jaw. TMJ. Teeth. Cheek. Head. Mind.
>
> **Main Functions:** Benefits the jaw. Dispels stasis. Alleviates pain. Calms the mind.

St-7 Xiaguan
下關

Below the Arch

Intersection of the Gallbladder and Stomach

In the depression of the mandibular notch, anterior to the condyloid process of the mandible and at the lower border of the zygomatic arch. Directly below GB-3. Situated in the lateral pterygoid muscle.

To aid location, place a finger on the condyloid process of the mandible with the patient's mouth open. When the mouth is closed, the finger will fall into St-7.

! This location can be extremely tender or painful to the slightest touch.

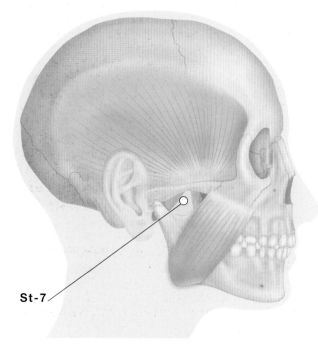

St-7

Best treatment positions
St-7 can be treated with the head facing upwards or sideways, depending on the treatment to be applied. It should be treated with the mouth closed, except when applying specific manual techniques.

Needling
• 0.3 to 0.5 cun perpendicular insertion angled slightly downward (St-7 can in certain cases be needled up to 1.5 cun, but this should not be attempted by practitioners without appropriate experience).
• 1 to 1.5 cun transverse insertion inferiorly toward St-6, posteriorly toward SJ-21, SI-19 or GB-2, or anteriorly along the lower border of the zygomatic toward SI-18.

!! Do not needle deeply, because this holds considerable risk of puncturing any of the vessels located here. Superficially lies the transverse facial artery and vein, and the zygomatic branches of the facial nerve. More deeply, the maxillary artery and vein. Also, do not puncture an enlarged parotid gland.

Moxibustion
Gentle indirect moxibustion can be used, although direct moxibustion is contraindicated.

Guasha
Gentle guasha can be effective, although it can cause bruising and is therefore rarely used here. However, guasha can be extremely effective for acute pain of the temporomandibular joint and toothache.

Magnets
Magnets can also be helpful.

Manual techniques and shiatsu
Similar to St-6. In order to achieve a stronger and deeper stimulation at this location, try applying stationary pressure carefully with the patient's mouth slightly open.

!! Avoid excessive unilateral pressure. This poses considerable risk of injuring the temporomandibular joint.

Stimulation sensation
Localised distension, numbness and aching spreading into the temporomandibular joint should be achieved. Deqi may also reach the ears, sides of the face, cheeks and gums. Strong stimulation can cause an electric or numb sensation.

Actions and indications
St-7 is a *very important point for disorders of the temporomandibular joint*. It *alleviates pain and stiffness of the jaw and benefits the ears, cheeks and teeth*.

Indications include temporomandibular joint pain and stiffness, difficulty opening and closing the mouth, facial paralysis and pain, trigeminal neuralgia, deviation of the eye and mouth, toothache, swelling of the cheek and parotitis. It has also been employed to improve hearing and treat deafness, tinnitus, otitis and Menière's disease.

Main Areas: Jaw. Ear. Cheek. Teeth.

Main Functions: Dissipates stasis. Alleviates pain and swelling. Benefits the TMJ.

St-8   Touwei

頭維

Head Corner

Intersection of the Gallbladder and Yang Wei Mai on the Stomach channel

In the shallow depression at the corner of the forehead, at the superior margin of the temporalis muscle, directly above St-7 and GB-3, 0.5 cun within the anterior hairline and 4.5 cun lateral to the anterior midline (Du-24).

To aid location, clench the jaw so as to define the border of the temporalis muscle, slide the tip of the finger directly upwards from St-7 and GB-3 to slip into the shallow depression formed by the superior border of the temporalis muscle and the bony cleft, defined by the superior temporal line on the coronal suture. On light palpation, the pulse of the temporal artery can be perceived.

Best treatment positions
St-8 can be treated with the head facing upwards or to the side, depending on the treatment to be applied. The patient may be lying down or sitting in a chair.

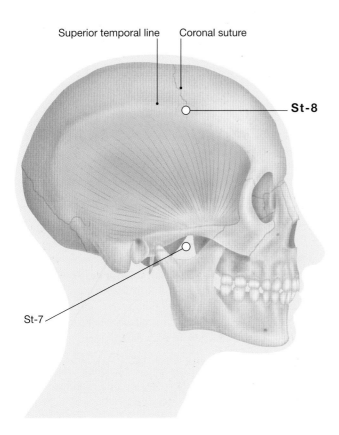

Superior temporal line   Coronal suture

St-8

St-7

Needling
• 0.5 to 1 cun transverse insertion downwards toward GB-4, or posteriorly.

Pick up the cutaneous tissue of the scalp (pinch the scalp) and insert the needle subcutaneously, under the epicranial aponeurosis parallel to the bone. If the scalp is very tight this may be difficult; therefore needle perpendicularly 0.1 to 0.2 cun.

However, because perpendicular needling is not as effective, consider applying moxibustion or massage to loosen the area or choose another technique.

! Do not puncture branches of the superficial temporal artery and vein.

Moxibustion
This location is traditionally contraindicated for moxibustion, but in practice, careful application can be effective in certain cases. Apply gentle indirect moxibustion for 3–5 minutes.

! Do not overheat this area because of underlying temporal vessels. Do not burn hair.

Manual techniques and shiatsu
Friction or sustained pressure may be applied carefully with the tips of the thumbs or fingers. This location can be extremely sensitive in certain cases, particularly if there is a lot of tension and tightness of the epicranial tissues. In such cases it is best to mobilise the scalp gently in a circular motion.

! This region can be extremely sensitive to pressure in cases where there is a lot of pain.

Stimulation sensation
Regional ache, numbness or distension. Deqi can extend to the Gallbladder channel.

Actions and indications
St-8 is an important point to *clear the head and brighten the eyes*. It helps *resolve dampness, expel wind, and stop excessive lacrimation*. Common indications include headache, migraine, muzzy or heavy feeling in the head, dizziness, vertigo, poor concentration, depression, mental and psycho-emotional disorders, facial paralysis, eye disorders, excessive lacrimation, twitching or spasm of the eye muscles and diminishing or blurred vision.

Main Areas: Head. Eyes. Mind.

Main Functions: Dispels wind and dampness.
Benefits the head, brain and eyes.
Stops lacrimation.

St-9 Renying

人迎

Man's Prognosis

Point of the Sea of Qi
Point of the Window of Heaven
Intersection of the Gallbladder on the Stomach channel

In the carotid triangle, anterior to the border of the sternocleidomastoid muscle, between the common carotid artery and thyroid cartilage, approximately 1.5 cun lateral to the tip of the laryngeal prominence (Adam's apple).

Situated at the lateral border of the omohyoid muscle. In its deep position lies the longus capitis and the anterior scalene muscle.

! In cases of thyroid enlargement, either relocate St-9 superiorly or choose another point (such as LI-18).

!! This is an extremely sensitive location and both massage or acupuncture treatment can be extremely dangerous if incorrectly applied.

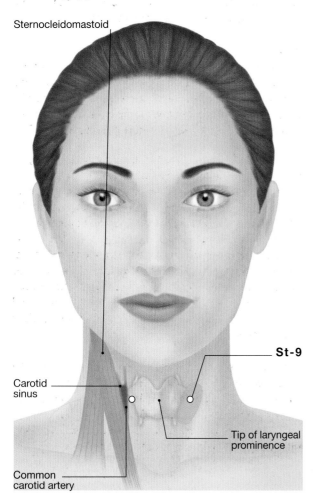

Sternocleidomastoid

St-9

Carotid sinus

Tip of laryngeal prominence

Common carotid artery

Contraindications
Ensure the client does not suffer from carotid sinus hypersensitivity syndrome before applying any form of treatment to the throat area.

!! If the person feels dizzy or faint during or after the treatment it could mean that the blood pressure has dropped below normal. Lie the patient down with the legs raised. Having a sweet drink (such as fruit juice) may also help. It is also possible that the person may feel nauseous or cold due to excessive sympathetic nerve stimulation. Allow the person to rest for at least 20 minutes, or, in severe cases, call an ambulance.

Best treatment positions
Acupuncture and manual treatment is best applied in a supine position without a pillow under the head so that the throat is in an 'open' position. However, manual techniques and shiatsu can also be applied in a side-lying or sitting position.

Needling
- 0.3 to 1 cun perpendicular insertion, medial to the artery. Push the artery toward the sternocleidomastoid with the fingers of one hand and insert the needle into the space between the thyroid cartilage and artery with the other hand.

!! This point is one of the most dangerous points and requires special skill in needling. Do not needle deeply and do not apply any manipulation other than very small rotation.

! Do not puncture any of the numerous vessels and nerves lying in the vicinity of this location: superficially, the anterior jugular vein and transverse cervical nerve. Deeper, the superior thyroid artery and vein, the superior laryngeal nerve, the superior root of the ansa cervicalis and slightly laterally the vagus nerve, not to mention the carotid artery and internal jugular vein.

! Do not puncture an enlarged thyroid gland.

Moxibustion
Contraindicated.

Manual techniques and shiatsu
There are a variety of manual techniques that can be effectively applied to St-9 for different purposes. As a general rule, manual techniques are more readily applied. This is partly because needling can be dangerous and requires special skill and partly because of the distinct therapeutic results obtained from manual techniques. However, manual techniques can also be extremely dangerous if incorrectly applied (see contraindications, above).

! Apply the pressure gently for a few seconds at a time. Do not apply pressure to both sides simultaneously, except for gentle pressure to the thyroid cartilage.

Sustained perpendicular pressure is applied carefully with the fingertips in a slightly medial direction onto the omohyoid muscle and thyroid cartilage. Additionally, very gentle pressure can be applied simultaneously to both sides of the thyroid cartilage with the fingers on one side and the thumb on the other. Furthermore, very gentle mobilisation of the thyroid cartilage to the left and right can also be effective.

Another technique is to apply the pressure laterally to the carotid artery and internal jugular vein, whilst stretching the sternocleidomastoid laterally. Pressure can be applied reasonably strongly in certain cases, but only by a skilled practitioner. The pressure can reach the transverse processes of C4–C5 through the deep muscles and nerves. This means that both or either the sympathetic or parasympathetic nerves to the heart may be affected, offering therapeutic results in a range of cardiovascular complaints, including high or low blood pressure, palpitations, tachycardia and bradycardia. However, this method can have unpredictable results in certain cases and should be used with extreme caution. Additionally, because the pressure increases in the internal jugular vein, the technique should be applied with great caution or not at all, in cases of circulatory-vascular problems.

This technique also stimulates the vagus nerve and sympathetic fibres that have an effect on many organs, areas and functions of the body. To access the vagus nerve, apply gentle pressure to the lateral side of the artery.

!! Do not apply the pressure for more than a few seconds at a time.

Carotid sinus massage
Apply gentle pressure-massage with the fingertips directly to the bifurcation of the artery where the carotid sinus is located. Locate the carotid bifurcation slightly superior to the level of the tip of the laryngeal prominence. Stimulation should be applied for 1 to 3 minutes on each side separately until the pulse rate starts to slow down and the patient's energy 'calms'. For indications see comments section (below).

Sternocleidomastoid release
Grasp the sternal head of the sternocleidomastoid, with the finger on its anterior border at St-9, and the thumb on its posterior border at LI-18 (or vice-versa). Press, stretch and lift the muscle outwards. This technique can be applied along the length of the sternal head of the muscle.

Omohyoid release
Grasp the superior belly of the omohyoid muscle with the finger on its posterior border at the St-9 location and the thumb on its anterior border slightly higher up (or vice-versa).

Anterior neck stretch
This stretch can be applied at different angles to open the entire region. Apply in a supine position or, as a self-stretch, sitting up. Keeping the cervical spine as straight as possible, extend the head a little so that the chin lifts up in a slightly contralateral direction to the side being treated. Then stretch the platysma muscle in an inferior direction by drawing it downwards with the palm of the hand at the infraclavicular area. Alternatively immobilise the platysma by holding it pressed against the chest wall and then lift the chin in a contralateral direction until the stretch is achieved.

Stimulation sensation
A distending, aching, tingling or electric sensation spreading out around the point, into the throat or upward to the submandibular area is often achieved. In many cases the sensation also extends downward toward the clavicle and shoulder and/or down into the chest.

Additionally, there should be a noticeable slowing of the pulse, which should feel calmer and softer.

Actions and indications
St-9 is *a very important point to clear heat, subdue excessive yang and descends rising qi.* It also *effectively regulates qi and Blood circulation and alleviates pain.* Furthermore, it is *important to moisten and open the throat, stop swelling and benefit the Lungs and breath.*

Indications include redness of the face and eyes, hot flushes, headache, fever, sweating, palpitations, tachycardia, dizziness, mental restlessness, fright, panic attack, high or low blood pressure, insomnia, pain in the lower back or anywhere in the body, pain or constriction of the chest, asthma, swelling or pain in the throat due to interior or exterior heat, wind or dampness, tonsillitis, goitre, diseases of the thyroid, oesophageal constriction, plum stone throat, difficulty swallowing, and speech impairment. St-9 is also *useful also for menopausal symptoms* such as hot flushes, hypertension, anxiety and insomnia.

Carotid sinus massage *increases the action of the parasympathetic division of the nervous system, relaxing the whole body, causing vasodilation and thus a decrease of blood pressure*, while it *simultaneously lowers the heart rate and output.* It has a *powerful calming and relaxing effect* on the entire body and mind.

Therefore, in such cases, it is more effective to apply manual pressure directly to the artery rather than needling the exact St-9 acupuncture location. The latter may be considered more effective in the treatment of *local disorders of the throat* including inflammation of the larynx and thyroid disease.

Manual pressure of the St-9 area is one of the most important *first aid manipulations* to be used in cases of symptoms due to excessive rising of yang qi, including hot flushes, palpitations, dizziness, hypertension, emotional upset, fright or panic.

> **Main Areas:** Throat. Thyroid gland. Face. Head. Brain. Heart. Blood vessels.
>
> **Main Functions:** Descends rising yang. Clears heat. Calms the mind and body. Increases PSNS activity. Lowers heart rate and output. Benefits the throat and thyroid.

St-10   Shuitu
Liquid Passage

水突

On the anterior border of the sternocleidomastoid muscle, midway between St-9 and St-11.

Best treatment positions
Treatment positions and manual techniques are similar to Renying St-9.

Needling
• 0.3 to 0.8 cun perpendicular insertion.

! Do not insert deeply. Do not puncture any of the numerous vessels of this region (see St-9).

Actions and indications
Although St-10 is not a commonly used point, it can be effective in cases of a *sore, swollen throat, disorders of the thyroid gland*, goitre, disorders of the vocal chords, difficulty breathing or swallowing and asthma.

> **Main Areas:** Throat. Thyroid gland.
>
> **Main Function:** Benefits the throat.

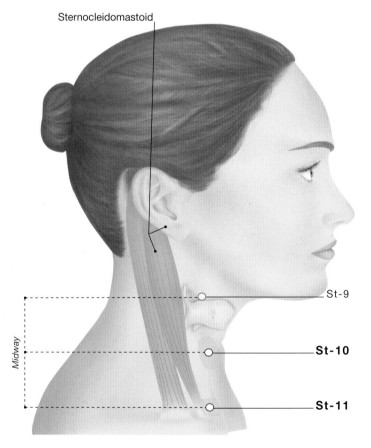

Sternocleidomastoid

Midway

St-9

St-10

St-11

St-11   Qishe

氣舍

Abode of Qi

Above the medial end of the clavicle, between the clavicular and sternal head of the sternocleidomastoid muscle, level with Ren 22.

Best treatment positions
Similar to St-9 and St-10.

Needling
• 0.3 to 0.5 cun perpendicular insertion.

!! Situated above major vessels and the lung apex. Deep insertion may cause a pneumothorax.

Actions and indications
St-11 is mainly used for *respiratory disorders* due to Lung qi counterflow and *diseases of the throat*.

> **Main Areas:** Throat. Thyroid gland.
>
> **Main Function:** Benefits the throat.

St-12   Quepen

缺盆

Empty Basin
(Supraclavicular Fossa)

At the midpoint of the supraclavicular fossa, 4 cun lateral to the midline (approximately level with Ren-22). Situated along the course of the subclavian vessels and lung apex.

Contraindications
All forms of treatment are contraindicated during pregnancy and heavy menstruation.

Best treatment positions
This location is best treated with pressure and manual techniques lying supine or sitting in a chair.

Needling
• 0.3 to 0.5 cun perpendicular insertion, directly behind the clavicle to avoid the needle tip going too far posteriorly and puncturing the lung apex.

St-12

4 cun

4 cun

!! Needling this location is potentially dangerous. Avoid deep insertion as there is considerable risk of puncturing the lung apex or the subclavian vessels. Superficially, do not puncture branches of the supraclavicular nerve.

Manual techniques and shiatsu
Pressure applied perpendicularly downwards is effective as a first aid treatment for coughing, dyspnoea and hypertension (it may be more effective if the patient is sitting up rather than lying down).

Pressure can be applied simultaneously behind and under the clavicle at St-12 and St-13. This is very effective for stiffness and pain of the surrounding area and shoulder.

Moxibustion
Moxibustion is rarely recommended at this location. However, light moxibustion can be applied for 3–10 minutes.

!! Direct or strong moxibustion is contraindicated.

Stimulation sensation

Effective deqi is easier to achieve at St-12 by manual pressure application rather than needling, because needling this site is tricky, and requires substantial experience and skill. See note on manual techniques and shiatsu, above.

Perpendicular pressure should produce a strong deqi sensation radiating down through chest and lungs. The sensation may even reach the stomach and abdomen.

Actions and indications

St-12, similar to St-9, is an important point for *descending excessive upward rising of qi as well as opening and relaxing the chest and benefiting the lungs and respiration.*

It has been widely employed to treat hypertension, hot flushes, redness of the face, dizziness, fullness of the chest, dyspnoea, cough, asthma, hiccup, swelling of the throat, lymphadenopathy, intercostal neuralgia and pain in the shoulder and neck.

Furthermore, St-12 is mentioned as one of the *Eight (bilateral) Points to Clear Heat from the Chest*, alongside Lu-1, Bl-11 and Bl-12 and is considered important to *clear heat from the upper jiao.*

Main Areas: Chest. Lungs. Shoulder.

Main Functions: Descends rising qi.
Lowers blood pressure. Clears heat.

St-13   Qihu
Qi Door
氣戶

In the depression directly below St-12, just under the inferior border of the clavicle, on the mid-mamillary line, 4 cun lateral to the midline. To aid location, it is approximately level with Ren-21 and Kd-27.

Best treatment positions

This point can be treated with the patient lying down in a supine position or sitting up.

Needling

• 0.4 to 1 cun transverse insertion medially, laterally or downward along the Stomach channel.
• 0.2 to 0.5 cun perpendicular insertion.
• 1 to 2 cun subcutaneously toward Lu-2 or Ren-21.

! Do not needle deeply as this poses considerable risk of puncturing the lung.

Manual techniques and shiatsu

Perpendicular pressure and friction techniques are applicable. A sitting or lying position can be used. Pressure can be applied simultaneously behind and under the clavicle at St-12 and St-13.

! Do not apply strong pressure to the rib cage.

Moxibustion

Moxibustion is rarely recommended at St-13. However, gentle moxibustion can be applied for 3–10 minutes.

! Direct or strong moxibustion is contraindicated.

Actions and indications

Treatment at St-13 is rarely employed, although it is applicable for *disorders of the chest and respiratory system* including heaviness and pain of the chest, dyspnoea, cough and hiccup.

It can also be effectively employed to *treat pain and stiffness of the infraclavicular area and shoulder* and disorders of the breasts.

Main Areas: Clavicle. Shoulder. Chest.

Main Functions: Alleviates pain and stiffness. Benefits the breathing.

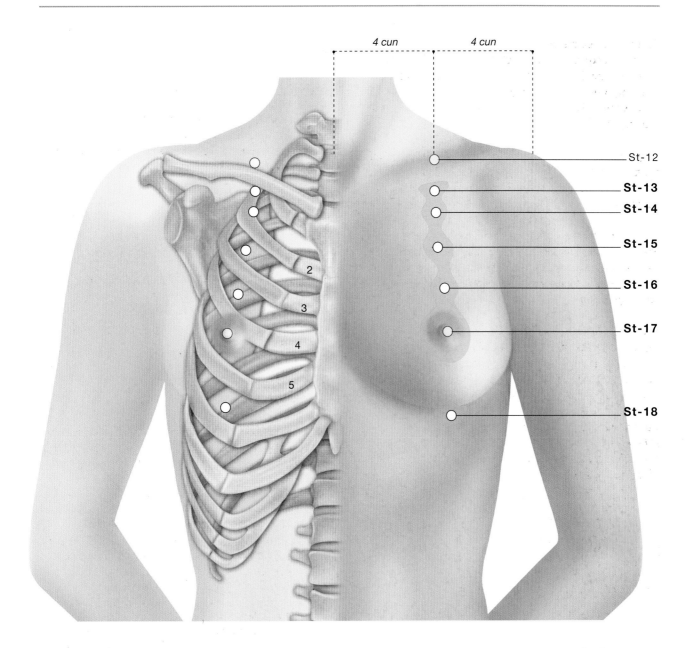

4 cun   4 cun

St-12
St-13
St-14
St-15
St-16
St-17
St-18

St-14   Kufang   庫房
Store Room

In a depression in the first intercostal space, directly below St-13, on the mid-mamillary line, 4 cun lateral to the anterior midline (approximately level with Ren-20 and Kd-26).

Best treatment positions
This point is best treated with the patient lying down in a supine position or sitting up.

Needling
- 0.4 to 0.8 cun transverse insertion medially, laterally or downward along the Stomach channel.
- 0.2 to 0.5 cun perpendicular insertion.

! Do not puncture underlying mammary glands.

!! Do not needle deeply as this poses considerable risk of puncturing the lung.

Manual techniques and shiatsu
Perpendicular pressure and friction is applicable to the intercostal spaces. Deep friction of the intercostal muscles is very effective to unbind the chest.

! Do not apply pressure to mammary glands. Do not apply strong pressure to the rib cage.

Moxibustion

Moxibustion is rarely recommended at this location. However, light indirect moxibustion can be applied for 3–10 minutes.

! Do not overheat the mammary glands.

Actions and indications

Treatment at *St-14, St-15 and St-16 helps expand and relax the chest and decrease counter-flow qi.*

It is applicable for fullness of the chest, dyspnoea, respiratory problems, intercostal neuralgia, localised stiffness or pain of the chest and ribs, swelling and pain of the mammary glands and mastitis. Choose between these points depending on which are more sensitive to pressure palpation.

> **Main Areas:** Chest. Breast.
>
> **Main Functions:** Alleviates pain and swelling. Benefits the breast and Lungs.

St-15　Wuyi　　　　屋翳
Roof

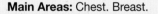

Directly below St-14, in the second intercostal space, on the mid-mamillary line, 4 cun lateral to the midline (approximately level with Ren-19 and Kd-25). The location of St-15 and St-16 varies depending on the structure of the mammary gland.

Treatment and applications
See St-14.

> **Main Areas:** Chest. Breast.
>
> **Main Functions:** Alleviates pain and swelling. Benefits the breast and Lungs.

St-16　Yingchuang　　腐窗
Breast Window

Directly below St-15, in the third intercostal space, on the mid-mamillary line, 4 cun lateral to the midline (approximately level with Ren-18 and Kd-24). See also location note for St-15.

Treatment and applications
See St-14.

> **Main Area:** Breast.
>
> **Main Function:** Alleviates pain and swelling.

St-17　Ruzhong　　　乳中
Breast Centre

At the centre of the nipple. Level with the fourth intercostal space, 4 cun lateral to the anterior midline (approximately level with Ren-17 and Kd-23).

Contraindications
Needling and moxibustion is contraindicated. This is a reference point and is not generally used to treat.

Note: Manual self-stimulation of the nipples, regularly applied, may *improve hormone levels* in conditions such as *amenorrhoea, infertility, uterine prolapse, loss of libido, frigidity or dysmenorrhoea.* The nipples can be stimulated regularly in the last 3 weeks of pregnancy to *stimulate the release of oxytocin* which can make the *delivery easier.* Additionally, stimulation of the nipples for the weeks following delivery will *help the uterus shrink to its normal size.* Also manual [reasonably strong] stimulation of the nipples (if the baby doesn't immediately suckle following delivery) can aid in the *expulsion of the placenta.*

Furthermore, strong stimulation of the nipples can help *revive consciousness* in cases of *fainting and coma.*

Soreness, pain, swelling or redness of the nipples are *signs that may be used diagnostically.* These signs point to Liver qi stagnation, Liver heat, Blood stasis and or phlegm accumulation in the breast and can be hormonal imbalances, breast disease or pregnancy.

> **Main Areas:** Nipple. Breast. Uterus. Mind.
>
> **Main Functions:** Lifts sinking qi. Resuscitates consciousness. Increases libido.

St-18　Rugen

Breast Root

乳根

In the fifth intercostal space directly below the nipple, on the mid-mamillary line, 4 inches lateral to the anterior midline (approximately level with Kd-22).

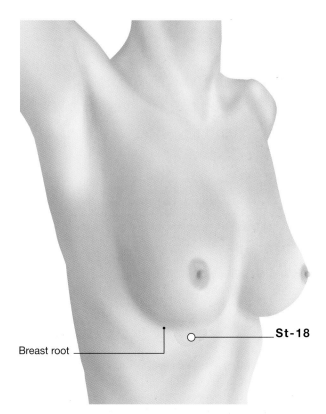

Breast root

St-18

Best treatment positions
Acupuncture and manual treatment is best applied in a supine position. Also, self-acupressure is effectively applied sitting up.

Needling
• 0.3 to 0.7 cun perpendicular insertion.
• 0.5 to 1.5 cun transverse medial or lateral insertion.

!! Do not needle deeply as this poses considerable risk of puncturing the lung.

Moxibustion
Moxibustion is rarely recommended at this location. However, light indirect moxibustion can be applied for 3–10 minutes.

! Direct moxibustion is contraindicated. Do not overheat the mammary glands.

Manual techniques and shiatsu
Perpendicular pressure and friction techniques are applicable and all the way along the intercostal space.

Self-acupressure applied regularly with the thumbs is most effective for disorders of the breast.

! Do not apply strong pressure to the rib cage.

Stimulation sensation
Regional ache, distension or tingling extending into the chest, upward to the breast or downward toward the liver and hypochondrial area.

Actions and indications
St-18 is an *important point to expand and relax the chest* and is a *major point for many disorders of the breast.*

It is commonly used to treat pain, swelling, fibrosis and many disorders of the mammary glands, insufficient lactation, mastitis, pain or tightness of the chest, hypochondrial distension and pain, asthma, bronchitis and cough.

Main Areas: Breasts. Lungs. Chest. Liver.

Main Functions: Dispels stasis.
Benefits the breasts.

St-19　Burong
不容
Not Contained

Just below the costal margin, 6 cun above the level of the umbilicus and 2 cun lateral to the midline, level with Ren-14 and Kd-21.

Note: In persons who have a narrow costal angle, a location of 2 cun lateral to the midline may fall on the costal cartilage. Therefore the 2 cun distance must be decreased, so that the point will be located closer to the midline. In some such cases, the first point below the rib cage is St-20 (level with Ren-13 and Kd-20) or even St-21 (level with Ren-12). Consequently, it could be considered either that St-19 and St-20 and/or St-21 fall at the same location, or that St-19 and/or St-20 are in fact inside the rib cage and cannot be accessed for treatment (in effect they do not 'exist'). This means that needling and massage at St-20 or St-21 would be the same as for St-19, and NOT the same as that for a "normal" St-20 or St-21 location further down. The simplest way to overcome this problem is to consider that treatment at this 'multiple point' would combine the functions of all these points.

Best treatment positions
Acupuncture and manual treatment is best applied in a supine position. However, self-acupressure is effectively applied sitting up.

Needling
• 0.5 to 1 cun perpendicular insertion.

!! Do not needle deeply, particularly if there is enlargement of the liver or heart, or if the patient is very thin.

!! Do not puncture the peritoneum.

Manual techniques and shiatsu
Gentle perpendicular pressure is effective as well as friction techniques applied to the costal margin.

! Do not apply strong pressure here.

Moxibustion
Cones: 3. Pole: 5–15 minutes.

Stimulation sensation
Regional aching and distension possibly extending upwards or downwards, toward the stomach, chest and hypochondrial area.

Actions and indications
St-19 is not a very commonly used point, because other points are more effective in the treatment of interior complaints (such as St-21, Ren-12 and St-25). It can however be employed to *harmonise the Stomach and ease stagnation in the middle jiao*. Indications include epigastric fullness and pain, indigestion, poor appetite, vomiting, abdominal distension, abdominal rumbling, hypochondrial pain, intercostal neuralgia, dyspnoea, cough and chest pain.

> **Main Areas:** Stomach. Abdomen. Heart.
>
> **Main Function:** Harmonises the middle jiao.

St-20　Chengman
承滿
Receiving Fullness

1 cun below St-19, 5 cun above the level of the umbilicus, 2 cun lateral to Ren-13. See note for St-19.

Treatment and applications
Similar to St-19 and St-21.

> **Main Areas:** Stomach. Abdomen. Heart.
>
> **Main Function:** Harmonises the middle jiao.

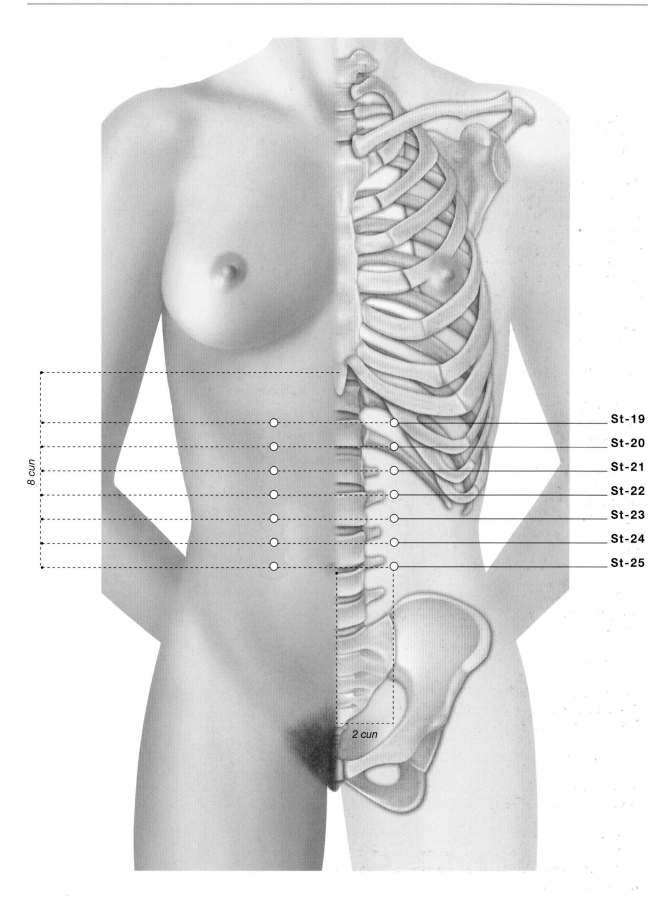

8 cun

St-19
St-20
St-21
St-22
St-23
St-24
St-25

2 cun

St-21 Liangmen 梁門
Ridge Gate

2 cun lateral to Ren-12, 4 cun above the level of the umbilicus. See note for St-19.

Best treatment positions
Treatment is best applied in a supine position with the hips flexed and the legs supported with cushions.

Needling
• 0.5 to 1.5 cun perpendicular insertion.

!! Do not needle deeply, particularly if there is enlargement of the liver or heart, or if the patient is very thin. Do not puncture the peritoneum.

Moxibustion
Cones: 3–5. Pole: 5–15 minutes.

Manual techniques and shiatsu
Perpendicular pressure or friction can be used. Self-acupressure can also be applied effectively, in a standing or sitting position while bending the trunk forward.

! Do not apply pressure in cases where there is nausea or excessive fullness of the stomach.

Stimulation sensation
Sensation may radiate up or down the channel, toward the stomach, chest and hypochondrial area.

Actions and indications
St-21 has similar functions to St-19 and St-20, but is much more commonly used. It *may be considered as a Stomach Alarm-Mu point but more for excess conditions compared to Ren-12.* It is especially useful in cases of *rebellious Stomach qi.*

St-21 is an important point to *harmonise the Stomach, ease stagnation from the middle jiao and descend rebellious qi.* Indications include epigastric fullness, heaviness, tightness and hardness, stomach pain, indigestion, heartburn, gastritis, gastric ulceration, hiatus hernia, nausea, vomiting, hypochondrial distension and pain, abdominal distension, loose stool, diarrhoea, undigested food in the stool, poor appetite and abdominal rumbling.

> **Main Areas:** Epigastrium. Abdomen. Heart.
>
> **Main Functions:** Descends rebellious qi. Relieves stagnation. Harmonises the Stomach.

St-22 Guanmen 關門
Shutting the Gate

1 cun below St-21, 3 cun above the level of the umbilicus, 2 cun lateral to Ren-11.

Needling
• 0.5 to 1.5 cun perpendicular insertion.

! Do not needle deeply, particularly if the patient is very thin. Do not puncture the peritoneum.

Manual techniques and shiatsu and moxibustion
Similar to St-21 and St-25.

Actions and indications
St-22 is not a very commonly used point but it can be employed in similar situations as adjacent Stomach channel points such as St-21, St-23 and St-24.

> **Main Areas:** Epigastrium. Abdomen. Chest.
>
> **Main Function:** Regulates Stomach qi.

St-23 Taiyi 太乙
Great Unity

1 cun below St-22, 2 cun above the level of the umbilicus, 2 cun lateral to Ren-10 and Kd-17.

Applications and treatment
Similar to adjacent Stomach channel points such as St-21 and St-25.

Needling
• 0.5 to 2 cun perpendicular insertion. See also St-21 and St-25.

> **Main Areas:** Stomach. Heart.
>
> **Main Functions:** Harmonises the middle jiao. Soothes the Heart and calms the mind.

St-24 Huaroumen 滑肉門

Slippery Flesh Gate
(Pylorus)

1 cun below St-22, 1 cun above the level of the umbilicus, 2 cun lateral to Ren-9.

Applications and treatment
Similar to adjacent Stomach channel points such as St-21 and St-25.

Needling
• 0.5 to 2 cun perpendicular insertion. See also St-21 and St-25.

> **Main Areas:** Stomach. Abdomen. Heart.
>
> **Main Functions:** Harmonises the Stomach and intestines. Calms the mind.

St-25 Tianshu 天樞

Celestial Pivot

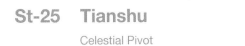

Alarm *Mu* point of the Large Intestine

2 cun lateral to Ren-8 (centre of the umbilicus) on the rectus abdominis muscle.

Best treatment positions
Treatment is best applied in a supine position with the hips slightly flexed and the legs supported with cushions, so that the abdomen can be as relaxed as possible (ensure the lower back is lying flat on the floor).

Needling
• 0.5 to 1.5 cun perpendicular insertion.

! Do not needle deeply, particularly in thin patients as this will puncture the peritoneum.

Moxibustion
Cones: 5–15. Pole: 10–20 minutes. Rice-grain moxa is also applicable. Also, burn the cones on ginger or garlic slices.

Cupping
Medium or small sized cups with light or medium suction are applicable.

Magnets
Stick-on magnets can be effectively employed.

Manual techniques and shiatsu
Sustained pressure applied perpendicularly with the fingertip or thumb helps harmonise the intestines and lower jiao. Bilateral pressure applied in a medial direction so that the rectus abdominis muscle belly is lifted and the umbilicus is slightly pressed, is more effective in cases where perpendicular pressure is painful. Circular or cross-fibre friction is also effective to relax the musculature. Pressure can also be applied with the heel of the hand.

Self-acupressure can be applied with the thumbs or fingers in a standing or sitting position while bending the trunk forward.

! Avoid pressure on St-25 and other abdominal points, if the abdomen is very painful and hard in cases of severe constipation, inflammation of the abdomen or pregnancy.

Stimulation sensation
Localised distension and warmth extending to the surrounding area or along the course of the channel should be achieved. A pulling sensation is also commonly obtained from needling abdominal points.

Actions and indications
St-25 is a *very important point* and is *widely used to alleviate abdominal pain and regulate the lower jiao*. It helps *clear dampness and heat and regulate the intestines* as well as *promote the descending of Stomach qi* and *relieve food retention*.

Indications include disorders of the intestines, abdominal distension, swelling and pain, rumbling, gastroenteritis, diarrhoea, dysentery, foul smelling stools, mucus or blood in the stool, appendicitis, Crohn's disease, dry stool, constipation, obstruction of the intestines, nausea, vomiting, retching, leucorrhoea, irregular menstruation, dysmenorrhoea and dysuria.

Moxibustion is particularly effective to clear dampness from the lower jiao.

> **Main Areas:** Intestines. Umbilicus. Abdomen. Uterus.
>
> **Main Functions:** Clears dampness and heat. Regulates qi in the lower jiao. Benefits the intestines.

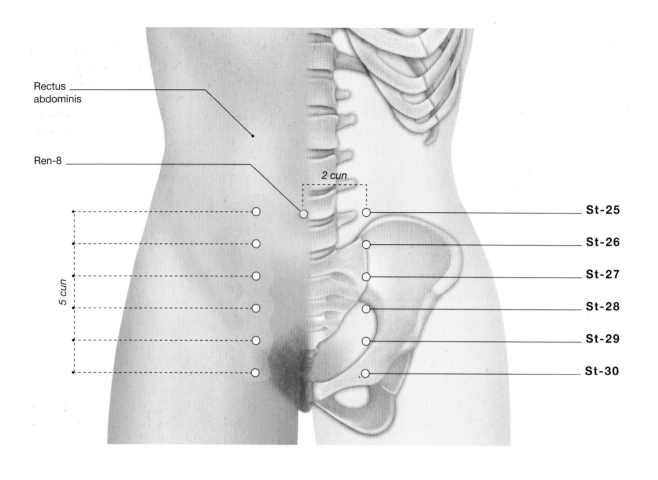

Rectus abdominis

Ren-8

2 cun

5 cun

St-25
St-26
St-27
St-28
St-29
St-30

St-26 Wailing

Outer Mound

外陵

1 cun below the umbilicus, 2 cun lateral to the midline, level with Ren-7. On the rectus abdominis muscle.

Best treatment positions
Similar to St-25.

Actions and indications
St-26 is not a very commonly used point although it can be employed in similar situations as adjacent Stomach channel points such as St-25, St-27 and St-28. All these points have an effect on the *lower abdomen, intestines, urinary bladder, and uterus* and are indicated in cases of distension, heaviness, swelling or pain of the abdomen, abdominal rumbling, diarrhoea, constipation, hernia, dysuria, cystitis, dysmenorrhoea, menstrual irregularities, infertility, and spermatorrhoea.

Main Areas: Intestines. Abdomen.

Main Function: Regulates the lower jiao.

St-27 Daju

Great Bulge

大巨

2 cun below the umbilicus, 2 cun lateral to the midline, level with Ren-5.

Needling
• 0.5 to 1.5 cun perpendicular insertion. On the rectus abdominis muscle.

! Do not needle deeply, particularly if the patient is very thin. Do not puncture the peritoneum or a full bladder.

Treatment and applications
Similar to St-26.

Main Area: Abdomen.

Main Function: Regulates the lower jiao.

St-28   Shuidao

Waterway

水道

3 cun below the umbilicus, 2 cun lateral to Ren-4.

Needling
• 0.5 to 1.5 cun perpendicular insertion.

! Do not needle deeply, particularly if the patient is very thin. Do not puncture the peritoneum or a full bladder.

Manual techniques and shiatsu
Similar to St-25.

Moxibustion
Cones: 3–5. Pole: 5–15 minutes.

! Do not burn pubic hair.

Actions and indications
St-28 *benefits the whole of the lower abdomen* and is particularly useful in the *treatment of urogenital disorders* and *problems of the reproductive organs and uterus.* Indications include distension, heaviness, swelling or pain of the lower abdomen, hernia, dysuria, haematuria, cystitis, urinary tract infections, dysmenorrhoea, frigidity, menstrual irregularities, prolapse of the uterus, infertility, spermatorrhoea, pelvic inflammatory disease, prostatitis, and erectile dysfunction.

> **Main Areas:** Urogenital system. Uterus.
>
> **Main Functions:** Clears dampness and heat. Regulates qi in the lower jiao. Benefits menstruation. Increases fertility.

St-29   Guilai

Return

歸來

4 cun below the umbilicus, 2 cun lateral to Ren-3.

Treatment
Similar to St-28 and St-30.

Needling
• 0.5 to 1 cun perpendicular insertion.

!! Do not needle deeply, particularly if the patient is very thin. Do not puncture the peritoneum or a full bladder.

Actions and indications
St-29 has similar actions to St-28 and St-30. It has been widely employed to treat *disorders of the reproductive and urogenital system.* It is particularly indicated for amenorrhoea, dysmenorrhoea and lower abdominal pain, cold in the lower abdomen, infertility, uterine prolapse, loss of libido, impotence and testicular swelling or pain.

> **Main Area:** Abdomen.
>
> **Main Function:** Regulates the lower jiao.

St-30   Qichong

Qi Surge

Intersection of the Chong Mai and Stomach
Point of the Sea of Nourishment
(Sea of Water and Grain)

2 cun lateral to the anterior midline (Ren-2), superior and slightly lateral to the pubic tubercle, on the medial side of the femoral artery and vein.

Best treatment positions
This point is best treated with the patient lying in a supine position with the hips flexed and the thighs and knees well supported with cushions.

Needling
• 0.5 to 1 cun perpendicular insertion.

! Do not needle deeply, particularly if the patient is very thin. Do not puncture the anterior cutaneous branch of the iliohypogastric nerve or branches of the superficial epigastric artery and vein; more deeply and slightly laterally, the femoral vein or artery.

Manual techniques and shiatsu
Stationary perpendicular pressure can be applied to both sides simultaneously with the thumbs. Self-acupressure is useful and can be applied lying supine or standing up. The latter is particularly indicated for chronic conditions and deficiency of the lower jiao.

Additionally, applying perpendicular pressure to the entire supra-pubic area is effective (pressing through Ren-2, Kd-11, Sp-13, Sp-12 and Liv-12). Friction is not as effective as perpendicular pressure at this location.

Moxibustion

Pole: 5–15 minutes. Direct moxibustion is not easily applicable to this location.

! Do not burn the pubic hair.

Magnets

Magnets can be applied to this location to help improve blood circulation and the condition of the vessel walls in the lower limbs and abdomen. For best results, alternate poles with other points along the course of the femoral artery and vein (including Liv-12 and Sp-12) or great saphenous vein (including Liv-8, Sp-11, Sp-8 and Sp-6).

Stimulation sensation

Regional aching, distension and tingling extending out around the point, toward the genitals and distally along the channel, or electricity giving way to numbness of the thigh. Also deqi can travel upward across the abdomen.

Actions and indications

St-30 is considered one of the most *important points to promote fertility and regulate menstruation*. It helps *regulate qi and Blood in the lower jiao and dispel stasis*. Indications include infertility, amenorrhoea, irregular menstruation, abnormal uterine bleeding, dysmenorrhoea, frequent miscarriage, leucorrhoea, prolapse of the uterus or rectum, haemorrhoids, pain of the external genitals, impotence, spermatorrhoea, frequent urination, lower abdominal pain, twisting abdominal pain, inguinal hernia, testicular retraction and pain. Additionally, it has been employed to treat difficulty in delivering the placenta and insufficient lactation.

According to classical texts, the Chong Mai emerges at the point where the femoral artery pulse is perceived at St-30. Treatment is applied here in order to *regulate the Chong Mai and descend rebellious Stomach qi*.

Additionally, it has been extensively used as a *mental focus point during qigong training*.

> **Main Areas:** Reproductive organs. Uterus. Testicles. Bladder. Intestines. Lower abdomen.
>
> **Main Functions:** Benefits the lower jiao. Regulates menstruation. Improves sexual function and fertility.

St-31 Biguan
Thigh Gate

髀關

Below the hip in the prominent depression, appearing when the thigh is flexed, between the sartorius and tensor fasciae latae muscles. Approximately level with the perineum and directly below the anterior superior iliac spine.

This is a large point, and may be accessed from a slightly wider area, extending both upwards toward the anterior superior iliac spine, and downward, lateral to the sartorius muscle.

Best treatment positions

St-31 is best treated with the patient lying sideways or supine. The thigh must be flexed and supported with cushions.

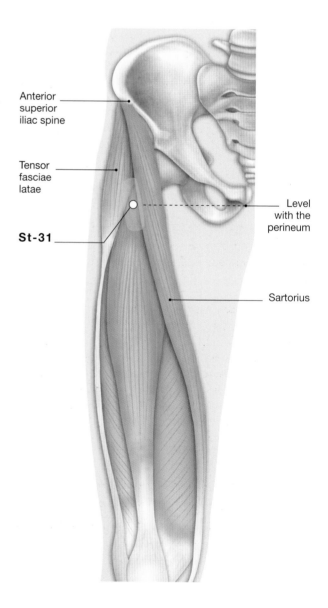

Anterior superior iliac spine

Tensor fasciae latae

St-31

Level with the perineum

Sartorius

Needling
• 1 to 2.5 cun perpendicular insertion.

Moxibustion
Cones: 5–7. Pole: 15–30 minutes.

Cupping
Medium or strong cupping with medium or small sized cups can be effective.

Guasha
Guasha can be applied distally along the channel and laterally or medially across the fibres of tensor fasciae latae and sartorius.

Manual techniques and shiatsu
Reasonably strong stationary perpendicular pressure is most effective and is best applied in a supine or side-lying position with the thigh flexed.

ST-31 may also be effectively stretched by extending the femur at the hip joint in a prone, side-lying or kneeling position (avoid hyper-extension of the lumbar spine).

Additionally, apply palm pressure onto the tensor fasciae latae to stretch it in a posterior direction to open this location. Self-stimulation with thumbs in standing and crouching positions is an effective exercise to benefit the hips and legs.

Stimulation sensation
Aching, distension, tingling or electricity giving way to numbness is often achieved distally along the channel.

Also, the deqi may extend across the front of the hip and abdomen or inwards to the hip joint and down the thigh toward the leg.

Actions and indications
St-31 is a *very powerful point to benefit the hips and improve flow of qi and Blood to the entire lower extremity.* It *dispels wind and dampness from the hips and lower limbs* and is commonly employed to treat restricted movement, stiffness, contraction, atrophy, paralysis, numbness and pain of the hips, knees and entire lower limb. It can also be effectively employed to alleviate lumbar and abdominal pain.

> **Main Areas:** Hips. Lower limbs.
>
> **Main Functions:** Dissipates stasis and alleviates pain and stiffness. Dispels wind and dampness.

St-32 Futu
伏兔
Crouching Rabbit

6 cun above the laterosuperior border of the patella, on the line joining the lateral border of the patella with the anterior superior iliac spine.

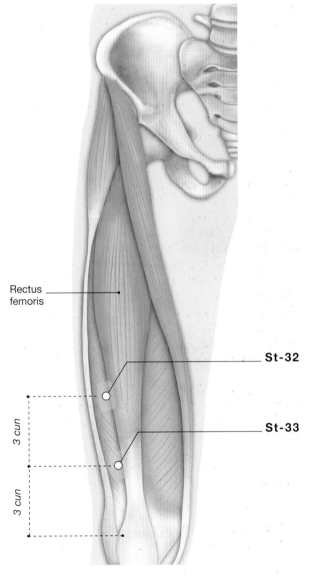

Rectus femoris

St-32

St-33

3 cun

3 cun

Best treatment positions
With the patient in a supine position, the knees flexed and the thighs well supported with cushions.

Needling
• 1 to 2 cun perpendicular insertion.

Moxibustion
Cones: 3–5. Pole: 5–15 minutes.

Cupping
Light or medium strength cupping with medium sized cups can be very effective. Moving cupping along the channel pathway is also useful.

Manual techniques and shiatsu
Both perpendicular pressure and friction techniques are effective. Friction along the length of the channel can also be beneficial.

Stimulation sensation
A tingling, aching or numb sensation spreading out around the point and downward or upward along the channel is usually achieved.

Actions and indications
St-32 is primarily used as a *local point to clear dampness, wind and cold from the channel and alleviate pain.*

> **Main Area:** Thigh.
>
> **Main Functions:** Dispels wind, dampness and cold. Alleviates pain.

St-33   Yinshi   陰市
Yin Market

3 cun (one hand width) above the laterosuperior border of the patella, on the line joining the lateral border of the patella with the anterior superior iliac spine. Midway between the lateral superior border of the patella and St-32.

Treatment and applications
Similar to St-32.

> **Main Area:** Thigh.
>
> **Main Functions:** Dispels wind, dampness and cold. Alleviates pain.

St-34   Lianqiu   梁丘
Ridge Mound

Accumulation Cleft-*Xi* point

In the depression 2 cun proximal to the laterosuperior border of the patella, between the rectus femoris and vastus lateralis muscles, on the line connecting the anterior superior iliac spine to the lateral border of the patella.

To aid location, a visible depression appears at St-34 when the leg is extended. Also, to ascertain the 2 cun distance, measure the patella, which is 2 cun in height.

Best treatment positions
Manual techniques can applied with the knee extended and the leg rotated slightly medially, or with the knee flexed (use cushion support). Needling, however, is best applied with the knee slightly flexed.

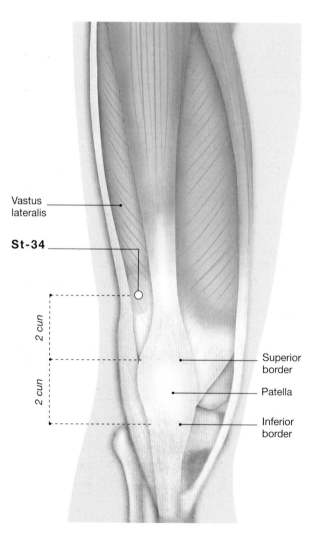

Vastus lateralis

St-34

2 cun

2 cun

Superior border

Patella

Inferior border

Needling
• 0.5 to 1.5 cun perpendicular insertion.
• 1 to 2 cun horizontal insertion toward Sp-10.

! Do not puncture the cutaneous branches of the femoral nerve and more deeply, the descending branch of the lateral circumflex femoral artery.

Moxibustion
Cones: 3–5. Pole: 5–15 minutes.

Cupping
Medium or strong cupping with medium or small sized cups can be very effective. Moving cupping is also extremely effective along the pathway of the Stomach channel on the thigh.

Guasha
Applicable.

Manual techniques and shiatsu
Stationary perpendicular pressure or friction is best applied in a supine position with the leg extended and rotated slightly medially.

Stimulation sensation
An aching sensation spreading out around the point and radiating to the knee is most common. However, a dull tingling or numb ache can be achieved upward toward the abdomen and epigastrium.

Actions and indications
St-34, the Accumulation Cleft-Xi point of the Stomach channel, is frequently treated in excess disorders to pacify the Stomach, alleviate pain and descend rebellious qi. Indications include acute stomach ache, spasm of the stomach, gastritis, heartburn, bitter taste, nausea and vomiting.

St-34 is also important to clear channel obstructions and benefit the knees. Symptoms include pain or swelling of the knee and thigh, stiffness and restricted movement of the knees and legs.

It has also been employed to treat a variety of other symptoms including diarrhoea, mastitis and palpitations.

Main Areas: Stomach. Epigastrium.
Lower limbs. Knees.

Main Functions: Pacifies the Stomach.
Descends rebellious qi. Alleviates pain.

St-35 Dubi (Waixiyan) 犢鼻
外膝眼

Calf's Nose
(Lateral Eye of the Knee)

Lateral to the patellar tendon, in the large depression appearing when the knee is flexed. In its deep position situated in the knee joint space between the articular surfaces of the femur and tibia.

Best treatment positions
St-35 is best treated with the patient in a supine position with the knee flexed and supported with cushions. However, treatment can also be applied in other positions.

Needling
• 0.5 to 1.5 cun perpendicular insertion, slightly medially, toward the centre of the knee joint.
• 1 to 1.5 cun horizontal insertion, through or under the patellar tendon to connect with the Medial Eye of the Knee, (M-LE-16).
• 1 to 2 cun oblique superior medial insertion under the patella.

! Do not puncture arteries and veins of the genicular network.

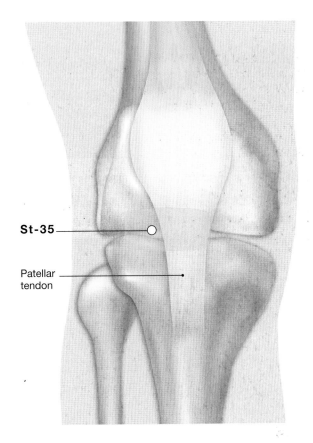

St-35

Patellar
tendon

Moxibustion

Cones: 3–7. Pole: 5–15 minutes. Rice-grain moxa is also applicable.

Cupping

Medium or strong cupping with small cups can be very effective.

Guasha

Effectively applied across the patellar tendon.

Magnets

Use opposite poles on the medial and lateral eye of the knee (Xiyan).

Manual techniques and shiatsu

Perpendicular pressure can be applied quite strongly to this location, and is most effective in a supine position with the knee flexed. However, a side-lying position can also be employed. Friction techniques are most effective if also applied to the patellar tendon and other soft tissues and insertions surrounding the knee joint.

Stimulation sensation

Localised aching or soreness extending into the knee joint or down the leg is commonly achieved. Treatment is most effective when a numbness or ache is felt deep inside the joint, or at the exact area of the complaint.

Actions and indications

This is a very *important point for the treatment of disorders of the knee* including pain, stiffness, swelling or restricted movement. It can be used in such conditions as chronic degenerative or rheumatoid arthritis of the knee, articular cartilage degeneration, chondropathy and lateral meniscus injury. Combine it with M-LE-16 (Inner Eye of the Knee).

Main Area: Knees.

Main Functions: Alleviates pain, stiffness and swelling. Strengthens the knees.

St-36   Zusanli   足三里
Leg Three Miles

Uniting Sea-*He*, Earth (Horary) point
Command point of the abdomen
Point of the Sea of Nourishment
One of the nine points for Returning Yang
Heavenly Star point

On the tibialis anterior muscle, approximately one finger width lateral to the tibial crest, level with the lower border of the tibial tuberosity, 3 cun (one hand width) below St-35. Approximately 1 cun anterior and inferior to GB-34.

To aid location, it is in a small opening between the fibres, on the high point of the tibialis anterior muscle belly. Ask the patient to dorsiflex and invert the foot to define the tibialis anterior.

! St-36 can be extremely painful and tight.

Best treatment positions

Treatment is best applied with the patient lying comfortably in a supine position. The knees should be slightly flexed, with cushion support. However, sitting in a chair or lying down sideways can also be employed.

Needling

• 0.5 to 1.5 cun perpendicular insertion.
• 1 to 3 cun oblique insertion directed inferiorly along channel.

! Deep insertion can injure the anterior tibial artery and veins, and the deep branch of the peroneal nerve.

Moxibustion

Cones: 3–10. Pole: 5–20 minutes.

Cupping

Medium or strong cupping with small cups can be effective. Also, moving the cups up and down the tibialis anterior muscle can be beneficial.

! Do not apply cupping to areas of distended veins.

Guasha

Guasha across and along the tibialis anterior fibres is also very beneficial.

! Do not apply guasha across distended vessels.

Manual techniques and shiatsu

Perpendicular pressure and friction techniques can be applied quite strongly to this location. Pressure is best applied in a supine position with the knee extended or slightly flexed (use cushion support under the knee and leg as necessary).

Perpendicular pressure is applied to the depression on the belly of the tibialis anterior muscle, where the fibres part under pressure. Additionally, pressure can be applied slightly further laterally on the lateral border of the muscle. Shiatsu pressure can also be successfully applied with the palms, elbows and knees.

If the muscle is very tight and painful, apply circular and cross-fibre friction to relax the muscle fibres. Stretching and rolling the tibialis anterior muscle fibres laterally, away from the tibia, with the palm or fingers also effectively relaxes and opens this area.

Furthermore, applying friction to break down nodules in the deep tissues surrounding this location is extremely effective for many disorders.

! Perpendicular pressure can be painful in certain cases. Avoid pressure on varicosities or thread veins.

Stimulation sensation

St-36 produces a strong tingling, electric or aching sensation with relatively minor stimulation (except in cases of extreme deficiency of qi and Blood). Deqi from St-36 usually extends down the leg toward the ankle and often reaches the toes. Also, it can extend upward across the knee and thigh, possibly reaching the abdomen and chest.

! Sometimes the sensation here can be very intense and cause a sudden electric pain shooting down the leg.

Actions and indications

St-36 is one of the most *dynamic and widely used points, and has been employed in almost every disorder. It strengthens the middle jiao qi and boosts the vital substances: qi, blood, fluids, yin and yang.* Treatment applied to St-36 is *important in most chronic disorders where there is weakness of the Stomach, Spleen and other organs.*

Its traditional functions are listed as follows: *Tonifies qi, Blood, yin and yang; boosts Stomach and Spleen qi; benefits the digestion and abdomen; resolves dampness; strengthens the central qi and raises sinking qi; warms and tonifies yang and restores collapsed yang (with moxa); regulates nutritive and defensive qi, strengthens the immune system and expels pathogenic factors; moistens Yin and generates fluids; tonifies the Lungs; dispels stagnation from the chest; descends rebellious Stomach qi; regulates the intestines; strengthens the legs and benefits the knees.*

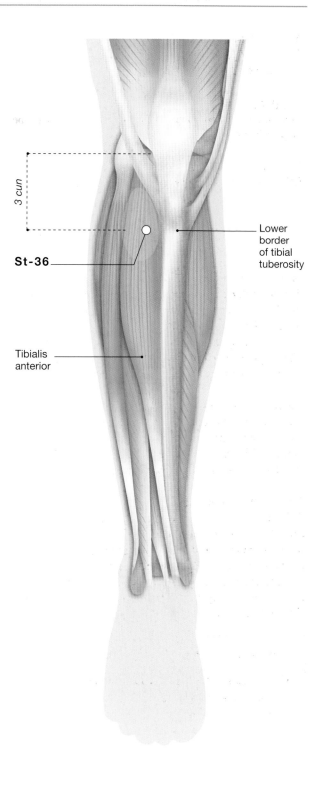

3 cun

St-36

Lower border of tibial tuberosity

Tibialis anterior

There is a wide range of indications for St-36 including tiredness, lack of vitality, weakness, debility, flaccidity of the flesh and muscles, dizziness, prolapse of organs, spontaneous sweating, shortness of breath, dyspnoea, weak immunity, recurrent colds and flus, asthma, poor appetite, indigestion, nausea, vomiting, morning sickness, epigastric pain, heartburn, belching, hiccup, difficulty swallowing, gastric ulceration, gastritis, oesophagitis, hiatus hernia, abdominal distension, loose stools, constipation, diarrhoea, abdominal rumbling, flatulence, undigested food in the stools, scanty menstruation, infertility, postpartum dizziness, floaters in the eyes, dry skin and hair, low or high blood pressure, anaemia, thirst, dry mouth, feeling of heat, fever, weakness of the tendons and muscles, back pain, tiredness and weakness of the legs, atrophy or paralysis of the lower limbs, knee disorders, stiffness and pain of the legs, disorders of the breast, insufficient lactation, hemiplegia, palpitations, chest pain, angina, depression and mood swings.

Furthermore, St-36 can be used in weight loss programmes to harmonise the Stomach and increase metabolism.

St-36 can be stimulated on athletes before and after exercising in order to strengthen the legs.

Additionally, St-36 can be used in *beauty treatments* in combination with other points that lift the qi (such as Du-20 and Ren-6) and local points on the face.

St-36 has also been traditionally employed to treat a variety of other symptoms and disorders including lockjaw, epilepsy, chills and fever, headache, sore throat, tinnitus, flank pain, wind stroke and loss of consciousness.

Main Areas: Entire body. Stomach and Spleen. Digestive system. Abdomen. Chest. Lower limb. Knee.

Main Functions: Tonifies and lifts qi. Blood. Fluids. Yin and yang. Boosts the Stomach and Spleen. Benefits the abdomen and chest.

St-37   Shangjuxu   上巨虛
Upper Great Hollow

Lower Sea point of the Large Intestine
Point of the Sea of Blood

3 cun below St-36, 6 cun below the knee crease, one finger's breadth lateral to the tibial crest. Situated on the tibialis anterior muscle.

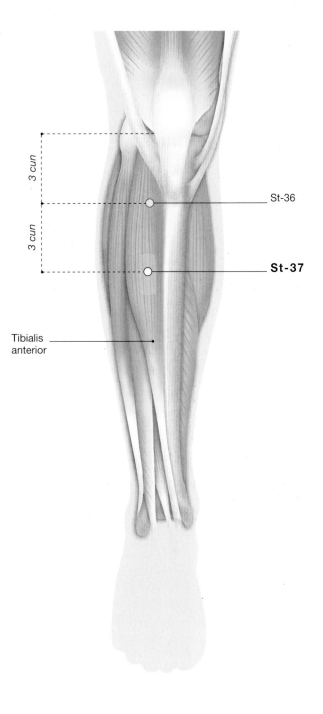

3 cun

3 cun

St-36

St-37

Tibialis anterior

Best treatment positions
Similar to St-36.

Needling
• 0.5 to 1.5 cun perpendicular insertion.

Moxibustion
Cones: 3–7. Pole: 5–20 minutes.

Guasha
Effective for channel problems.

Manual techniques and shiatsu
Similar to St-36.

Stimulation sensation
A sensation extending upwards is most effective for disorders of the abdomen.

Actions and indications
St-37 is an *important point to clear dampness and heat from the Large Intestine, alleviate diarrhoea and regulate Spleen and Stomach qi.* It is useful in any *acute or chronic disorder affecting the intestines.* Symptoms include loose stools, dysentery, undigested food in the stool, abdominal rumbling, abdominal distension and pain, constipation and umbilical pain.

Additionally, treatment at St-37 *clears the channel* and alleviates pain and stiffness of the lateral aspect of the leg.

Traditionally, St-37 has been employed to treat a variety of other symptoms such as fullness and pain of the chest, dyspnoea, shortness of breath, flank pain, stomach pain and swelling of the face.

> **Main Areas:** Large Intestine. Digestive system. Abdomen.
>
> **Main Functions:** Regulates the Large Intestine. Dispels dampness. Alleviates pain. Diarrhoea.

St-38　Tiaokou
Ribbon Opening
條口

8 cun above the lateral malleolus, in the depression approximately one finger's breadth lateral to the tibial crest. On the tibialis anterior muscle.

To aid location, it is midway between St-35 and St-41.

Best treatment positions
Similar to St-36 and St-37.

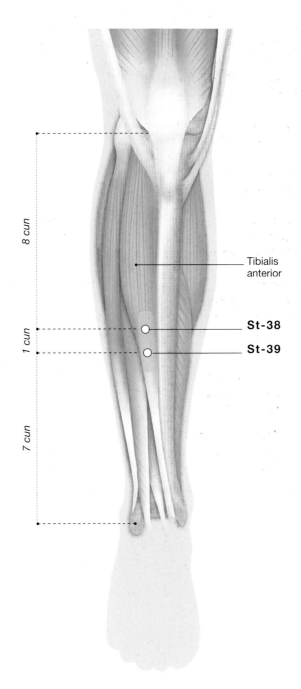

8 cun

1 cun

7 cun

Tibialis anterior

St-38

St-39

Needling
• 0.5 to 1.5 cun perpendicular insertion.

Actions and indications
St-38 has *similar internal functions to St-37 and St-39*. Additionally, it *expels wind, cold and damp from the stomach channel, alleviating pain and benefitting the shoulder.*

Its main indications include pain or numbness of the leg or knee, stomach ache, and pain and stiffness of the shoulder.

For best results when treating shoulder problems, mobilize the joint at the same time as stimulating St-38.

Main Areas: Shoulder. Digestive system.

Main Functions: Dispels wind. Damp and cold. Alleviates pain. Benefits the shoulder.

St-39 Xiajuxu
Lower Great Hollow

Lower Uniting-Sea-*He* point of the Small Intestine
Point of the Sea of Blood

1 cun below St-38 (9 cun below the knee crease), one finger's breadth lateral to the tibial crest.

Treatment and applications
The functions and treatment of St-39 are *similar to St-37 and St-38* although it has a greater effect on the *Small Intestine*. It is mainly used for symptoms such as abdominal distension and pain, abdominal rumbling, diarrhoea and pain or stiffness of the lower limbs.

Main Areas: Small Intestine. Digestive system. Abdomen.

Main Functions: Regulates the intestines. Alleviates pain.

St-40 Fenglong
Abundant Bulge

豐 隆

Connecting *Luo* point

On the anterolateral aspect of the leg, 8 cun below the knee crease, two finger width's lateral to the tibial crest (one finger's width lateral to St-38).

Situated in the extensor digitorum longus. Alternatively, locate it between the extensor digitorum longus and peroneus brevis muscles.

! This is a very strong point and should be stimulated gently in deficient patients.

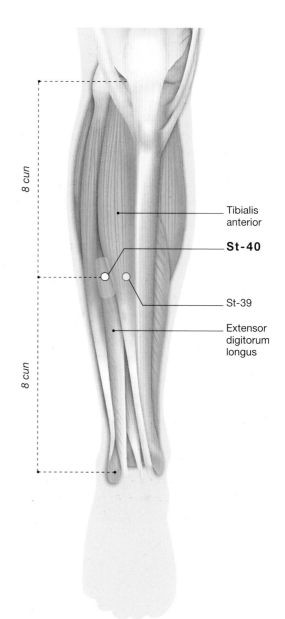

8 cun

8 cun

Tibialis anterior

St-40

St-39

Extensor digitorum longus

Best treatment positions
With the patient in a supine position. Palpate gently with the fingertip to find the depression on the lateral border of the extensor digitorum longus.

Needling
• 0.5 to 1.5 cun perpendicular insertion.

Moxibustion
Cones: 7–15. Pole: 5–20 minutes.

Guasha
Effectively applied for channel problems.

Manual techniques and shiatsu
Similar to St-36.

! This location is often sensitive or tender and pressure should be applied carefully.

Stimulation sensation
A strong sensation is often achieved spreading upward and/or downward along the channel pathway.

Actions and indications
St-40 is *possibly the most important point used to resolve phlegm* from any part of the body, and is particularly important for the *digestive and respiratory systems*. It effectively *transforms dampness, opens and relaxes the chest and alleviates cough*. Furthermore, it *clears heat* and *calms and clears the mind*.

Indications include productive cough, dyspnoea, tightness, heaviness and pain of the chest, asthmatic wheezing, bronchitis, pneumonia and other diseases accompanied by heavy phlegm build-up, palpitations, vomiting, epigastric pain, mental restlessness and anxiety, epilepsy, insomnia, depression and other psychological disorders, dizziness, Menière's disease, vertigo, feeling of muzziness and heaviness, headache, numbness of the legs and body, lumps, cysts, lipomas and tumours.

Main Areas: Chest. Head. Mind. Lungs. Stomach. Heart.

Main Functions: Resolves phlegm and transforms damp. Opens the chest. Relieves cough. Calms and clears the mind. Benefits the digestive system.

St-41   Jiexi 解谿
Dividing Cleft

River-*Jing*, Fire (Tonification) point

On the front of the ankle, at the junction of the dorsum of the foot and the leg, in the depression between the tendons of extensor digitorum longus and extensor hallucis longus.

To aid location, it is level with the prominence of the lateral malleolus, when the foot is flexed at right angles to the leg.

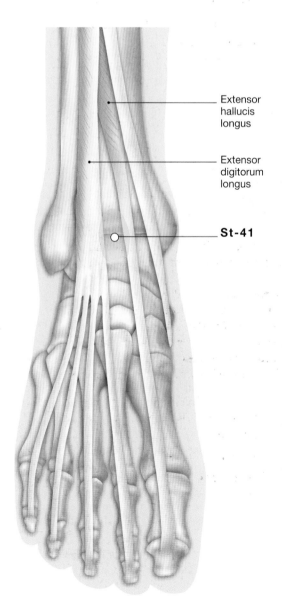

Extensor hallucis longus

Extensor digitorum longus

St-41

Best treatment positions
St-41 is best treated with the patient in a supine position. However, other positions may also be employed.

Needling
- 0.5 to 1.5 cun perpendicular insertion.
- Oblique insertion medially under the tendon of extensor hallucis longus toward Sp-5.
- Oblique insertion laterally under the tendon of extensor digitorum longus toward GB-40.

! Do not puncture the anterior tibial artery or the peroneal nerve usually passing just medial to this location.

Moxibustion
Cones: 3–5. Pole: 5–15 minutes Rice-grain moxa is also applicable.

Guasha
Effective for disorders of the ankle and pain.

Manual techniques and shiatsu
Extend the toes to define the tendons, and dorsiflex the foot to reach perpendicular pressure deeper into the point if necessary. Rubbing and friction techniques are effective applied directly onto the tendons. Mobilisation techniques to open and stretch the front of the ankle are also very useful.

Stimulation sensation
A reasonably strong sensation radiating into and around the ankle joint and/or up the leg is often achieved.

Actions and indications
St-41 is an important point for many disorders of the ankle. Furthermore, it clears Stomach heat, dispels wind, clears the head, brightens the eyes and calms the mind.

Indications include swelling and pain of the ankle and dorsum of the foot, weakness of the lower limbs, burning pain in the stomach, thirst, constipation, abdominal distension, dizziness, headache, redness and pain of the eyes, vertigo, mental restlessness and insomnia.

This location is very important because it is where the gravity line passes through the ankle. As such, it is a reference point for ensuring vertical alignment within standing Qigong.

> **Main Areas:** Ankle. Foot. Stomach. Head.
>
> **Main Functions:** Alleviates pain. Clears heat.

St-42 Chongyang 衝陽
Surging Yang

Source-*Yuan* point

On the highest point of the dorsum of the foot at the pulse of the dorsalis pedis artery, approximately midway between the tuberosity of the navicular and the base of the fifth metatarsal bone. In the small depression between the bases of the second and third metatarsal bones and the lateral and intermediate cuneiform bones, just lateral to the tendon of the extensor digitorum communis that attaches to the second toe.

! The dorsalis pedis artery causes this location to be sensitive to all forms of treatment.

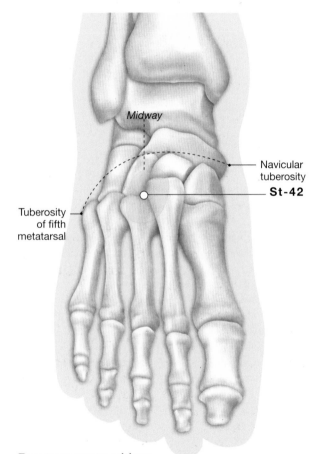

Best treatment positions
St-42 is best treated with the patient lying down supine. However, sitting or side-lying can also be employed.

Needling
- 0.3 to 0.5 cun perpendicular insertion. The needle tip should enter the small gap between the bones.

! Do not puncture the dorsalis pedis artery or veins of the dorsal cutaneous network.

Manual techniques and shiatsu
Stationary pressure and friction techniques are effective. Mobilisation techniques applied to the tarsal bones are effective to open St-42 and its surrounding area.

! Do not rub or apply friction to the artery.

Moxibustion
Cones: 3. Pole: 5–10 minutes. Light stimulation only. Rice-grain moxibustion is also applicable.

! Do not overstimulate St-42 because of the numerous cutaneous vessels at this site.

Stimulation sensation
A spreading sensation extending over the dorsum of the foot and/or to the second and third toes, or upward toward St-41 should be achieved. Deqi can also extend up the leg following the course of the channel.

Actions and indications
Although St-42 is the Source-Yuan point and therefore tonifies the Stomach and Spleen qi it is not as commonly employed for this purpose as other points (such as St-36, Sp-6 and Sp-3). It can however be employed in cases of *weakness and deficiency of the Stomach and Spleen* and treats a variety of *digestive symptoms* such as poor appetite, vomiting, loose stools and epigastric pain.

St-42 can also be used to *calm the mind* and *treat poor concentration*, tiredness, weakness, exhaustion, mental restlessness and fright.

St-42 also helps *unblock the channel pathway and alleviate pain*. Symptoms include deviation of the mouth, facial pain, toothache and atrophy, swelling or pain of the dorsum of the foot and toes.

Traditionally, the *strength and quality of the pulse* at Chong Yang St-42 (dorsalis pedis artery) is considered to indicate the state of the body's yang qi, whereas the St-8 pulse (temporal artery) is related to the state of the jing. The pulse at Ren Ying St-9 (carotid artery) discloses the general prognosis. Also, the 3 pulses: at the wrist (radial artery at Lu-9 and Lu-8), neck (common carotid at St-9) and dorsum of the foot (dorsalis pedis artery at St-42) are known as the Heaven, Earth and Man pulses.

> **Main Areas:** Stomach. Middle jiao. Foot. Mind.
>
> **Main Functions:** Tonifies qi and yang. Alleviates swelling and pain.

St-43 Xiangu
Sunken Valley

陷谷

Stream-*Shu* point, Wood point

On the dorsum of the foot, between the second and third metatarsal bones, in the depression distal to the junction of their bases.

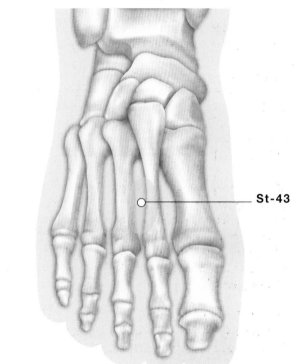

St-43

Needling
• 0.3 to 0.5 cun perpendicular insertion.

! Do not puncture cutaneous veins of the dorsal network, or the dorsal cutaneous branches of the superficial peroneal nerve and the dorsal metatarsal artery.

Manual techniques and shiatsu
Sustained perpendicular pressure and gentle friction techniques are applicable with the fingers and thumbs.

Actions and indications
St-43 is rarely used for interior Stomach disorders, because other Stomach channel points are more effective. It is, however, useful for *regional disorders* such as injury and pain of the dorsum of the foot and metatarsals.

> **Main Area:** Foot.
>
> **Main Functions:** Regulates qi and Blood. Alleviates swelling and pain.

St-44   Neiting
Inner Court

内庭

Spring-*Ying* Water point
Heavenly Star point

Between the second and third toes, proximal to the margin of the web (at the end of the crease), between the metatarsophalangeal joints.

! This is a strong point and care should be taken not to overstimulate it in deficient patients.

Best treatment positions
This point can be treated easily with the patient sitting or lying.

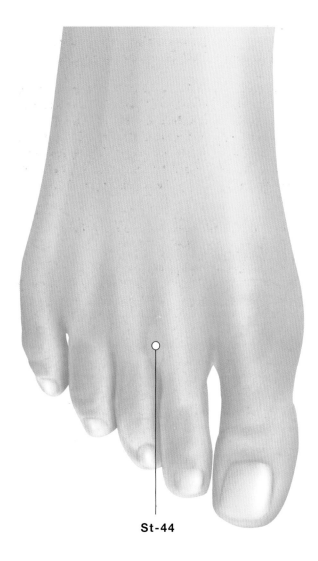

St-44

Needling
• 0.3 to 0.5 cun perpendicular insertion between the second and third metatarsophalangeal joint.

Moxibustion
Cones: 3–5. Pole: 5–7 minutes. Rice-grain moxibustion is also applicable.

Manual techniques and shiatsu
Deep perpendicular pressure is most effective. Flexing the second and third toes stretches them downwards opening St-44.

Stimulation sensation
An aching, numb or tingling sensation radiating around the location and spreading out across the dorsum of the foot should be achieved.

Actions and indications
St-44 is a *dynamic and widely employed point*. Its primary functions are to *clear heat from the Stomach, dispel wind and clear heat from the face and head, calm the mind*. However, it is also employed to benefit the digestion, clear damp heat from the Stomach and eliminate food stagnation.

Indications include burning epigastric pain, abdominal distension and pain, diarrhoea, dysentery, enteritis, constipation, gastritis, heartburn, halitosis, bleeding gums, mouth abscesses, periodonditis, dental caries, toothache, nosebleed, headache due to Stomach heat (particularly frontal headache), red, swollen painful eyes, conjunctivitis, chills and fever, febrile diseases, thirst, facial pain or paralysis, trigeminal neuralgia, deviation of the mouth, pain along the course of the Stomach channel, swelling and pain of the dorsum of the foot and toes, arthritis and injury to the second and third toes.

As a *local point, St-44 helps* alleviate swelling, stiffness and pain of the metatarsophalangeal joint and toe.

Main Areas: Stomach. Digestive system.
Face. Mouth. Eyes. Head.

Main Function: Clears heat.

St-45 Lidui 厲兌
Running Point

Well-Jing, Metal (Sedation) point

On the lateral side of the second toe, 0.1 cun proximal to the corner of the nail. At the intersection of two lines following the lateral border of the nail and the base of the nail.

Best treatment positions
This point can be treated easily with the patient sitting or lying.

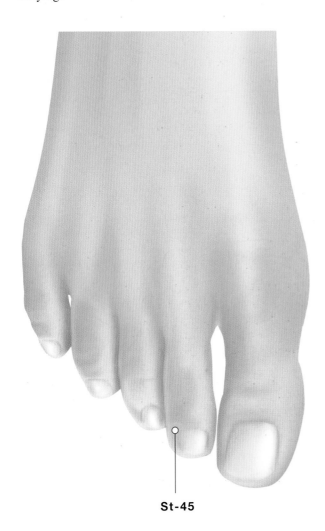

St-45

Needling
• 0.1 cun perpendicular insertion.

Moxibustion
Cones: 3. Pole: 2–5 minutes. Rice-grain moxa is also applicable.

Manual techniques and shiatsu
Friction or sustained pressure may be applied quite strongly with the thumb or fingertip until symptoms improve. Rubbing is also an effective technique applied to all the Well-Jing points at the ends of the fingers and toes.

Stimulation sensation
This location (in common with the other Well-Jing points) is often painful and strong stimulation can engender a very powerful sensation reaching the chest.

Actions and indications
St-45 has *similar functions to the other Well-Jing points* as it *calms the mind and resuscitates consciousness.*

Additionally, it is employed to *clear heat from the yang ming and Stomach channel* and *clear the eyes and head.* Common indications include toothache, deviation of the mouth, swelling of the face, sinusitis, epistaxis, tonsillitis, pharyngitis, facial paralysis, cold in the leg and foot, abdominal distension and fullness, mental restlessness and agitation, insomnia, epilepsy, fainting and coma.

> **Main Areas:** Face. Eyes. Mouth. Stomach. Stomach channel. Mind.
>
> **Main Function:** Resuscitates.

Chapter 13

Points of the

Leg Tai Yin
Spleen Channel

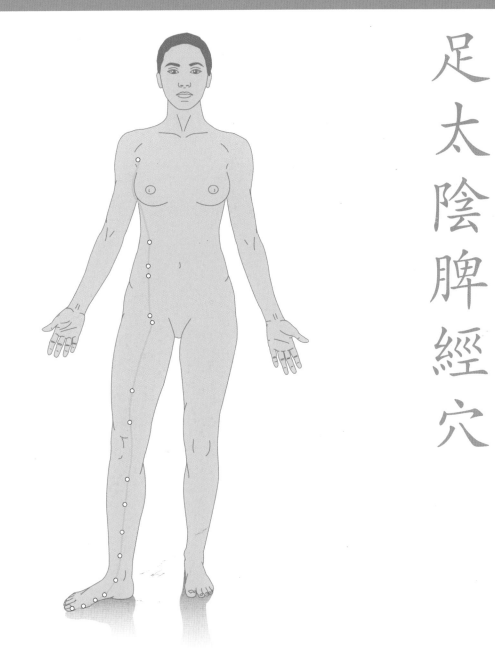

足太陰脾經穴

Sp-1 Yinbai
Hidden White

隱白

Well-*Jing*, Wood point
Third Ghost point

On the medial side of the big toe, approximately 0.1 cun proximal to the corner of the nail.

To aid location, it is the intersection of two lines following the medial border and the base of the nail.

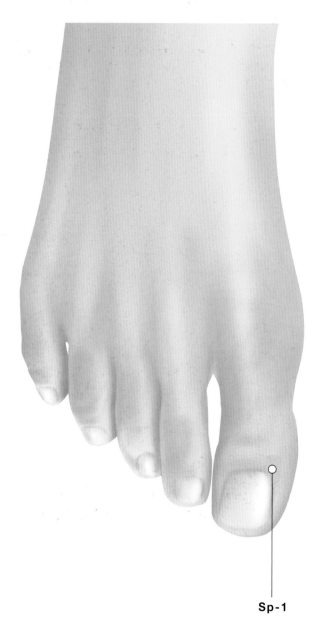

Sp-1

Best treatment positions
Needling and manual techniques are applied in a similar way to the other Well-Jing points. However, moxibustion is the treatment of choice for this location.

Needling
• 0.1 cun perpendicular insertion.

Moxibustion
Cones: 5–10. Pole: 5–20 minutes. Rice-grain moxa is also applicable.

Treatment with a moxa pole can be applied by the patient at home, for 5–15 minutes on each side, three times a day, until the bleeding ceases. In severe cases, apply every two hours.

Additionally, moxa Liv-1 if the bleeding is primarily due to Blood stasis.

Actions and indications
Sp-1 is possibly the most important point to *arrest bleeding* anywhere in the body because it aids the Spleen function of *holding Blood* and *raising qi*. It also *invigorates Blood* and *dispels stasis*. For these purposes it is usually treated with moxibustion.

Moxibustion at this location is particularly useful in the treatment of *disorders of the lower jiao*, including excessive uterine bleeding, dysmenorrhoea, threatened miscarriage, postpartum haemorrhage, chronic vaginal discharge, prolapse of the uterus or rectum, haemorrhoids, blood in the stool or urine, abdominal distension and varicose veins.

Moxibustion at Sp-1 has also been employed as a first aid procedure to arrest haemorrhage anywhere in the body.

Sp-1 also *clears the Heart* and *calms the mind* and can be used in such cases as dizziness, vertigo, fainting, loss of consciousness, depression and insomnia.

Main Areas: Uterus. Blood vessels. Mind.

Main Functions: Arrests bleeding. Lifts qi. Calms and clears the mind.

Sp-2 Dadu
Great Pool

大都

Spring-*Ying*, Fire (Tonification) point

On the medial aspect of the big toe in the small depression distal and inferior to the first metatarsophalangeal (MTP) joint.

To aid location, it is at the junction of the skin of the plantar and dorsal surface, between the flesh and bone.

Best treatment positions
Similar to Sp-3.

Needling
• 0.3 to 0.5 cun perpendicular insertion.

Manual techniques and shiatsu
Stationary pressure and friction is applicable with the fingertips or thumbs.

Moxibustion
Cones: 5–10. Pole: 5–15 minutes. Rice-grain moxa is also applicable.

Actions and indications
Although Sp-2 is not as commonly used as other Spleen points, it can be effective to *harmonise the Spleen and Stomach*, *resolve dampness* and *clear heat*, particularly from the digestive system. Symptoms include chills and fever, stomach pain, vomiting, diarrhoea, abdominal distension, chest pain and insomnia.

Additionally, moxibustion helps *warm yang* and *lift sinking qi*.

As a local point, Sp-2 is useful in cases of swelling, pain, arthritis, gout, deformity or injury of the first metatarsophalangeal joint.

> **Main Areas:** MTP joint. Toe. Digestive system.
>
> **Main Function:** Clears dampness and heat.

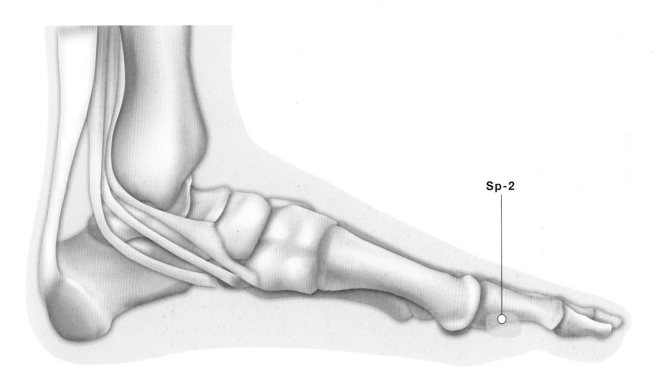

Sp-2

Sp-3   Taibai
Great White

太白

Stream-*Shu*, Earth (Horary) point
Source-*Yuan* point

On the medial aspect of the foot in the small depression proximal and inferior to the head of the first metatarsal bone, at the junction of the skin of the plantar and dorsal surface.

Between the abductor hallucis tendon and first metatarsal bone. In its deep position lies the flexor hallucis brevis muscle.

To aid location, slide your fingertip proximally over the medial aspect of the first metatarsophalangeal joint into the depression formed between the flesh and bone.

Best treatment positions
This location is best treated with the medial surface of the foot facing upward and the patient in a supine or side-lying position. However, lying face down or sitting in a chair can also be employed.

Needling
• 0.3 to 1 cun perpendicular insertion under the bone.

!! Ensure the needle does not penetrate the tendon of abductor hallucis. Also, if the needle is deeply inserted (through the flexor hallucis brevis muscle), the tip may reach the tendon of flexor hallucis longus. In both cases it will feel very tight and painful.

! Do not puncture cutaneous veins of the dorsal network of the foot or the medial tarsal artery. On the plantar surface, do not puncture the digital branch of the medial plantar nerve to the big toe, and deeper, the medial plantar artery.

Manual techniques and shiatsu
Stationary pressure is applied with the fingertip or thumb into the space between the muscle and bone. Friction can be applied across the abductor hallucis tendon, and deeper into the flexor hallucis brevis muscle fibres.

Stretching the tendon and muscle away from the bone in a plantar direction will help open this area. Additionally, mobilising the first metatarsophalangeal joint and stretching the toe helps to relax the soft tissues.

Moxibustion
Cones: 3–10. Pole: 5–15 minutes. Rice-grain moxa is also effectively applied.

Magnets
Magnets are effectively employed.

Stimulation sensation
Localised soreness, distension, warmth or tingling possibly extending distally toward the toe, or proximally along the channel.

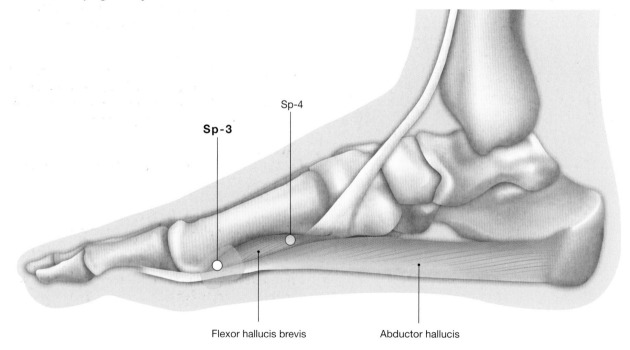

Flexor hallucis brevis   Abductor hallucis

Actions and indications

Sp-3 is a major point to *fortify the Spleen* and *Earth element*. It *boosts transformation and movement*, *regulates the middle jiao* and *benefits the digestive system*. It is one of the most important points to *resolve dampness*, *reduce swelling* and *clear damp heat*. Moreover, it *promotes qi and Blood circulation*, *relieves stasis* and *alleviates pain*.

Common indications include tiredness, weakness and heaviness of the limbs and body, poor appetite, desire to eat sweets, obesity, cellulite, fluid retention, oedema, hypothyroidism, diabetes, abdominal distension and pain, abdominal rumbling, stomach ache, heartburn, indigestion, nausea, vomiting, gastroenteritis, dysentery, candidiasis, loose stools, diarrhoea, constipation, haemorrhoids, blood in the stool, vaginal discharge, vaginitis, frequent urination, dysuria, cystitis, headache, cough with profuse sputum and fluid in the lungs.

Additionally, Sp-3 helps the *Spleen House Thought (Yi)* and improves mental functions and concentration in such cases as poor memory, sleepiness, feeling of heaviness and muzziness, depression, mental confusion, arteriosclerosis and declining mental faculties.

Another usage of Sp-3 is to strengthen the muscles, limbs and spine, and it has been employed to treat chronic lower back ache, spinal disorders and weakness, atrophy or paralysis.

As a local point, it may be used to treat gout, arthritis or injury of the big toe and first metatarsophalangeal joint.

The Sp-3 location also corresponds to reflexology and sujok points that treat the spine.

Main Areas: Digestive system. Intestines. Urinary system. Muscles. Mind.

Main Functions: Transforms dampness. Tonifies Spleen qi and yang.

Sp-4   Gongsun

Grandfather Grandson
(Yellow Emperor)

公孫

Connecting *Luo* point
Opening (Master) point of the Chong Mai

On the medial aspect of the foot, in the depression distal and inferior to the base of the first metatarsal bone, at the junction of the skin of the plantar and dorsal surface. Between the abductor hallucis tendon and first metatarsal bone. In its deep position lies the flexor hallucis brevis muscle.

Locate by sliding your fingertip proximally from Sp-3 along the shaft of the first metatarsal, into the depression formed between the flesh and the base of the bone.

Treatment
Similar to Sp-3.

Needling
• 0.5 to 1.5 cun perpendicular insertion, under the bone.

! Ensure the needle does not go into the abductor hallucis tendon as it can be very tight and painful. Furthermore, when needling deeply, avoid the flexor hallucis longus tendon.

! Do not puncture veins of the dorsal cutaneous network of the foot, or the cutaneous branches of the saphenous nerve and the superficial peroneal nerve. On the plantar surface, when needling deeper, do not puncture the digital branch of the medial plantar nerve of the big toe, and more deeply, the medial plantar artery and vein.

Manual techniques and shiatsu
Similar to Sp-3. Combine stationary pressure and friction with mobilisation techniques. Deep friction of the abductor hallucis tendon and flexor hallucis brevis muscle is effective to help dissipate stagnation

Moxibustion
Cones: 3–8. Pole: 5–15 minutes. Rice-grain moxa is also applicable.

Magnets
Magnets are also effectively employed at this location.

Use the north pole on Sp-4 and the south pole on contralateral P-6, or vice-versa, to regulate the Chong Mai and the Yin Wei Mai.

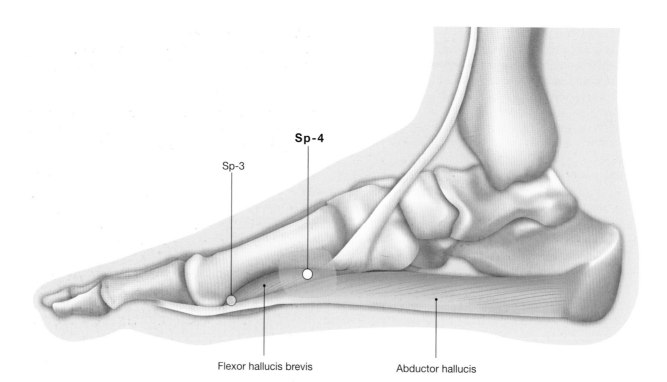

Sp-4

Sp-3

Flexor hallucis brevis

Abductor hallucis

Stimulation sensation

Deqi can be reasonably difficult to achieve, partly because this location is often quite tight and painful and because the epicentre of the point is difficult to locate in the small gap under the bone.

The most common sensation achieved at Sp-4 is soreness, ache, distension or electricity perceived locally or extending across the sole of the foot. However, the most effective systemic therapeutic results seem to be achieved when the sensation is felt going up the leg and reaching the abdomen or chest, following the course of the Spleen Luo channel or Chong Mai.

Actions and indications

Sp-4 is a very important and widely used point for a variety of therapeutic purposes. Its primary functions are to *regulate the Chong Mai* and *dispel stasis* from the three jiao. Additionally it is extensively employed to *regulate the middle jiao*, *boost the Stomach and Spleen* and *augment Blood production*. Furthermore, it helps *transform dampness* and *dispel swelling*.

In relation to the *digestive system,* Sp-4 has been widely employed in the treatment of chronic or acute abdominal pain, distension, fullness or heaviness, abdominal rumbling, flatulence, constipation, irritable bowel syndrome, Crohn's disease, gastroenteritis, dysentery, epigastric pain, gastritis, hiatus hernia, heartburn, oesophagitis, nausea, vomiting and morning sickness during pregnancy.

Sp-4 can also be useful to *alleviate nausea* and digestive symptoms caused by heavy medication, including chemotherapy, particularly in combination with P-6 Neiguan and St-36 Zusanli.

Sp-4 is very *important in gynaecology* because it regulates menstruation and benefits the uterus. Indications include irregular menstruation, premenstrual syndrome, dysmenorrhoea, endometriosis, polycystic ovaries, amenorrhoea, excessive menstrual bleeding and infertility.

Furthermore, Sp-4 is very important to *relieve stasis from the chest, regulate the Heart* and *calm the mind.* It has been extensively employed to treat chronic or acute pain and heaviness of the chest, angina pectoris, vascular disease, anaemia, psychosomatic disorders, insomnia and depression.

Main Areas: The three jiao. Stomach. Abdomen. Uterus. Heart. Mind.

Main Functions: Opens the Chong Mai. Regulates qi. Dispels Blood stasis. Benefits menstruation.

Sp-5 Shangqiu

商丘

Metal Hill

River-Jing, Metal (Sedation) point

In the depression anterior and inferior to the medial malleolus. Midway between the navicular tuberosity and the prominence of the medial malleolus.

Best treatment positions
Treatment is best applied in a supine or side position with the medial surface of the foot facing upwards.

Needling
• 0.3 to 0.5 cun perpendicular insertion.
• 1 to 1.5 cun oblique insertion to join with St-41.

! Do not puncture the great saphenous vein, the cutaneous branch of the saphenous nerve, the medial tarsal artery or the branch of the superficial peroneal nerve.

Manual techniques and shiatsu
Combine stationary pressure and gentle friction with mobilisation techniques to loosen the tarsal joints.

Moxibustion
Cones: 3–5. Pole: 5–10 minutes. Light-medium stimulation only. Rice-grain moxa is also applicable.

Guasha
Gently applied guasha is applicable.

Actions and indications
Sp-5 is mainly used for *disorders of the ankle, foot,* leg and knee in combination with other local and adjacent points.

However, it also effectively treats interior conditions by virtue of its functions of *boosting the Spleen and Stomach, drying dampness* and *regulating qi and Blood.*

Symptoms include abdominal distension and pain, diarrhoea, abdominal rumbling, stomach ache, indigestion, heartburn, vomiting, constipation, haemorrhoids, heaviness of the limbs, oedema, breast pain, infertility, dysmenorrhoea and endometriosis.

Sp-5 has also been traditionally used to treat a variety of other disorders including tiredness and lethargy, depression, insomnia, excessive thinking, chills and fever, jaundice, stiffness of the tongue, convulsions and swelling of the throat.

> **Main Areas:** Ankle. Abdomen.
>
> **Main Functions:** Dries dampness. Regulates qi and Blood. Benefits the lower jiao.

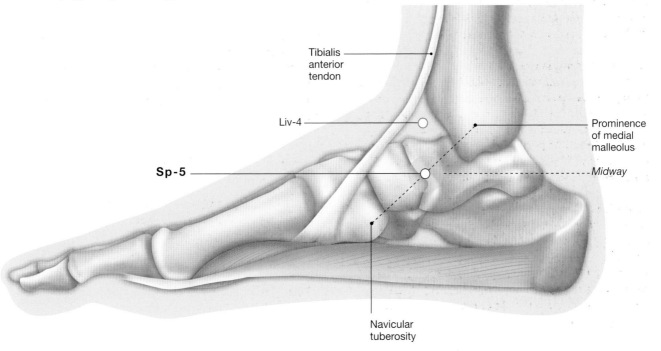

Tibialis anterior tendon

Liv-4

Sp-5

Prominence of medial malleolus

Midway

Navicular tuberosity

Sp-6   Sanyinjiao

三陰交

Three Yin Intersection

Intersection of the Spleen, Liver and Kidney
One of the nine points to Return Yang

In the soft depression 3 cun superior to the prominence of the medial malleolus, posterior to the medial tibial border. In the flexor digitorum longus muscle, and more deeply, the tibialis posterior muscle. Deeper still, the flexor hallucis longus muscle.

To aid location, Sp-6 is approximately one hand-width proximal to the medial malleolus. Palpate the large, trench-like depression (often larger and softer in women) gently and carefully to ascertain the most reactive point(s).

Alternative locations
It could be considered that a slightly more anterior location affects the Liver more, a posterior one the Kidney, and a central one the Spleen.

! Sp-6 can be extremely sensitive and painful, particularly during the premenstrual phase.

Contraindications
Do not treat Sp-6 during pregnancy and heavy menstrual bleeding.

! Strong stimulation can bring on menstruation early, particularly in Spleen deficient patients.

Best treatment positions
Treatment is best applied in a supine position with the knee flexed and the thigh laterally rotated so that the Spleen channel is exposed properly. Ensure that the outside of the thigh, knee and leg are adequately supported with cushions. Moreover, Sp-6 can be treated supine with the leg extended.

Alternatively, lying down prone, sideways or sitting up in a chair can be employed.

Needling
• 0.5 to 2 cun perpendicular insertion toward GB-39.
• 0.3 to 1.5 cun perpendicular insertion in a slightly posterior or proximal direction.

! Anteriorly, do not puncture the great saphenous vein and the cutaneous branch of the saphenous nerve; deeper and slightly posteriorly, the posterior tibial artery and veins and the tibial nerve; deeper still, and in a slightly anterior direction, the peroneal artery and veins.

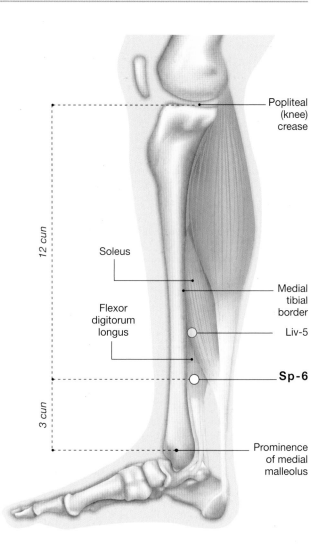

Popliteal (knee) crease

12 cun

Soleus

Flexor digitorum longus

Medial tibial border

Liv-5

Sp-6

3 cun

Prominence of medial malleolus

Manual techniques and shiatsu
Sustained perpendicular pressure is applicable with a variety of 'tools' including the fingers, thumbs and palms. However the latter may, in many cases, be more appropriate because this site can be very painful. Gentle friction can also be effective.

Additionally, rubbing Sp-6 and the surrounding area superficially helps warm and tonify the yang qi.

If the area seems very tight and painful, apply cross-fibre stretching to the soleus and flexor digitorum longus muscles first. Stretch the muscle bellies in a posterior direction with the palm of the hand.

! This location can be extremely sensitive and painful, particularly during the premenstrual phase.

Moxibustion

Cones: 3–8. Pole: 10–20 minutes. Use light-medium stimulation only. Rice-grain moxa is also effective.

! Direct moxibustion is not recommended at this location in patients with varicosities.

Magnets

Magnets can be effectively used at this location. For Spleen and Stomach deficiency, as well as Qi and Blood deficiency, use the north pole on Sp-6 and the south pole on St-36, or vice-versa. For Blood-Yin deficiency use the south pole on Sp-6 bilaterally and the north pole on Ren-4, or vice-versa.

Stimulation sensation

Regional soreness, ache and distension, possibly extending proximally up the channel toward the knee, medial aspect of the thigh and abdomen. Additionally, electricity may be felt spreading down toward the sole of the foot and toes.

Deqi perceived in a proximal direction is more effective for internal disorders and seems essential for promoting labour.

Actions and indications

Sp-6 is one of the most widely used points and is of utmost importance in any treatment aiming to *nourish Blood and Yin, calm and cool the body and mind* and *strengthen the Spleen, Liver* and *Kidneys*, whose channels converge here.

Additionally, Sp-6 is important to *regulate qi and Blood, dispel stasis* and *alleviate pain*.

Sp-6 is an important point to benefit the *digestive system*, and is widely employed to *resolve dampness* and *damp heat*, particularly from the middle and lower jiao. It is extensively employed in cases of poor appetite and digestion, stomach ache, abdominal rumbling, abdominal distension and pain, loose or rough stools, gastroenteritis, diarrhoea, constipation and irritable bowel syndrome.

Furthermore, it is widely employed to *resolve dampness* and *damp heat*, particularly from the middle and lower jiao.

It is also of primary importance in gynaecology because it *regulates the uterus and menstruation* and *induces labour*. Indications include dysmenorrhoea, amenorrhoea, irregular or delayed menstruation, delayed and difficult labour, difficulty in discharging the placenta, infertility, frigidity, vaginal discharge, impotence, genital itching or pain, dysuria, frequent urination, cystitis, urethritis and incontinence.

Sp-6 *cools and nourishes yin* and *calms the mind* and is beneficial in such cases as dizziness, tinnitus, vertigo, headache, feeling of heat, skin diseases, dry mouth and throat, night sweats, hypertension, palpitations, restlessness, insomnia and depression.

Sp-6 has also been widely employed in a variety of other disorders including chronic tiredness, exhaustion, blurred vision, tinnitus, emaciation, obesity, bulimia, swelling, oedema, diabetes and liver disease.

As a *local point* it effectively treats weakness, atrophy or paralysis of the lower limb, oedema or pain of the ankle or foot.

Main Areas: Entire body, particularly the abdomen. Liver. Spleen. Kidney.

Main Functions: Boosts the Spleen and Stomach. Transforms dampness. Nourishes Blood and yin. Calms the mind. Regulates qi and Blood. Benefits menstruation. Promotes labour.

Sp-7   Lougu
Leaking Valley

漏谷

3 cun proximal to Sp-6, in a depression immediately posterior to the medial tibial border.

Best treatment positions
Similar to Sp-6 and Liv-5.

Needling
• 0.5 to 1.5 cun perpendicular insertion.

Actions and indications
Sp-7 is not a very commonly employed point, although it has been traditionally used to *fortify the Spleen*, *promote urination*, *resolve dampness* and *reduce swelling*. Symptoms include abdominal distension, abdominal rumbling, dysuria, urinary retention, arthritis, swelling and cold pain of the leg and knee.

Sp-8   Diji
Earth's Cure

地機

Accumulation Cleft-*Xi* point

5 cun inferior to the knee crease, in the depression posterior to the medial tibial border. Between the soleus muscle and the tibia.

The depression of Sp-8 is formed between the medial tibial border (just superior to the medial end of the soleal line), the soleus muscle (inferiorly), and the insertion of the popliteus muscle (superiorly).

To aid location, Sp-8 is one third of the distance between the popliteal (knee) crease and the prominence of the medial malleolus, or 3 cun (one hand width) distal to Sp-9.

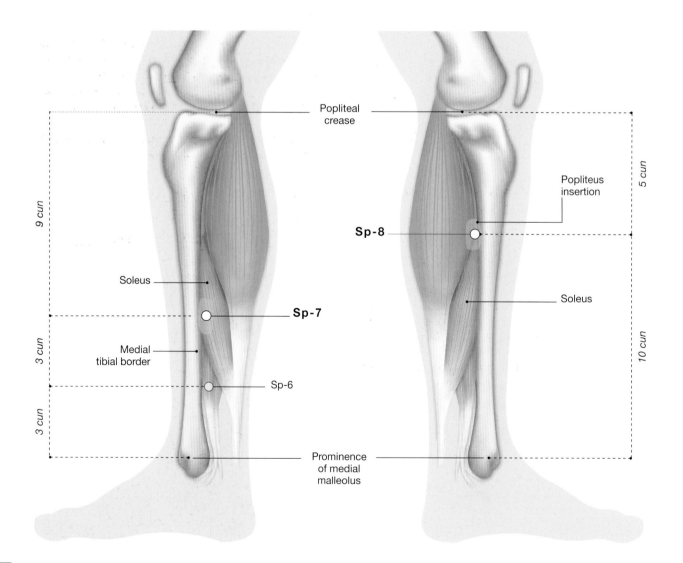

! Sp-8 is a very powerful point, and should be stimulated lightly in deficient patients. Also, strong treatment at this location can bring on early menstruation, particularly in Spleen-deficient patients.

Best treatment positions
Similar to Sp-6. If this location is very tight and painful, apply needling and manual techniques with the knee flexed and the thigh laterally rotated so that the Spleen channel is exposed properly. Ensure that the outside of the thigh, knee and leg are well supported by cushions. However it can also be treated with the leg extended.

Needling
• 0.5 to 2 cun perpendicular insertion.

! Do not puncture the greater saphenous vein or the cutaneous branch of the saphenous nerve. More deeply and slightly posteriorly, avoid the posterior tibial artery and veins and the tibial nerve. Deeper still and in a slightly anterior direction, avoid the peroneal artery and veins.

Manual techniques and shiatsu
Similar to Sp-6. Reasonably light friction is often the best choice initially, because perpendicular pressure can be very painful. However, sustained perpendicular pressure is very effective applied between the muscle and bone.

If the area seems very tight and painful, apply cross-fibre stretching to the soleus muscle first. Stretch it in a posterior direction with the palm.

! Sp-8 can be very painful and tight. Also, it can bruise easily, especially in predisposed patients.

Moxibustion
Cones: 3–8. Pole: 5–15 minutes.

Magnets
Magnets can also be effectively used at this location. For Spleen-Stomach and Qi and Blood deficiency use the north pole on Sp-6 and the south pole on St-36, or vice-versa. For Blood-Yin deficiency use the south pole on Sp-6 bilaterally, and the north pole on Ren-4, or vice-versa.

Guasha
Lightly applied guasha can be beneficial.

! Do not rub across the greater saphenous vein.

Stimulation sensation
Local ache, soreness and distension extending distally down the leg toward the medial ankle area, or proximally along the channel. The sensation can be very powerful and reach the abdomen.

Actions and indications
Sp-8 is an important and powerful point to *resolve stasis, alleviate pain* and *regulate the flow of Qi and Blood* in the abdomen and along the entire course of the Spleen channel. In common with the other Cleft-Xi points, it helps to *moderate acute conditions* and *arrest bleeding*.

It is also very important to *regulate the uterus and menstruation*. Common indications include dysmenorrhoea, excessive or abnormal uterine bleeding, irregular menstruation, ovarian cysts, uterine fibroids and endometriosis.

Furthermore, Sp-8 has been employed to *harmonise the Spleen* and *resolve dampness* from the middle and lower jiao. Symptoms include abdominal distension and pain, poor appetite, diarrhoea, rectal bleeding, haemorrhoids, seminal emissions, retention of urine and oedema.

In addition, Sp-8 treats *acute pain* anywhere along the channel, but especially in the knees and legs.

> **Main Areas:** Uterus. Abdomen. Knee.
>
> **Main Functions:** Invigorates Blood. Dispels stasis. Regulates menstruation.

Sp-9   Yinlingquan
Yin Mound Spring

陰陵泉

Uniting Sea-*He*, Water point

In the depression below the medial tibial condyle, between the tibial border and the gastrocnemius muscle. The popliteus muscle is situated in its deep position. Locate with the knee flexed.

To aid location, run your fingertip upwards along the groove posterior to the medial border of the tibia until it naturally comes to a halt at the lower border of the medial tibial condyle.

Best treatment positions
Treatment is best applied in a supine position with the knee flexed and the thigh laterally rotated so that the medial aspect of the knee faces upwards. Ensure that the hip, thigh and knee is adequately supported with cushions.

Needling
• 0.5 to 1 cun perpendicular insertion along the posterior tibial border toward, or to join with, GB-34.

! In an anterior direction, do not puncture the greater saphenous vein or the cutaneous branch of the saphenous nerve. More, the medial inferior genicular artery and vein. Deeper still and in an anterior direction, the peroneal artery and veins. Deeper and posteriorly, avoid the posterior tibial artery and veins and the tibial nerve.

Manual techniques and shiatsu
Stationary pressure or gentle friction can be applied with the palm, fingertips or thumbs. Additionally, stretching the muscles in a posterior direction (with the palms) is also an effective technique.

Moxibustion
Cones: 3–10. Pole: 5–15 minutes. Rice-grain moxa can also be employed at Sp-9 and surrounding points.

Magnets
Magnets can also be effectively used at this location. For dampness in the lower jiao or oedema due to Spleen deficiency, use the south pole on Sp-9 and the north pole on Sp-6, or vice-versa. For urinary dysfunction use the north pole on Sp-9 and the south pole on Ren-3, or vice-versa.

Cupping
Medium or light cupping can, in certain cases, be beneficial for disorders of the knee.

Stimulation sensation
Local ache, soreness, warmth or tingling, possibly extending distally or proximally along the course of the channel. Electricity is also sometimes perceived spreading distally toward the ankle and toes.

Actions and indications
Sp-9 is one of the most powerful points to *open the water passages*, *drain dampness* and *regulate the lower jiao*, particularly in relation to the *intestines* and the *urogenital systems*. Its main indications include dysuria, cystitis, urethritis, urinary retention, incontinence, vaginal discharge, irregular menstruation, abdominal distension, abdominal pain, diarrhoea, undigested food in the stool, mucus in the stool, dysentery, enteritis, oedema, swelling of the lower limbs and abdomen.

It is also very effectively employed in the treatment of *channel disorders*, including pain or swelling at the medial aspect of the knee, pain of the thigh and lumbago.

> **Main Areas:** Lower jiao. Urogenital system. Intestines. Abdomen. Knee.
>
> **Main Functions:** Drains dampness. Regulates the lower jiao.

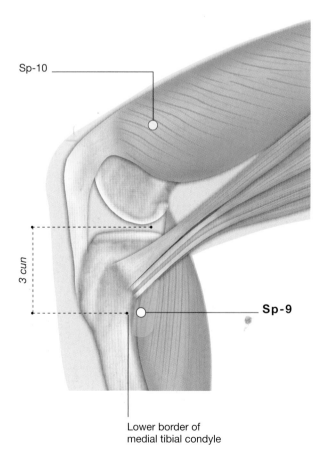

Sp-10

3 cun

Sp-9

Lower border of medial tibial condyle

Sp-10 Xuehai
Sea of Blood

血海

In the depression on the protuberance of the vastus medialis muscle, 2 cun proximal to the medial superior border of the patella. Directly above Sp-9 and level with St-34. Locate and treat with the knee flexed.

To aid location, place the (left) palm over the (right) knee so that the fingers are on the lateral side and point upwards. The tip of the thumb will lie on Sp-10, approximately.

Needling
• 0.5 to 1.5 cun perpendicular insertion.

! Do not puncture branches of the anterior femoral cutaneous nerve. More deeply, the muscular branches of the femoral artery, vein and nerve.

Manual techniques and shiatsu
Perpendicular pressure or friction techniques with the fingers, thumbs or palms is applicable.

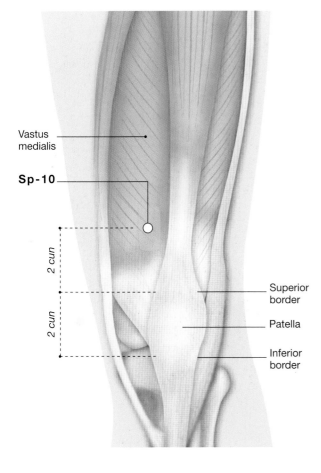

Vastus medialis

Sp-10

2 cun

2 cun

Superior border

Patella

Inferior border

Moxibustion
Cones: 3–5. Pole: 5–10 minutes. Rice-grain moxa is also effectively applied.

Magnets
Magnets are also effectively employed at this location. For disorders of the knee, use opposite poles on Sp-10 and St-34 and at the Eyes of the Knee (Xiyan, page 341).

Actions and indications
Sp-10 is a major point for *many disorders of Blood*. It *regulates and cools Blood*, *removes stasis* and *arrests bleeding*, with its broadest application in *gynaecological and skin diseases*. It helps *regulate menstruation* and dispel stasis from the uterus as well as having a powerful soothing effect on the skin, particularly if there is inflammation and itching.

Common indications include abnormal uterine bleeding, irregular menstruation, excessive menstruation, dysmenorrhoea, haematuria, amenorrhoea, genital sores, dermatitis, inflamed or itchy skin, ulceration, eczema, psoriasis, urticaria, herpes zoster, allergies and other skin disorders.

Additionally, Sp-10 can be employed to *dispel dampness* and treat symptoms such as dysuria, vaginal discharge and nausea.

As a *local point*, Sp-10 can be used to treat pain of the medial side of the knee and thigh.

Note
For skin diseases, use Baichongwo M-LE-34 (also known as Sp-10 and a Half) instead of, or additionally to Sp-10, particularly if it is more reactive on pressure palpation.

> **Main Areas:** Skin. Gynaecological system. Genitals.
>
> **Main Function:** Invigorates and cools Blood. Dispels dampness.

Sp-12   Chongmen   衝門
Surging Gate

Intersection of the Liver and the Yin Wei Mai on the Spleen channel

On the inguinal groove, in the depression of the saphenous hiatus, just lateral to the femoral artery, approximately 3.5 cun lateral to Ren-2.

To aid location, Sp-12 is slightly more than one hand's width lateral to the anterior midline. Furthermore, it is about one finger's width lateral to the palpable femoral artery and approximately 1 cun lateral to Liv-12.

Best treatment positions
Similar to Liv-12.

!! Do not apply any form of treatment to this area if there is any suspicion of thrombosis.

Important note
Traditionally, this location was treated by moxibustion rather than needling, because the latter was considered dangerous. However, moxibustion is not recommended at this location, except in very rare cases, and direct moxibustion is contraindicated. As a general rule, pressure techniques are easier to apply, and are therefore more readily recommended.

Needing
• 0.5 to 1 cun perpendicular insertion. See also Liv-12.

! Do not puncture the femoral artery medially, or the femoral nerve laterally.

Manual techniques and shiatsu
There is a variety of manual techniques that may be applied to this location (see Liv-12).

! Do not apply friction to the saphenous hiatus area. Also, do not apply any form of pressure to enlarged lymph nodes.

Stimulation sensation
Deqi at this location is usually experienced as a tingling or electric sensation spreading distally along the medial aspect of the thigh and leg. Additionally, numbness and tingling may extend medially or upwards into the pelvis and abdomen.

Actions and indications
Sp-12 has comparable actions to Liv-12, helping *regulate qi and Blood circulation, dispel stasis* and *alleviate pain*. Both these points have similar effects on the entire blood circulation and are particularly beneficial for *disorders of the lower limbs, groin and lower abdomen*. Indications include poor circulation, vascular disorders, cold legs and feet, hernia, testicular pain or swelling, impotence, dysmenorrhoea and uterine prolapse.

Sp-12 also helps *drain dampness* and *regulate urination* and has been used to treat dysuria, urinary retention or pain, swelling and cold in the lower abdomen.

As a *local point*, Sp-12 can be used to treat muscle strain and sciatica.

> **Main Areas:** Lower limbs. Groin. Vessels.
>
> **Main Functions:** Improves qi and blood circulation. Alleviates pain.

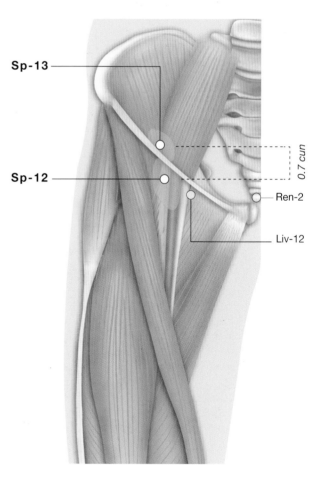

Sp-13　Fushe

府舍

Bowel Abode

Intersection of the Liver and the Yin Wei Mai on the Spleen channel

Approximately 0.7 cun superior and slightly lateral to Sp-12, 4 cun lateral to the anterior midline.

Needing
• 0.5 to 1 cun perpendicular insertion.

! Do not needle deeply, particularly if the patient is very thin. Needling deeply poses a considerable risk of puncturing the peritoneum. Do not puncture branches of the superficial epigastric artery and vein, and more deeply, the inferior epigastric artery and vein.

Manual techniques and shiatsu
Stationary perpendicular pressure or gentle friction techniques are applicable with the fingers or thumbs.

Moxibustion
Pole: 5–10 minutes. Direct moxibustion is not recommended at this location.

Actions and indications
Sp-13 is not a very commonly employed point, although it can be useful in cases of lower abdominal or groin pain, tightness and hernia. Its primary function is to regulate and relax the intestines.

> **Main Areas:** Lower abdomen. Groin.
>
> **Main Function:** Regulates qi in the intestines.

Sp-14　Fujie

腹結

Abdominal Bind

In a depression approximately 1.3 cun inferior to Sp-15 and 4 cun lateral to the anterior midline.

According to certain classical sources, Sp-14 is located slightly further laterally, at a 4.5 cun distance from the anterior midline.

Use Sp-14 instead of Sp-15 if it is more sensitive or reactive on pressure palpation.

Best treatment positions
Similar to Sp-15.

Actions and indications
Sp-14 is not very commonly used, although treatment can be successfully applied here for *similar purposes to Sp-15*. Its primary functions are to *regulate the intestines*, *dispel cold* from the lower jiao and *descend rebellious qi* from the chest. It is particularly indicated for diarrhoea and abdominal tightness and pain.

> **Main Areas:** Intestines. Abdomen.
>
> **Main Functions:** Regulates qi in the intestines. Descends rebellious qi.

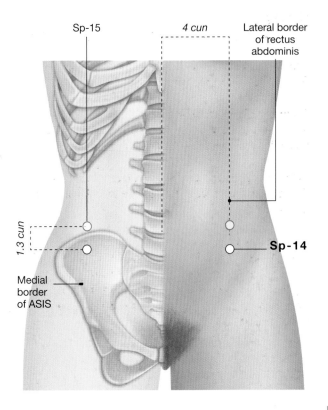

Sp-15　　4 cun　　Lateral border of rectus abdominis

1.3 cun

Sp-14

Medial border of ASIS

Sp-15 Daheng
Great Horizontal

Intersection of the Yin Wei Mai and Spleen

In the depression on the lateral border of the rectus abdominis muscle, 4 cun lateral to the centre of the umbilicus. In a large and soft shallow depression on the long crease crossing the centre of the abdomen horizontally. To aid location, the 4 cun can be measured from the lateral border of the rectus abdominis and from the medial border of the anterior superior iliac spine.

Alternative location
Sp-15 may also be located slightly further laterally, at a 4.5 cun distance from the anterior midline.

Best treatment positions
Treatment is applied in a supine position with the hips slightly flexed and the knees and legs well supported by cushions so that the abdomen can be as relaxed as possible (ensure the lower back is lying flat on the floor).

Needing
• 0.5 to 1.5 cun perpendicular insertion.

! Do not needle deeply, particularly if the patient is very thin. This poses a considerable risk of puncturing the peritoneum or an enlarged liver or spleen.

Manual techniques and shiatsu
Similar to St-25. Self-acupressure can also be very effective if applied regularly. Use the thumb or fingertips to apply the pressure, in a standing or sitting position while bending the trunk forward. Apply the pressure during exhalation.

! Avoid pressure on Sp-15 and other abdominal points if the abdomen is very painful and hard in cases of severe constipation, inflammation of the abdomen or pregnancy.

Moxibustion
Cones: 5–15. Pole: 10–20 minutes. Rice-grain moxa is also applicable.

Magnets
Magnet therapy can be helpful. To tonify the Spleen and intestinal qi, use the south poles on Sp-15 bilaterally and the north pole on Ren-8 or Ren-6, or vice-versa. To loose inches around the waist, alternate poles on points level with the umbilicus, including St-25, Ren-8, GB-26, Bl-23 and Du-4.

Cupping
Cupping with light or medium suction or empty cupping can be employed. Use a medium or large cup size. Also, apply circular movements of the cups around Sp-15.

Actions and indications
Sp-15 is a very useful point for the treatment of many *disorders of the intestines and abdomen*. Its functions are similar to those of St-25 (the Alarm Mu point for the Large Intestine), although it is used more often in the treatment of *chronic deficiency conditions*, particularly *constipation*.

It has been extensively employed to treat a variety of *digestive disorders* including irritable bowel syndrome, flatulence, loose stools, chronic diarrhoea, dysentery, abdominal distension and lower abdominal pain due to weakness of the Spleen.

Sp-15 has also been used for an assortment of other symptoms and disorders, including weakness and heaviness of the limbs and body, chronic tiredness, heat or cold in the abdomen and depression.

Main Areas: Intestines. Abdomen.

Main Functions: Tonifies the Spleen.
Regulates the intestines and treats constipation.

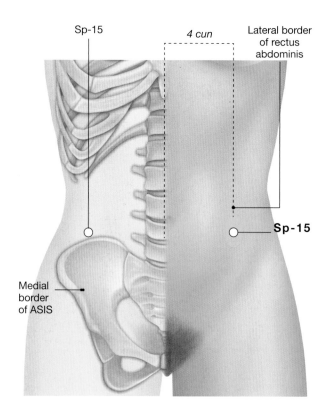

Sp-15   4 cun   Lateral border of rectus abdominis

Sp-15

Medial border of ASIS

Sp-16 Fuai
Abdominal Lament

Intersection of the Yin Wei Mai and Spleen

In the large depression directly below the costal arch, lateral to the margin of the rectus abdominis muscle. Approximately 4 cun lateral to the midline, 3 cun above Sp-15, level with Ren-11 and St-22.

Sp-16 is located slightly more medially, and/or inferiorly, in patients who have a narrow subcostal angle.

Note: Some classical texts place Sp-16 slightly further laterally, at a 4.5 cun distance from the midline.

Best treatment positions
Treatment is best applied in a supine position.

Needling
• 0.5 to 1.5 cun perpendicular insertion.

! Do not needle Sp-16 deeply in thin patients. This poses a considerable risk of puncturing the peritoneum and injuring the liver, spleen or colon, particularly if there is enlargement.

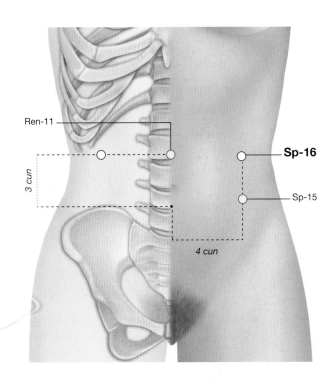

Manual techniques and shiatsu
Stationary pressure can be applied under the costal arch reasonably deeply with the fingertips or thumbs. Also, friction along the inferior border of the costal arch is applicable.

Self-acupressure can also be applied with the thumbs or fingertips, under the ribs in a standing or sitting position while bending the trunk forward.

! Sp-16 can be tender and should always be approached carefully. Avoid pressure on Sp-16 (and other abdominal points) if the abdomen is very painful and hard in cases of severe constipation or inflammation of the abdomen.

Moxibustion
Cones: 3–10. Pole: 5–20 minutes.

Cupping and magnets
Small or medium sized cups can be used with light or light-medium suction. Also, stick-on magnets can be effective.

Stimulation sensation
Localised distension, aching and warmth extending around the location and possibly upwards under the ribs and across the epigastrium, intestines or down across the abdomen.

Actions and indications
Sp-16 has been traditionally employed in the treatment of digestive disorders, caused by *disharmony of the Spleen and Large Intestine*. Symptoms include indigestion, abdominal distension and pain, periumbilical pain, abdominal rumbling, diarrhoea, dysentery and constipation.

Main Areas: Hypochondrium. Abdomen.

Main Functions: Harmonises the Spleen and Large Intestine.

Sp-17   Shidou
Food Cavity

食竇

Approximately 6 cun lateral to the anterior midline, three intercostal spaces below Sp-20, lateral to the mammary glands.

To aid location, it is level with the sixth rib or ICS, depending on the individual structure of the rib cage. Most acupuncture texts describe the location of Sp-17 in the fifth intercostal space, which is misleading because it is the sixth, not the fifth, that is situated here. The possible reasons for this discrepancy are discussed in detail in the section on Lu-1.

Best treatment positions
Similar to Sp-20, and P-1.

Needling
• 0.4 to 1 cun transverse insertion, laterally along the intercostal space.
• For disorders of the breast, needle under the glands medially toward the nipple 0.5 to 1.5 cun.

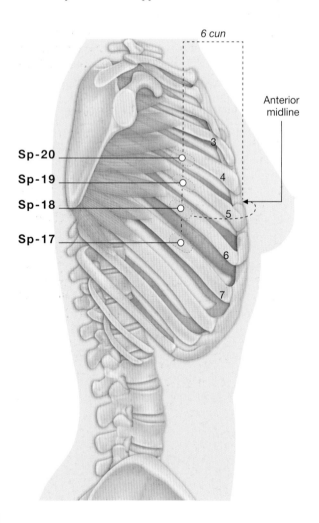

! Do not puncture the thoracoepigastric vein, or the mammary glands.

!! Do not needle deeply as this poses a considerable risk of puncturing the lung and inducing a pneumothorax.

Moxibustion
Pole: 5–15 minutes. Light stimulation only. Direct moxibustion is not recommended.

Actions and indications
Sp-17 was traditionally considered an important point to treat a variety of ailments, including postpartum abdominal distension, insufficient lactation, ascites, jaundice, malaria and urinary retention.

Its indications emphasise *digestive disorders* and *food retention* caused by *dysfunction of the Spleen*. Symptoms include indigestion, nausea, vomiting, inability to eat, fullness of the chest and abdomen, heartburn, difficulty swallowing and stomach ache. Additionally, moxibustion at this location was considered to *cure life-threatening conditions*.

In the modern-day practice, however, it is seldom used for these purposes and is mainly indicated for *disorders of the ribs and mammary glands* including rib pain, intercostal neuralgia, mastitis and fibrocystic breast disease.

> **Main Areas:** Chest. Ribs. Breast.
>
> **Main Function:** Regulates qi and Blood.

Sp-18   Tianxi
Celestial Cleft

天谿

Approximately 2 cun lateral to the nipple, two intercostal spaces below Sp-20, lateral to the mammary glands.

To aid location, it is approximately level with the nipple. Depending on the size and shape of the mammary glands, Sp-18 may have to be located further laterally.

Most acupuncture texts describe the location of Sp-18 in the fourth intercostal space, which is misleading because it is the fifth, not the fourth, that is situated here. The possible reasons for this discrepancy are discussed in detail in the section on Lu-1.

Best treatment positions

Similar to Sp-20 and other adjacent points.

Needling

• 0.4 to 1 cun transverse insertion laterally, following the contour of the rib cage.

For breast pain and fibrocystic breast disease needle medially under the mammary glands toward the nipple 0.5 to 1.5 cun.

! Do not needle into the mammary glands. Do not puncture the thoracoepigastric vein.

!! Do not needle deeply as this poses a considerable risk of puncturing the lung.

Actions and indications

Sp-18 is not very commonly employed, although it can be useful in the treatment of *disorders of the breast, ribs and thoracic cage*. It helps stimulate lactation and treats tightness, pain and constriction of the chest.

> **Main Areas:** Chest. Ribs. Breast.
>
> **Main Function:** Regulates qi and Blood.

Sp-19   Xiongxiang   胸鄉
Chest Village

Lateral and superior to the nipple, one intercostal spaces below Sp-20, lateral to the mammary glands.

Treatment and applications

Similar to Sp-18 and Sp-20.

Sp-20   Zhourong   周榮
Complete Nourishment

On the chest, one intercostal space below Lu-1, approximately 6 cun lateral to the anterior midline.

To aid location, it is inferior to the insertion of the pectoralis minor muscle, depending on the individual structure of the thoracic cage.

Most acupuncture texts describe the location of Sp-20 in the second intercostal space, which is misleading because it is the third, not the second, that is situated here. The possible reasons for this discrepancy are discussed in detail in the section on Lu-1.

Best treatment positions

Sp-20 is best treated with the patient lying in supine.

See also Lu-1.

Needling

• 0.4 to 1 cun oblique or transverse insertion laterally, following the contour of the rib cage.

! Do not puncture the lateral cutaneous branches of the third intercostal artery, vein or nerve medially, or the muscular branch of the long thoracic nerve or the lateral thoracic artery and vein.

!! Do not needle deeply as this poses a considerable risk of puncturing the lung. Do not puncture lymph nodes. See also cautionary note for Lu-1.

Manual techniques and shiatsu

Perpendicular pressure and friction techniques are applicable to the intercostal space with the tips of the fingers or thumbs. Deep friction of the pectoralis major and intercostal muscles can be effective to unbind the chest. See also Lu-1.

! Do not apply strong pressure to the rib cage.

Moxibustion

Pole: 5–15 minutes. Light stimulation only.

! Although direct moxibustion is not traditionally contraindicated, it is not recommended in this area and should never be used on, or close to, mammary glands.

Actions and indications

Sp-20 is not a very commonly used point, although it can be useful to treat *disorders of the chest and ribs* including intercostal neuralgia, lymphadenopathy, swelling and pain of the breasts, dyspnoea, cough and lung diseases.

> **Main Areas:** Chest. Ribs. Breast.
>
> **Main Function:** Regulates qi and Blood.

Sp-21 Dabao

大包

Great Embrace

Great Connecting *Luo* point of the Spleen

On the mid-axillary line, midway between the centre of the axilla and the lower border of the eleventh rib. Sp-21 usually falls in the seventh intercostal space, but in some cases it may be in the sixth.

To aid location, it is approximately one hand's width below the axilla.

Best treatment positions
This location can be treated unilaterally with the patient in a side-lying position or bilaterally with the patient lying down supine or sitting up.

Needling
• 0.3 to 0.5 cun oblique insertion laterally, following the contour of the thorax.

! Do not needle deeply. This poses a considerable risk of puncturing the lung and inducing a pneumothorax.

Manual techniques and shiatsu
Perpendicular pressure and friction techniques are applicable to the intercostal space with the tips of the fingers or thumbs. Deep friction of the intercostal muscles is effective to unbind the chest.

A useful technique is to apply superficial rubbing over this location with the palms, until the heat is felt extending outwards.

Also, pressure can be applied with the palms on exhalation so as to compress the rib cage and expel more air from the lungs. This technique can be employed unilaterally in a side-lying position or bilaterally with the patient lying down supine or sitting up.

! This location can be quite sensitive or tender. Do not apply strong pressure to the rib cage.

Moxibustion
Cones: 3–10. Pole: 5–15 minutes. Moxibustion is very effective to treat pain and circulation disorders.

Cupping
Light or medium cupping can be effective at Sp-21 and surrounding area. Apply ample skin lubricant and use a medium sized cup.

Magnets
Stick-on magnets can also be useful.

Actions and indications
Sp-21 is not a very commonly used point, although it can be very effective to *invigorate Blood* and *dispel stasis* and is specifically indicated to *treat pain of any cause or location.*

It is indicated for a variety of *disorders of the chest, Heart, Lungs and Spleen.* It has been widely employed to treat such cases as thoracic fullness, tightness and pain, intercostal neuralgia, rib pain, coughing, dyspnoea, circulation disorders, exhaustion, cold body and limbs, shivering, pain or flaccidity of the joints and weakness of the limbs and body.

> **Main Areas:** Ribs. Thorax. Breast.
>
> **Main Functions:** Invigorates Blood and dispels stasis. Warms the body.

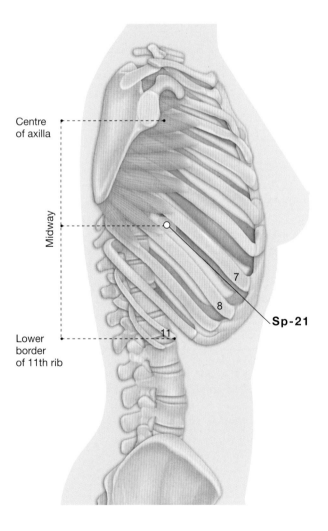

Centre of axilla

Midway

Lower border of 11th rib

7

8

11

Sp-21

Chapter 14

Points of the

Arm Shao Yin
Heart Channel

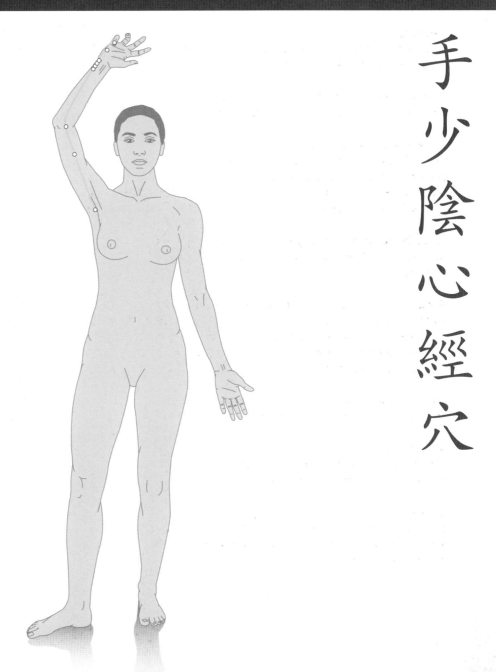

手少陰心經穴

He-1   Jiquan

極泉

Highest Spring

At the centre of the axilla, medial to the axillary artery. Locate and treat with the arm lifted above the head.

To aid location palpate the lateral inferior border of the pectoralis major muscle.

! This location is very sensitive and all forms of treatment should be applied carefully.

Best treatment positions

He-1 is usually treated with the patient in a supine posture, although manual techniques can be applied in a side-lying or sitting position, with the arm raised above the head.

Needling

• 0.5 to 1 cun perpendicular insertion.
• 0.5 to 1.5 cun perpendicular oblique insertion directed toward GB-21.

!! Do not puncture any of the numerous axillary vessels.

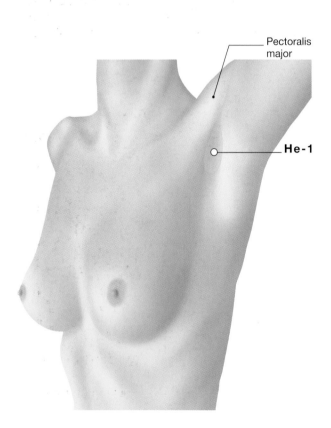

Pectoralis major

He-1

Manual techniques and shiatsu

Carefully applied sustained perpendicular shiatsu pressure is the most effective technique for this location and is best applied with the palms. The patient should be in a supine position with the arm lifted above the head. This is the most effective position to cool and calm the Heart and nourish the Yin.

Stretching open the axilla in a supine, side-lying or sitting position is effective for dispersing excessive heat from the Heart and removing Qi and Blood stasis from the shoulder joint. Stretching the axilla will also improve lymph circulation and ease swollen glands.

Another effective technique is to grasp the pectoralis major muscle with pressure applied to He-1 and Lu-1 simultaneously with the thumb and fingers. Cross-fibre stretching and friction can be effectively applied to the inferior lateral border of the pectoralis major muscle.

! This location can be particularly sensitive or 'ticklish', so it is important to apply pressure techniques very cautiously to begin with. Friction is not generally recommended. Also, using classic finger or thumb pressure may be too invasive. Do not apply pressure directly to the affected area in cases of inflamed glands or painful lumps.

Alternative acupressure location
Pressure can be applied directly to the axillary artery. Palpate deeply (carefully) to apply pressure to the nerves passing through the axilla. When a nerve is palpated there should be a tingling or electric sensation spreading along its course down the arm, possibly reaching the fingertips.

Moxibustion

Pole: 5–10 minutes with light or medium stimulation. Direct moxibustion is contraindicated at this location.

Stimulation sensation

Localised ache, tingling or numbness spreading into the axilla and chest, or down the arm. It can cause an electric sensation radiating down the entire arm toward the fingers, indicating the axillary nerves are being stimulated.

Actions and indications

Although He-1 *is a powerful point*, it is not very commonly employed in the modern day acupuncture practice, because needling the axilla can be awkward. However, the manual techniques described above can be applied much more easily.

He-1 can be effectively used to treat *disorders of the axilla, shoulder joint, heart and chest.*

Firstly, it treats *diseases of the axillary area* caused by *heat and fire in the Liver or Heart.* Symptoms include axillary pain, swelling or lumps, skin diseases, excessive sweating, inflammation of the sweat glands, intercostal neuralgia, lymphadenopathy and mastitis.

Secondly, He-1 affects the *mobility of the shoulder and arm* and is used in the treatment of frozen shoulder, inability to raise the arm, paralysis of the upper limb and cold pain of the arm and elbow.

Thirdly, it can be used for *diseases of the chest and Heart* caused by heat and fire or blood stasis causing symptoms such as fullness and pain of the chest, hypochondrial pain, mental agitation, arrhythmia and palpitations.

> **Main Areas:** Axilla. Shoulder. Chest. Heart.
> **Main Functions:** Clears heat. Regulates sweat. Regulates Heart qi.

He-3   Shaohai   少海

Lesser Sea

Uniting Sea-*He*, Water point

In the depression anterior to the medial epicondyle of the humerus near the medial end of the transverse cubital crease. Locate and treat with the elbow in flexion. Situated in the pronator teres muscle (superficially) and the brachialis muscle (deeper).

To aid location, it is approximately one finger-width diagonally anterior to the tip of the epicondyle.

Best treatment positions
With the patient in a supine position with the arm abducted and the elbow slightly flexed.

Needling
• 0.3 to 1 cun perpendicular insertion.

! Do not puncture the basilic vein or the medial brachial and medial antebrachial cutaneous nerves; more deeply, branches of the inferior ulnar collateral artery and vein, and inferiorly, the anterior branch of the ulnar recurrent artery. Furthermore, the median nerve and brachial artery are situated deeper and laterally.

Manual techniques and shiatsu
Sustained perpendicular pressure or gentle friction can be applied with the fingers and thumbs.

! This location is sensitive, so pressure should be applied carefully.

Moxibustion
Pole: 5–15 minutes. Light or medium stimulation only.

Although 3 to 5 cones are prescribed in many texts, direct moxibustion is not recommended. According to certain traditional sources, moxibustion is contraindicated.

Stimulation sensation
Local ache, distension, tingling, electricity or numbness spreading down the channel through the forearm toward the hand and fingers (particularly the fourth and fifth).

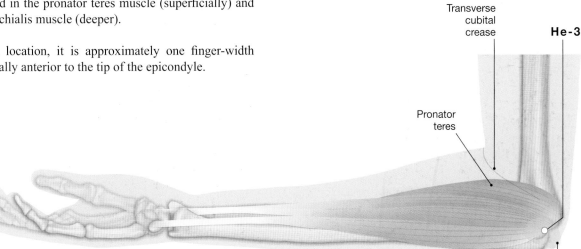

Transverse cubital crease

He-3

Pronator teres

Medial epicondyle

Actions and indications

He-3 is an important and widely used point to *clear both full and empty heat* and *transform phlegm* whilst having a *calming and soothing effect on the Heart and the mind.*

Indications include insomnia, mental agitation, depression, poor memory, psychological disturbances, madness, epilepsy, dizziness, chest pain, palpitations, lymphadenopathy, vomiting, toothache, headache and fevers.

As a *local point*, He-3 effectively treats pain and stiffness of the medial aspect of the elbow and forearm, tendinitis, golfer's elbow, weakness, trembling or numbness of the forearm and atrophy of the medial forearm muscles (flexors).

Main Areas: Elbow. Chest. Heart.

Main Functions: Clears heat. Transforms phlegm. Soothes the heart.

He-4 Lingdao

靈道

Spirit Path

River-*Jing*, Metal point

On the radial side of the tendon of flexor carpi ulnaris, 1.5 cun proximal to He-7 on the transverse wrist crease.

In the depression between the flexor carpi ulnaris and flexor digitorum superficialis. The pronator quadratus is situated in its deep position. To aid location, He-4 is level with Lu-7.

Best treatment positions
Similar to He-6 and He-7.

Needling
• 0.3 to 0.5 cun perpendicular insertion.
• 0.5 to 1 cun oblique insertion distally down the channel to join with He-5 or He-6.

! Do not puncture the cutaneous branches of the ulnar nerve or the medial antebrachial cutaneous nerve. More deeply, the ulnar artery, veins and nerve.

Actions and indications

He-4 is not as commonly used as other heart channel points; however it does have similar functions such as *calming the mind and regulating Heart qi.*

Treatment at He-4 is primarily employed in *channel disorders* of the forearm, wrist and elbow. It is particularly indicated for hypertonicity of the ulnar wrist flexors, stiffness of the wrist or elbow and contraction of the fingers. Although these therapeutic properties are also obtained from treating He-5, He-6 and He-7, He-4 may be more effective in such cases. Apply pressure palpation to determine which of these points is most reactive.

Main Areas: Forearm. Wrist. Heart.

Main Functions: Regulates qi and Blood. Alleviates pain. Calms the mind.

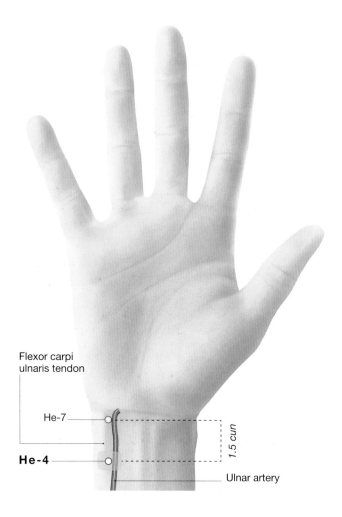

Flexor carpi ulnaris tendon

He-7

He-4

1.5 cun

Ulnar artery

He-5   Tongli   通里

Inward Connection

Connecting *Luo* point

On the radial side of the tendon of flexor carpi ulnaris, 1 cun proximal to He-7 on the transverse wrist crease.

Best treatment positions
Similar to He-7.

Needling
• 0.3 to 0.5 cun perpendicular insertion.
• 0.5 to 1 cun oblique insertion proximally along the channel to join with He-4, or distally to join with He-6 and He-7.

! Do not puncture the cutaneous branches of the ulnar nerve or the medial antebrachial cutaneous nerve; or more deeply, the ulnar artery, veins and nerve.

Actions and indications
He-5 is an important and widely used point to *regulate and tonify Heart Qi* and *calm the mind*.

Indications include palpitations or chest pain on exertion, spontaneous sweating, painful throat, mental tiredness, depression, dizziness, epilepsy, sadness, fright, shock and even hysteria or madness.

He-5 is extensively used in the treatment of *disorders of the tongue and speech* including paralysis or stiffness of the tongue, stuttering, aphasia and other speech difficulties.

Another traditional function of He-5 is to *clear heat and benefit the urinary system* and lower jiao via the relationship of the Heart with the Small Intestine and Uterus. Symptoms include dysuria, haematuria and excessive menstruation due to heat in the lower jiao.

Additionally, He-5 can be effectively treated for similar *channel disorders* to He-4 and He-7.

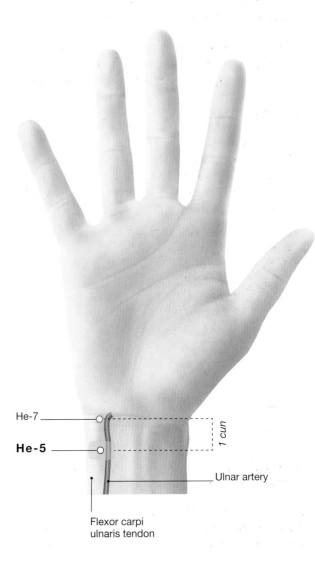

He-7 ——

He-5 ——

1 cun

—— Ulnar artery

Flexor carpi
ulnaris tendon

> **Main Areas:** Wrist. Heart. Tongue. Bladder.
>
> **Main Functions:** Regulates and tonifies Heart qi. Calms the mind. Benefits the tongue. Regulates speech.

He-6 Yinxi

陰郄

Yin Cleft

Accumulation Cleft-*Xi* point

On the radial side of the tendon of flexor carpi ulnaris, 0.5 cun proximal to He-7 on the transverse wrist crease.

Best treatment positions
Similar to He-7.

Needling
• 0.3 to 0.5 cun perpendicular insertion.
• 0.5 to 1 cun oblique insertion proximally along the channel to join with He-5 and/or He-4.
• 0.5 to 1 cun oblique insertion distally down the channel to He-7.

Alternative needling location
Insert the needle lateral to the tendon of flexor carpi ulnaris, so that it passes under the tendon sheath.

! Do not puncture the cutaneous branches of the ulnar nerve or the medial antebrachial cutaneous nerve; or more deeply, the ulnar artery, veins and nerve.

Actions and indications
He-6 is a *very important* and extensively used point because it effectively *clears heat and fire from the Heart and helps reduce excessive sweating and night sweating by securing the exterior*. Furthermore, it *cools Blood, nourishes Heart Yin and calms the mind*.

Indications include excessive sweating, particularly night sweating, steaming bone syndrome, pain or fullness of the chest, angina pectoris, palpitations, tachycardia, arrhythmia, insomnia, mental restlessness, agitation, dizziness, epistaxis, haemoptysis and sore throat.

He-6, He-4, He-5 and He-7 are all effective treatment sites for various *channel disorders and pain*. He-6 is particularly indicated for acute, stabbing pain along the channel pathway. Apply pressure palpation to determine which of these points is most reactive.

In cases of swelling of the wrist choose He-6, He-5 or He-4.

Main Areas: Exterior. Heart. Mind. Wrist.

Main Functions: Clears heat and fire. Calms the mind. Secures sweat.

He-7 Shenmen

神門

Spirit Gate

Source-*Yuan* point
Stream-*Shu*, Earth (Sedation) point

On the transverse wrist flexion crease, in the small depression proximal to the pisiform bone on the radial side of the tendon of flexor carpi ulnaris.

In the depression between the flexor carpi ulnaris and flexor digitorum superficialis. The pronator quadratus is situated in its deep position.

To aid location, He-7 is level with the proximal border of the pisiform bone when the wrist is flexed. This usually falls on the distal wrist flexion crease. Also, it is approximately level with Lu-9.

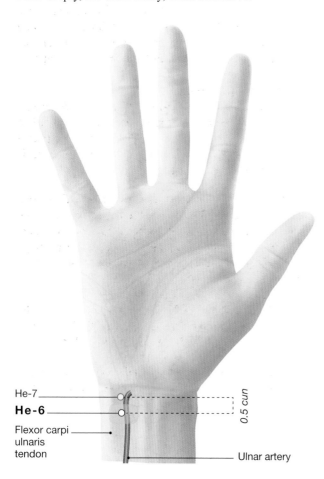

He-7
He-6
0.5 cun
Flexor carpi ulnaris tendon
Ulnar artery

Best treatment positions

He-4, He-5, He-6 and He-7 can be effectively treated in most positions, although supine is probably the most common. The hand and fingers should be relaxed during treatment. In cases where there is tightness of this area, the palm should be placed so that the wrist is in slight flexion.

Needling

- 0.3 to 0.5 cun perpendicular insertion, directed slightly toward the ulnar side so that the needle passes on the ulnar side of the ulnar artery, vein and nerve.
- 0.5 to 1 cun oblique insertion proximally up the channel to join with He-6 and/or He-5.
- 0.3 to 0.5 cun oblique insertion distally under the pisiform bone, directed toward its ulnar side.

If the surrounding soft tissues are very tight, or if there is substantial deformity of the wrist due to swelling, hypertonicity or other pathology, it is not possible to needle the standard He-7 location.

- 0.5 to 0.8 cun oblique insertion on the ulnar side of the flexor carpi ulnaris. The needle should pass under the tendon just proximal to the pisiform bone. Furthermore, He-7 can also be accessed by inserting the needle obliquely at He-6 or SI-5.

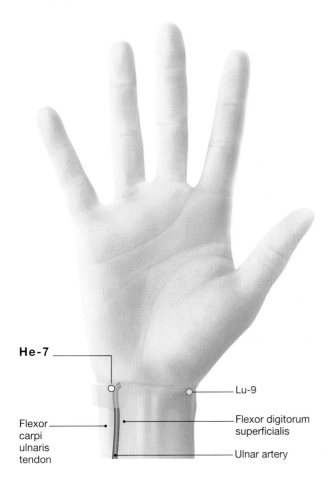

He-7

Flexor carpi ulnaris tendon

Lu-9

Flexor digitorum superficialis

Ulnar artery

! Do not puncture the cutaneous branches of the ulnar nerve or the medial antebrachial cutaneous nerve. More deeply, the ulnar artery, vein and nerve.

Manual techniques and shiatsu

Carefully applied sustained perpendicular pressure or gentle friction can be applied with the fingers and thumbs. An effective shiatsu technique is to press these four points simultaneously with the four fingers by squeezing with the thumb on the posterior aspect of the ulna. Another is to press into the depression of He-7 while simultaneously flexing and mobilising the wrist with the other hand.

Self-acupressure is very effective if applied regularly throughout the day and before sleeping.

Moxibustion

Cones: 1–3. Pole: 5–20 minutes. Rice-grain moxa is also effective. Light stimulation only.

Magnets

Stick-on magnets and specially designed bracelets that can stimulate these points may be used effectively to treat palpitations, angina, anxiety, insomnia, night sweats and other symptoms.

Stimulation sensation

Soreness or ache, tingling, electricity or numbness extending around the location and proximally or distally along the channel, through the wrist and hand toward the fingers (particularly to the third, fourth and fifth digit).

Actions and indications

He-7 is one of the *most commonly used and important points*. It is extensively employed to *calm the mind, reduce anxiety and regulate the Heart* and is primarily used in *deficiency conditions*, particularly if there is *depletion of Blood and Yin*.

Common indications include palpitations, tachycardia, arrhythmia, chest pain, angina pectoris, dull complexion, dizziness and psychological disorders including insomnia, anxiety, worry, stress, depression, panic attacks, stage fright, hysteria, tendency to laugh too much, poor memory and tiredness.

He-7 is also effective to treat *disorders of the wrist* such as pain, swelling and stiffness, ulnar flexor tendinitis, spasticity of the fingers and atrophy of the forearm.

Additionally, it has been traditionally used for a diversity of symptoms and conditions including heat in the five hearts, burning of the palms, spitting blood, swollen painful throat, dyspnoea, loss of voice, epilepsy, speech impairment, drooling, redness of the face, enuresis, dysuria and urinary tract infections.

He-7 is also effective to treat *disorders of the wrist* such as pain, swelling and stiffness, ulnar flexor tendinitis, spasticity of the fingers and atrophy of the forearm.

> **Main Areas:** Heart. Mind. Wrist.
>
> **Main Functions:** Calms the mind. Nourishes Heart Blood. Soothes the Heart. Clears heat.

He-8 Shaofu 少府

Lesser Mansion

Spring-*Ying*, Fire (Horary) point

On the palm, in the depression between the fourth and fifth metacarpal bones proximal to the distal transverse palmar crease (known as the "heart line"). The tip of the little finger touches this point when a fist is made.

Needling
• 0.3 to 0.5 cun perpendicular insertion.

This location can be very painful. It may be necessary to use a thicker needle if the palmar skin is hard and tight.

Although He-8 is a very important point, needling is mainly applied for channel disorders, and only if this is really necessary, because it is usually very painful.

! Do not puncture the palmar digital artery, vein or nerve.

Moxibustion
Cones: 3. Pole: 5–10 minutes. Rice-grain moxa can be effectively employed at He-7.

Manual techniques and shiatsu
Friction or sustained perpendicular pressure is applicable with the thumbs or fingertips.

Stimulation sensation
Aching, tingling or electricity giving way to numbness is perceived extending across the palm toward the fingers.

Actions and indications
He-8 is a useful point to treat excess conditions caused by heat and fire in the Heart. Symptoms include palpitations, tachycardia, sore swollen throat, thirst, fever, ulceration of the tongue, itching, dysuria, heat in the palms, convulsions, insomnia, mental agitation and even delirium.

In practice, however it is not commonly used for these complaints. Its sphere of action lies mainly in the treatment of channel disorders such as inflammation and pain of the fingers and palm, hypertonicity of the little finger and pain and stiffness of the forearm, arm and axilla.

> **Main Areas:** Heart. Mind. Excess conditions.
>
> **Main Functions:** Clears Heart fire. Cools and calms the heart. Benefits the palms.

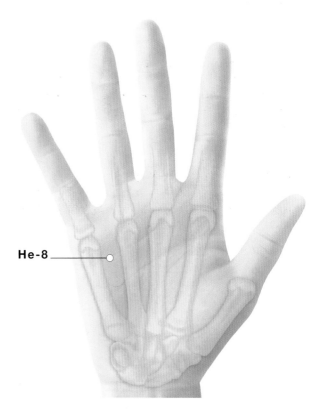

He-8

He-9   Shaochong

少衝

Lesser Surge

Well-*Jing*, Wood (Tonification) point

On the lateral (radial) side of the little finger, 0.1 cun proximal to the corner of the nail. At the intersection of two lines following the radial border of the nail and the base of the nail.

! Do not overstimulate in very deficient patients.

Best treatment positions
This point can be treated easily with the patient sitting or lying. A strong stimulation is most effective if applied regularly until symptoms subside.

Needling
• 0.1 cun perpendicular insertion. Prick to bleed.

Manual techniques and shiatsu
Dispersing type stimulation or sustained pressure may be applied with the tip of the finger or thumb.

Self-acupressure applied daily at this location is effective for chronic cardiac patients.

Moxibustion
Cone: 1. Pole: 3–10 minutes. Rice-grain moxa is also applicable.

First aid for syncope, shock, fainting or coma
If strong pressure with the fingers is not effective, use an object to tap the point (for example a pen or book). If tapping doesn't work, hit the point harder or prick to bleed.

Stimulation sensation
Similarly to the other Well-Jing points, He-9 is often painful, and strong stimulation here can engender a very powerful sensation reaching the chest. The breathing and pulse rate may change immediately.

Actions and indications
He-9 is a *powerful point to open the orifices, clear the mind, resuscitate consciousness, regulate Heart qi and clear heat.* Indications include arrhythmia, bradycardia, tachycardia, palpitations, angina pectoris, convulsions, throat pain and swelling, pain at the root of the tongue, fever, fainting, shock, coma, syncope, wind stroke and mental tiredness.

Main Areas: Mind. Heart. Chest.

Main Functions: Resuscitates consciousness. Regulates Heart qi.

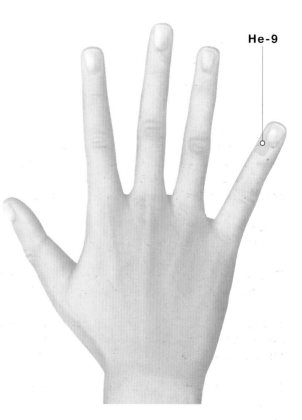

He-9

Chapter 15

Points of the

Arm Tai Yang
Small Intestine Channel

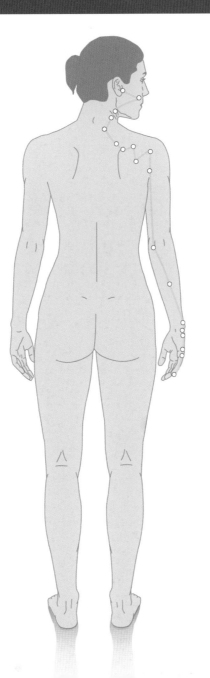

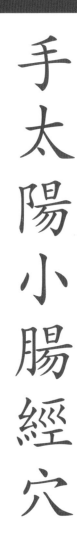

SI-1   Shaoze

Lesser Marsh

少澤

Well-*Jing*, Metal point

On the ulnar side of the little finger, about 0.1 cun proximal to the base of the nail, at the intersection of two lines following the ulnar border and the base of the nail.

Best treatment positions
Similar to the other Well-Jing points.

Moxibustion
Cones: 2–3. Pole: 5–10 minutes. Moxibustion is used to promote lactation. Rice-grain moxa is also effective.

Actions and indications
SI-1 is not very commonly used, although it has been traditionally employed to *release the exterior, clear wind and heat, calm the mind and restore consciousness.*

Another, important traditional use for this point is to *clear the chest, benefit the breasts and promote lactation.*

> **Main Areas:** Breast. Mind.
>
> **Main Functions:** Promotes lactation. Restores consciousness. Releases the exterior.

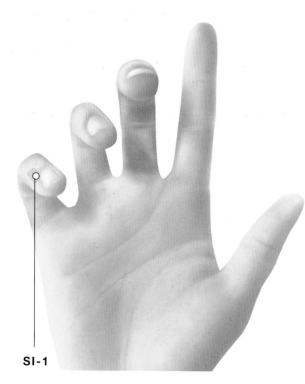

SI-1

SI-3   Houxi

Back Stream

後谿

Stream-*Shu*, Wood (Tonification) point
Opening (Master) point of the Du Mai

When a loose fist is formed, this point is found at the ulnar end of the distal transverse palmar crease in the depression between the flesh and bone, just proximal to the head of the fifth metacarpal bone.

To aid location, SI-3 is in the visible depression formed slightly proximal and dorsal to the skin fold.

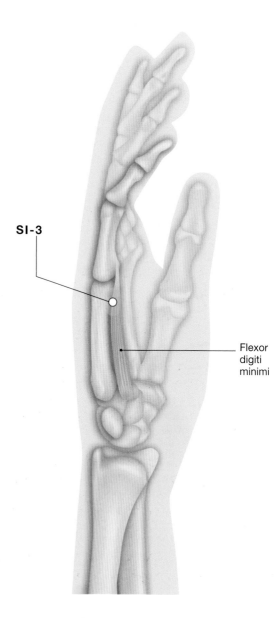

SI-3

Flexor digiti minimi

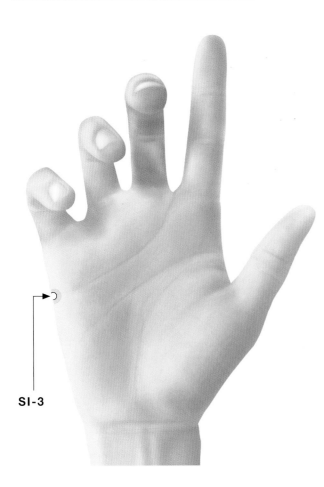

SI-3

Needling

Needle with the palm in a relaxed position so that the fingers are slightly flexed.

- 0.3 to 0.7 cun perpendicular insertion into the space between the bone and the hypothenar muscles.
- 1 to 2 cun insertion. The needle should be directed toward the centre of the palm in the direction of LI-3 or LI-4.

! When needling deeply, direct needle slightly dorsally to follow the contour of the palm, into the interosseous muscles, dorsal to the tendons of flexor digitorum, so as not to puncture the palmar vessels and nerves, lying anterior to, and between these tendons.

Manual techniques and shiatsu

Sustained perpendicular pressure is best applied into the space between the muscle and bone with the fingertip. Friction applied to the hypothenar muscles is also effective.

Additionally, opening the ulnar side of the palm by stretching the little finger toward the palm is beneficial.

Moxibustion

Cones: 1–3. Pole: 5–10 minutes. Rice-grain moxa is also effective.

Guasha

Guasha is applicable.

Magnets

Use opposite poles on SI-3 and Du-14 for pain and stiffness of the neck, and with Bl-62 (the coupled point for the Governing Vessel) to treat unilateral pain, stiffness or paralysis of the limbs or trunk.

Stimulation sensation

A sore, distending sensation should be achieved extending around the point and possibly throughout the hand. Deqi can also be achieved proximally along the channel.

Actions and indications

SI-3 is a very *important and widely used point* for a variety of disorders. Its primary function is to *regulate the yang qi*, whether it is excessive or deficient, and to *benefit the Du Mai*.

It is effective to *descend excessive yang, clear heat, calm the mind and benefit the neck, spine and sense organs*. However, SI-3 can also be used to *tonify and warm the Yang qi*. Furthermore, it *releases the exterior and dispels wind, cold and heat*.

Indications include pain and stiffness of the spine in general, particularly the neck, upper back and shoulders, lumbar pain, headache, occipital headache, chills and fever, tinnitus, inflammation of the eyes, migraine, dizziness, vertigo, spasms, convulsions, epilepsy, hypertension, palpitations, tachycardia, mental restlessness and insomnia.

As *a local point*, SI-3 can treat pain and stiffness of the wrist and fingers.

> **Main Areas:** Hand. Neck. Spine. Sense organs. Mind. Brain. Nervous system. Heart.
>
> **Main Functions:** Descends yang. Clears heat. Opens the Du Mai. Benefits the spine.

SI-4 Wangu 腕骨
Wrist Bone

SI-5 Yanggu 陽谷
Yang Valley

Source-*Yuan* point

On the ulnar border of the hand, in the depression between the base of the fifth metacarpal and the process of the triquetral bone. Locate with the hand in a loose fist.

In its deep position it is located between the triquetral and hamate bones.

Needling
Needle with the palm in a relaxed position so that the fingers are slightly flexed.

• 0.3 to 1 cun perpendicular insertion. The needle should be directed into the joint space between the process of the triquetral and the hamate bone.

! Do not puncture cutaneous dorsal veins of the hand, the posterior carpal artery or the dorsal branch of the ulnar nerve.

Manual techniques and shiatsu
Similar to SI-3. Another effective shiatsu technique applied to both the SI-4 and SI-5 locations, is to apply the pressure whilst simultaneously mobilising the hand in an ulnar direction. Also, stretching can be applied by radially flexing the palm.

Moxibustion
Cones: 1–3. Pole: 5–10 minutes. Rice-grain moxa can also be used.

Guasha
Guasha is applicable.

Magnets
Stick-on magnets can be used.

Actions and indications
SI-4 is an excellent point for *pain and stiffness of the fingers, wrist and forearm*, although it is not often employed for its traditional indications that include such diverse conditions as jaundice, cholecystitis, gastritis, diabetes, emaciation, tinnitus, toothache, sore throat, thirst and febrile diseases.

Main Areas: Wrist. Hand.

Main Function: Alleviates swelling and pain.

River-*Jing*, Fire (Horary) point

On the ulnar border of the wrist, in the depression of the wrist joint space between the ulna and the triquetral bone, slightly anterior to the styloid process of the ulna. On the transverse wrist crease formed when the wrist is flexed in an ulnar direction.

SI-5 can also be treated simultaneously to He-7. Additionally, He-7 can be accessed by needling the SI-5 location.

Best treatment positions
See SI-4.

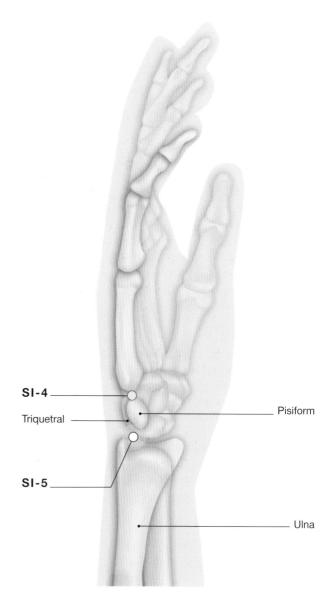

SI-4 — Pisiform
Triquetral
SI-5 — Ulna

Needling
- 0.3 to 1 cun perpendicular insertion. The needle should be directed into the joint space between the ulna and the triquetral bone.

! Do not puncture the posterior carpal artery or the dorsal branch of the ulnar nerve.

Actions and indications
Similar to SI-4. SI-5 is particularly effective for *problems of the wrist* such as stiffness, pain and arthritis.

However, it also *clears heat and calms the mind* and can be used in psychosomatic disturbances.

> **Main Areas:** Wrist. Hand.
>
> **Main Function:** Alleviates swelling and pain.

SI-6 Yanglao
Support the Aged

養老

Accumulation Cleft-*Xi* point

On the posterior aspect of the head of ulna, in the bony cleft appearing when the palm faces the chest, between the ulna and the tendon of extensor digiti minimi.

To aid location, place your index finger on the head of the ulna and slowly turn the palm toward the chest. The narrow cleft between the tendons of extensor digiti minimi and extensor carpi ulnaris becomes palpable on the head of the ulna. Extending the little finger and wrist defines these tendons.

Needling
- 0.3 to 0.5 cun perpendicular insertion into the small space between the ulna and tendon of extensor digitorum longus.
- 0.5 to 1.5 cun oblique proximal insertion.

! Do not puncture cutaneous vessels of the dorsal carpal network or the branches of the posterior antebrachial cutaneous nerve and the ulnar nerve, and more deeply, the posterior interosseous artery and vein.

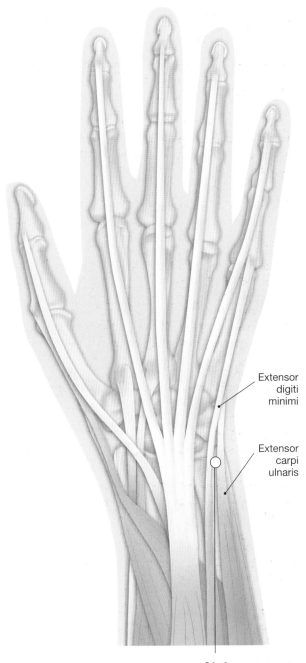

Extensor digiti minimi

Extensor carpi ulnaris

SI-6

Manual techniques and shiatsu
Sustained perpendicular pressure can be applied into the small space of the radio-ulnar joint with the fingertips or thumbs. Friction across the tendon of extensor carpi radialis and extensor digiti minimi can also be effective. Additionally, stretching of this area can be achieved by flexing the wrist and little finger.

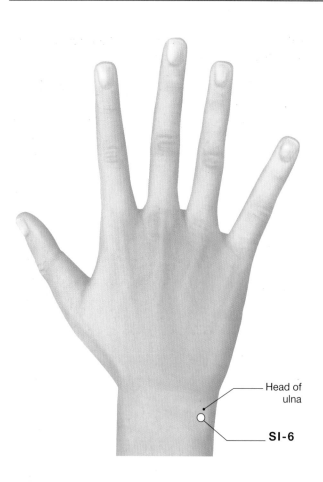

Head of
ulna

SI-6

Moxibustion

Cones: 1–3. Pole: 5–10 minutes. Rice-grain moxa is also very effective.

Stimulation sensation

A sore distending or electric sensation is often achieved extending around the point and proximally along the channel.

Actions and indications

SI-6 is a particularly effective point to *stop pain anywhere along the Small Intestine channel*, particularly the wrist, elbow and shoulder.

It has also been traditionally used to *increase vitality in the elderly* and alleviate symptoms such as lumbar pain, failing vision and deafness. Additionally, it has been employed to treat hernia pain, appendicitis and hemiplegia.

> **Main Areas:** Arm. Wrist. Shoulder.
>
> **Main Functions:** Regulates qi and Blood. Alleviates pain.

SI-8 Xiaohai

Small Sea

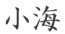

Uniting Sea-*He* point, Earth (Sedation) point

In the shallow depression of the flat area between the olecranon process of the ulna and the medial epicondyle of the humerus. Locate with the elbow flexed.

Needling

• 0.3 to 0.5 cun perpendicular insertion.
• 0.5 to 1 cun oblique distal insertion.

! Do not puncture the ulnar nerve.

Manual techniques and shiatsu

Sustained pressure is applicable with the fingers or thumbs. Friction can also be applied gently.

Moxibustion

Cones: 3–5. Pole: 5–15 minutes.

Actions and indications

SI-8 is an effective point for *disorders of the ulnar nerve, elbow, forearm and shoulder*.

> **Main Areas:** Elbow. Forearm.
>
> **Main Functions:** Regulates qi and Blood. Alleviates pain.

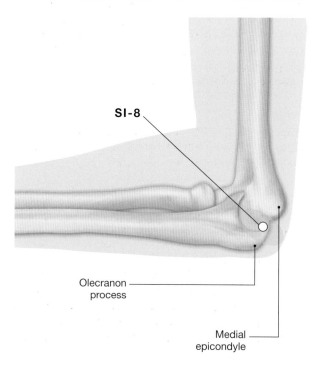

SI-8

Olecranon
process

Medial
epicondyle

SI-9   Jianzhen

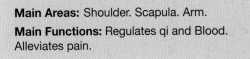

True Shoulder

On the posterior aspect of the shoulder in a depression below the posterior border of the deltoid muscle, approximately 1 cun above the superior end of the posterior axillary crease, when the is arm adducted.

Below the infraglenoid tubercle, in the teres major muscle.

Best treatment positions
Different positions can be used depending on the mode of treatment to be applied. Acupuncture is best with the patient lying down sideways or prone. However, manual techniques, moxa pole therapy and cupping can also be effectively applied sitting up.

Needling
• 0.5 to 1.5 cun perpendicular insertion.

! Do not puncture the cutaneous branches of the humeral circumflex vein or artery, the circumflex scapular artery and vein or the branch of the axillary nerve.

Manual techniques and shiatsu
Pressure is applied deep into the point with the arm in various positions (depending on flexibility of shoulder). Friction techniques can be applied across the fibres of teres major.

Furthermore, flexing the shoulder joint stretches open this location. Mobilisation techniques, combined with stretching the arm at various angles is most effective.

Moxibustion
Cones: 3–5. Pole: 5–20 minutes.

Cupping
Medium and small sized cups are used with medium or strong suction at SI-9, SI-10, SI-11, SI-12 and other regional points. Using cups with a curved rim is best.

Guasha
Effectively applied across the deltoid, teres major and teres minor muscles.

Actions and indications
SI-9, SI-10, SI-11 and SI-12 are all very *useful points for many disorders of the shoulder and arm*. They are primarily used to treat impaired mobility, difficulty in abducting and lifting the arm, frozen shoulder, atrophy, paralysis, pain and inflammatory conditions of the shoulder and arm.

Pain and stiffness should be reduced after treatment at SI-9, SI-10, SI-11, SI-12, and SI-13.

Main Areas: Shoulder. Scapula. Arm.

Main Functions: Regulates qi and Blood. Alleviates pain.

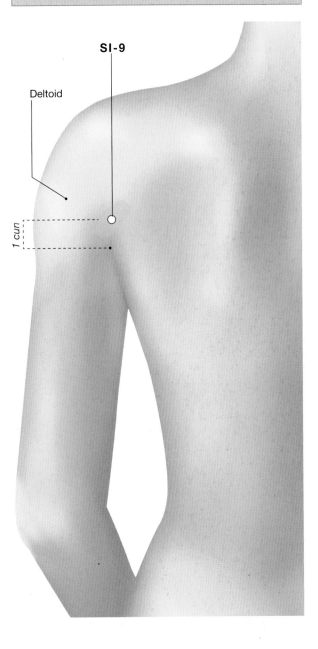

SI-10 Naoshu 臑俞

Upper Arm Shu Point

Intersection of the Yang Wei Mai and Yang Qiao Mai on the Small Intestine channel

Directly above SI-9 in the depression directly below the scapular spine. In the posterior portion of the deltoid muscle and in its deep position, situated in the infraspinatus.

To aid location, a visible depression appears when the arm is raised above the head (abducted).

Best treatment positions
Similar to SI-9 and SI-11.

Needling
• 0.5 to 1.5 cun perpendicular insertion angled slightly downward.

! Do not puncture the posterior circumflex humeral artery and vein or more deeply, the suprascapular artery, vein or nerve and the axillary nerve.

Actions and indications
Similar to SI-9. Additionally, SI-10 has an effect on the *axillary lymph glands* and helps *reduce swelling.*

> **Main Areas:** Shoulder. Scapula. Arm.
>
> **Main Functions:** Regulates qi and Blood. Alleviates pain.

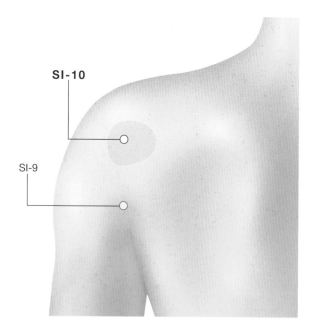

SI-11 Tianzong 天宗

Heavenly Gathering

At the centre of the scapula. Midway between its medial and lateral border, one-third of the distance along the line joining the midpoint of the lower border of the scapular spine to the inferior angle of scapula.

To aid location, create an equilateral triangle between SI-9, SI-10 and SI-11. In practice, SI-11 is best located by applying pressure palpation, to determine the most tender spot in the region of the centre of the scapula.

Best treatment positions
Similar to SI-9, SI-10 and SI-12.

Needling
• 0.5 to 1.5 cun perpendicular or oblique insertion in various directions.

! Do not puncture branches of the circumflex scapular artery and vein or the suprascapular nerve.

Manual techniques and shiatsu
Mobilisation techniques, combined with stretching the shoulder at various angles to release stagnation, is most effective applied together with sustained pressure and/or friction.

Moxibustion and cupping
Moxibustion and cupping treatment is very successful in the treatment of frozen shoulder and stiffness due to cold and stasis of Blood.

! Do not apply moxibustion if there is acute inflammation of the shoulder joint capsule. Cups, however, can be applied to clear the heat caused by the inflammation.

Guasha
Guasha can be very effective for stiffness, pain and other disorders of the shoulder.

Magnets
Magnet therapy can also be beneficial. Use opposite poles on SI-11 and surrounding ashi points on the infraspinatus, or on SI-10, SI-12 and other adjacent points.

Actions and indications
Similar to SI-9 and SI-10. SI-11 is probably the most commonly used of these points having a *very powerful relaxing effect on the entire shoulder.*

SI-11 also has a *calming effect on the digestive system*, particularly the stomach, oesophagus, intestine, liver and gallbladder when there are symptoms such as indigestion, acid reflux, abdominal pain, irritable bowel, diarrhoea, dysphagia and hypochondrial pain.

Additionally, it can be used for complaints of the breasts such as pain and insufficient lactation. It has also been traditionally used for breathing difficulty and coughing.

> **Main Areas:** Shoulder. Scapula. Arm. Chest.
>
> **Main Functions:** Regulates qi and Blood. Alleviates pain. Relaxes the chest.

SI-12   Bingfeng

Grasping the Wind

Intersection of the Gallbladder, Sanjiao and Large Intestine on the Small Intestine channel

At the centre of the suprascapular fossa, directly above SI-11.

To aid location, a visible depression is formed at SI-12 when the arm is abducted.

Best treatment positions
Similar to SI-9, SI-10 and SI-11.

Needling
- 0.5 to 1 cun oblique insertion, medially along supraspinal fossa toward SI-13.
- 0.3 to 1 cun perpendicular insertion into the belly of the supraspinatus muscle, in a slightly posterior direction.

! Do not puncture the suprascapular nerve, artery or vein.

!! Do not needle deeply in an anterior direction, because of danger of puncturing the lung apex.

Actions and indications
Similar to SI-9, SI-10, SI-11, SI-13 and SI-14.

> **Main Areas:** Scapula. Supraspinatus.
>
> **Main Functions:** Regulates qi and Blood. Alleviates pain.

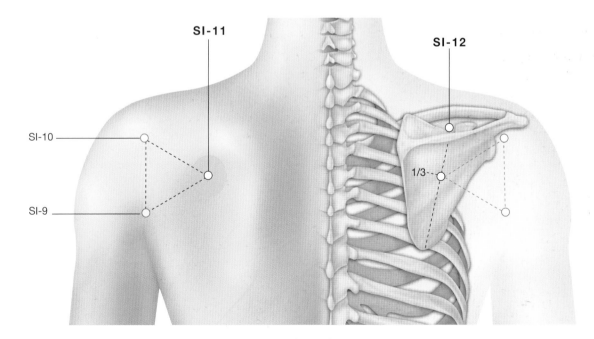

SI-13   Quyuan

Crooked Wall

曲垣

SI-14   Jianwaishu

Outer Shoulder Point

肩外俞

At the medial end of the suprascapular fossa, in the trapezius muscle, and deeper, the supraspinatus.

To aid location, it is approximately midway between SI-10 and the spinous process of T2.

Treatment and applications
Similar to SI-9, SI-10, SI-11, SI-12 and SI-14.

3 cun lateral to the lower border of the spinous process of the first thoracic vertebra (Du-13) on the line of the medial border of scapula.

Situated in the trapezius and serratus posterior superior. In its deep position lies the iliocostalis muscle and the levator scapulae insertion.

Best treatment positions
Manual techniques, cupping and moxibustion should be applied until an aching or distending sensation extending throughout the surrounding area is perceived. Pain and stiffness should be diminished after the treatment, which is best applied in a sitting or side position (see also SI-9, SI-10, SI-11, SI-12).

Needling
• 0.3 to 0.5 cun perpendicular insertion.
• 0.5 to 1 cun oblique medial insertion.

! Do not puncture the medial cutaneous branches of the posterior rami of the first and second thoracic nerves, the accessory nerve and deeper the dorsal scapular nerve and the transverse cervical artery and vein.

!! Do not needle deeply at a perpendicular angle. This holds a considerable risk of puncturing the lung.

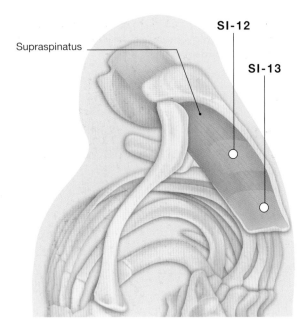

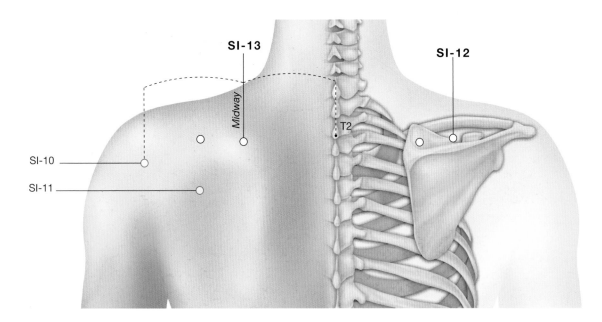

Actions and indications

SI-13 and SI-14 have similar actions to the other surrounding Small Intestine points. They effectively improve the flow of qi and Blood and stop pain in the shoulder and arm, upper back and neck.

SI-14 can also be used as a levator scapulae muscle trigger point.

> **Main Areas:** Shoulder. Neck. Levator scapulae.
>
> **Main Functions:** Regulates qi and Blood. Alleviates pain.

SI-15   Jianzhongshu   肩中俞

Middle Shoulder Point

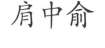

2 cun lateral to the lower border of C7 (Du-14), approximately at the end of the transverse process of T1. Situated in the trapezius and levator scapulae muscles.

Best treatment positions

Similar to Bl-11 and adjacent Small Intestine points.

Needling

• 0.3 to 0.5 cun perpendicular insertion.
• 0.5 to 1 cun oblique insertion in medial direction.

! Do not puncture the transverse cervical artery or vein, the branches of the third and fourth cervical nerves, and, more deeply, the accessory nerve.

!! Do not needle deeply perpendicularly, to avoid puncturing the lung.

Actions and indications

SI-15 is primarily used to treat *disorders of the neck, shoulder, upper limb and lungs.*

Symptoms include stiffness of the neck, asthma, cough, chills and fever and absence of sweating in exterior diseases (see also SI-14).

> **Main Areas:** Neck. Shoulder. Chest.
>
> **Main Functions:** Regulates qi and Blood. Alleviates pain. Relaxes the chest.

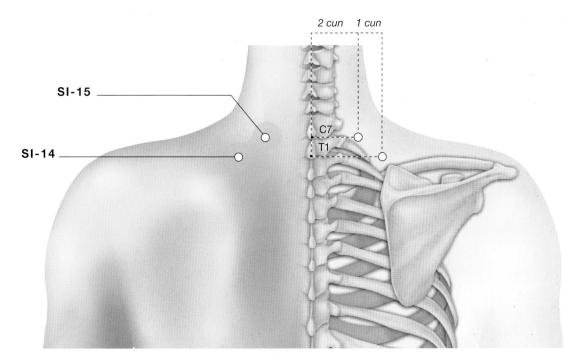

SI-17   Tianrong

Celestial Hood

天容

In the depression immediately posterior to the angle of mandible, at the anterior border of the sternocleidomastoid muscle, where the carotid pulse can be palpated. Situated at the inferior margin of the posterior belly of the digastric muscle (deeper) and deeper still, anterior to the carotid artery.

Define the sternocleidomastoid muscle by asking the person to turn their head away from the side to be palpated, whilst applying resistance to the chin.

Needling
• 0.5 to 1 cun perpendicular insertion toward the root of the tongue, anterior to the carotid vessels.

!! Do not needle deeply, because of danger of puncturing the numerous vessels located at this site: the anterior branch of the greater auricular nerve, the retromandibular and facial vein, the facial artery, the carotid artery, a cervical branch of the facial nerve, the vagus nerve and the superior cervical ganglion of the sympathetic trunk.

Manual techniques and shiatsu
Acupressure should be applied carefully with the fingertip into the space between the sternocleidomastoid and the angle of mandible. The digastric muscle can be palpated and pressed lightly in this space. Also apply the pressure in an anterior direction under the bone on the medial side of the mandible.

! Do not apply strong pressure.

Moxibustion
Cones: 3. Pole: 5–10 minutes. Rice-grain moxa is applicable.

Stimulation sensation
Often a sore, distending or electric sensation extends to the affected areas, particularly the throat and tongue.

Actions and indications
SI-17 is a *very effective point for disorders of the ear, cheek, throat and tongue* and is particularly indicated for pain or swelling and nodules in these areas.

Main Areas: Throat. Ears.

Main Functions: Regulates qi and Blood. Alleviates pain. Relieves swelling.

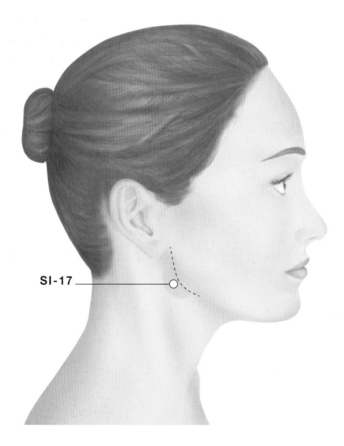

SI-17

SI-18   Quanliao   顴髎

Cheek Bone Hole

Intersection of the Small Intestine and Sanjiao channels

In the depression at the lower border of the zygomatic arch, directly below the outer canthus of the eye. Situated at the anterior border of the masseter muscle.

To aid location, SI-18 is approximately level with LI-20.

Needling
• 0.2 to 0.6 cun perpendicular insertion.
• Transverse or subcutaneous insertion in various directions. Medially toward the nose, laterally along the curve of the zygomatic arch toward St-7 and inferiorly or posteriorly toward St-6.

! Do not puncture the branches of the transverse facial artery and vein, the facial nerve, or the infraorbital nerve. Inferiorly the facial artery and vein and the buccal artery, vein and nerve. Laterally, the parotid duct and the accessory parotid gland.

Manual techniques and shiatsu
Gentle finger pressure or friction techniques can be applied to the zygomatic major (and minor) muscles perpendicularly or upward against the zygomatic crest. Deep friction is effective applied to the anterior margin of the masseter muscle, slightly lateral to this location.

Also, picking up, squeezing and rolling the zygomatic muscles and tapping applied with the fingertips can tonify flaccid cheeks giving a 'lifting' effect.

Moxibustion
Traditionally moxibustion is contraindicated at this location. However, gentle moxibustion with a moxa boat can help bring colour to a pale face and help certain dry skin conditions. Moxibustion is generally contraindicated in heat conditions. However, it can be employed to treat certain skin conditions caused by heat because it helps open the pores and release pathogenic heat and dampness. However it should not be used in cases of empty heat and red thread veins. Additionally, moxibustion can be employed in cases of *facial paralysis* caused by invasion of wind and cold.

Actions and indications
SI-18 is *effective for problems of the cheeks, eyes and teeth*, including facial paresis, trigeminal neuralgia, spasm of the cheek muscles and inflammatory conditions such as sinusitis, otitis, parotitis and swelling of the cheeks.

SI-18 *clears heat* and can be used for *aesthetic problems* of the skin such as redness, thread veins and acne. Applying manual techniques at this location, tens or electroacupuncture can help *tonify the zygomatic muscles, giving a face lifting effect.*

> **Main Areas:** Throat. Ears.
>
> **Main Functions:** Regulates qi and Blood. Alleviates pain. Relieves swelling.

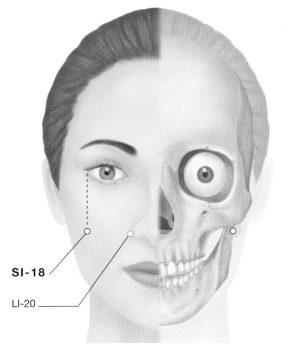

SI-18

LI-20

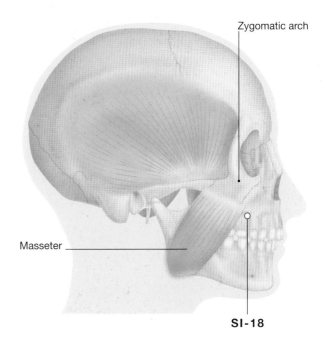

Zygomatic arch

Masseter

SI-18

SI-19　Tinggong

聽宮

Palace of Hearing

Intersection of the Sanjiao and Gallbladder on the Small Intestine channel

Anterior to the tip of the tragus in the depression formed when the mouth is opened, above GB-2 and below SJ-21.

To aid location, when the patient opens their mouth, the condyloid process of the mandible slides forward to reveal the depression.

Best treatment positions
Similar to GB-2.

SI-19 is often chosen instead of, or in addition to, GB-2 and SJ-21 and vice-versa. It is best to palpate these three points in order to ascertain which is most reactive.

Needling
• 0.5 to 1 cun perpendicular needling directed slightly posteriorly. Insert the needle with the patient's mouth open. After insertion, the patient can close the mouth.
• Join SJ-21, SI-19 and GB-2 (subcutaneous needling).

! Do not puncture the auriculotemporal nerve or the superficial temporal artery and vein and more deeply the facial nerve.

Manual techniques and shiatsu
For unilateral problems, apply simultaneous finger pressure to SI-19 and other adjacent points, such as GB-2 and SJ-21. Joining some or all of these points with qi projection techniques is most effective.

For bilateral complaints apply sustained perpendicular pressure to both sides. The patient can allow the jaw muscles to relax during the treatment so that the mouth will be slightly open.

! Administer the pressure very gradually, particularly if there is pain and inflammation. Excessive pressure can exacerbate pain.

Moxibustion
Pole: 5 to 15 minutes. Light or medium stimulation only. Direct moxibustion is not recommended.

! Neither overheat this area nor apply moxibustion if there is acute inflammation of the ear.

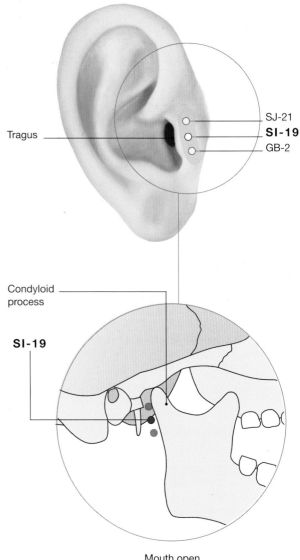

Mouth open

Magnets
Stick-on magnets can be very effective for pain and other disorders of the ears. Alternate poles on GB-2, SI-19 and SJ-21 or other adjacent points.

Actions and indications
Similar to GB-2. SI-19 is very effective for many problems of the ears including acute inflammation, tinnitus and deafness.

SI-19 is also traditionally considered to *calm the mind*.

Main Areas: Ears. Temple. Jaw.

Main Functions: Regulates qi and Blood and alleviates pain. Clears heat. Improves hearing.

Chapter 16

Points of the

Leg Tai Yang
Bladder Channel

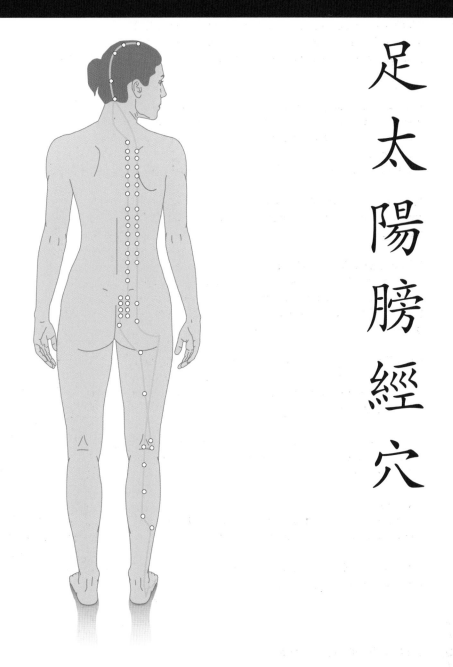

足
太
陽
膀
經
穴

BI-1   Jingming

睛明

Bright Eyes

Intersection of the Small Intestine, Stomach, Gallbladder, Sanjiao, Yin Qiao and Yang Qiao Mai on the Bladder channel

Approximately 0.1 cun medial and superior to the inner canthus of the eye. Locate and treat with the eyes closed.

Superior to the medial palpebral ligament. In its deep position situated in the medial rectus muscle and the superior oblique muscle.

To aid location, the best needling site is usually at the centre of the visible depression just above the inner canthus.

Best treatment positions
A supine position with head supported comfortably with pillows. Needling and pressure should be applied with the patient's eyes closed.

! Remove contact lenses before treatment.

!! This is one of the most sensitive and dangerous points. Great care should be taken in the application of all forms of treatment.

Needling
• 0.3 to 1 cun perpendicular insertion. Support the medial side of the eyeball with the index finger and push it laterally holding it gently but firmly. Insert the needle slowly with the other hand. Do not manipulate the needle.

!! Needling this location is potentially dangerous and requires special skill and experience. Great care should be taken as wrongly angled insertion can damage the eye.

Use the thinnest needle possible (gauges: 36–40 mm: 0.18–0.14).

The patient should keep the eyes as relaxed and still as possible during needle retention and avoid unnecessary blinking. It is best that the eyes remain closed for the duration of the treatment, until after the needle is removed, to avoid the skin being pulled.

Apply pressure with a cotton pad after removing the needle for up to one minute.

! Bl-1 can bruise easily. If any slight swelling is observed remove the needle immediately and apply pressure and a cold compress. If bruising occurs, apply the cold compress for 2 to 5 minutes. The patient can take an arnica homeopathic remedy of 30 ch or 200 ch, followed by 12 ch or 30 ch per day for a week (in some cases a higher potency may be given). The bruising should disappear within a week and will not affect the eyesight.

!! Do not puncture branches of the angular artery and vein; in its deep position, the branches of the supraorbital and the nasociliary nerve, the supratrochlear artery, the opthalmic artery and nerve, and the optic nerve.

Manual techniques and shiatsu
Stationary perpendicular pressure is best applied with the tip of the finger. In some cases, using the little finger is best. The pressure can be applied in three directions: (a) perpendicularly into the small space between the eyeball and the medial orbital margin, (b) medially onto the medial orbital margin, and (c) superiorly onto the superior orbital margin (trochlear fovea).

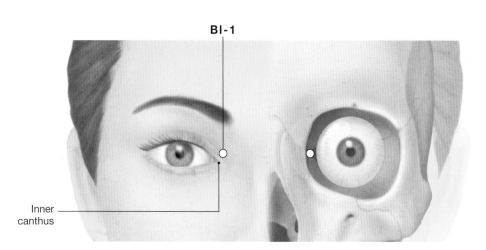

BI-1

Inner canthus

Gentle friction applied in very small circles can also be helpful. Additionally, gentle circular massage can be applied to a wider area, using a skin lubricant such as natural plant oil or specialised eye care product.

Self-acupressure can be applied daily in cases of chronic eye disorders, fatigue and to improve the appearance of the surrounding area.

! Ensure lubricants do not get into the eye.

Moxibustion
Contraindicated.

Actions and indications
Bl-1 is a *very important point*, used in a wide variety of eye disorders. Its primary functions are to *clear and brighten the eyes, dispel wind and heat, moisten and cool the eyes, nourish yin and improve vision.*

Symptoms include tired, dry, inflamed, sensitive eyes, itching or inflammation of the inner canthus, excessive lacrimation, chronic or acute eye pain, disorders of the optic nerve, poor or diminishing vision, blurred vision, colour blindness, night blindness, and diseases of the eye including conjunctivitis, keratitis, irregular refraction and iritis.

It is also a *major beauty point* and *helps improve the appearance of the surrounding skin.* It effectively treats dark circles, visible capillaries, bags and swollen eyelids.

> **Main Area:** Eyes.
>
> **Main Functions:** Clears and brightens the eyes. Improves vision. Dispels wind and clears heat. Alleviates pain. Nourishes yin.

Bl-2 Zanzhu
Gathered Bamboo

攢竹

Near the medial end of the eyebrow, in a small depression superior to the inner canthus and Bl-1.

The frontalis, orbicularis oculi and depressor supercilii muscles all converge at Bl-2. More deeply it is situated in the corrugator muscle.

To aid location, feel for the tender spot by palpating laterally from the medial end of the eyebrow.

Best treatment positions
A supine position is usually employed. Use appropriate cushion under the patient's head.

Needling
• 0.2 to 0.3 cun perpendicular or oblique insertion.
• 0.3 to 0.5 cun transverse insertion medially toward the base of the nose (nasion) or Yintang M-HN-3.
• 0.5 to 1 cun transverse insertion inferiorly toward Bl-1.
• 1 to 1.5 cun lateral transverse insertion toward Yuyao M-HN-6.

After removing the needle, apply pressure to the point with a cotton pad.

! Do not puncture the medial branch of the supraorbital nerve or the supratrochlear artery and vein. Bl-2 bruises easily if a lot of manipulation is applied. See note on first aid for bruising for Bl-1, opposite.

Manual techniques and shiatsu
Pressure and gentle friction is applicable with the tip of the fingers or thumbs.

Bl-2

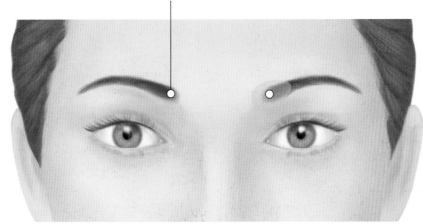

Deep pressure and friction of a tight corrugator muscle helps relieve tension from the area in between and surrounding the eyebrows and is useful to *improve appearance*. Furthermore, pinching and lifting the muscle mass at the medial end of the eyebrow is very effective.

A useful technique for *pain and headaches* is to apply perpendiclular pressure rhythmically in an outward direction along the entire eyebrow from Bl-2, through Yuyao M-HN-6, reaching SJ-23.

Moxibustion
Pole: 1–3 minutes, gentle stimulation. Use smokeless moxa only. Direct moxibustion is contraindicated.

Actions and indications
Bl-2 is a *major point for disorders of the eyes and forehead* because it *dispels wind, clears heat, regulates qi and Blood* and *alleviates pain*.

It has been extensively employed in such cases as frontal headache, migraine, sinusitis, facial paralysis, chronic or acute pain and other disorders of the eyes.

> **Main Areas:** Eyes. Forehead.
>
> **Main Functions:** Regulates qi and Blood. Alleviates pain. Dispels wind. Clears heat.

! Do not puncture the supratrochlear artery and vein, the supraorbital nerve or the frontal branch of the superficial temporal artery and vein.

Manual techniques and shiatsu
Perpendicular pressure and friction is applicable with the tips of the fingers or thumbs.

Moxibustion
Pole: 1–5 minutes, gentle stimulation. Use smokeless moxa only. Direct moxibustion is contraindicated.

Magnets
Magnets can be effectively employed to treat pain.

Actions and indications
Although Bl-3 is primarily used as a *local point*, to *dispel wind, clear the head and relieve stasis and pain*, it also has more internal functions including *clearing heat and calming the mind*. Indications include headache, sinusitis, epilepsy, dizziness, disorders of the eyes and facial paralysis.

> **Main Area:** Head.
>
> **Main Functions:** Dispels wind. Clears heat. Alleviates pain.

Bl-3   Meichong   眉衝
Eyebrow Ascension

Directly superior to Bl-2, 0.5 cun within the anterior hairline, level with Du-24 and Bl-4.

Needling
• 0.3 to 1 cun transverse posterior insertion.

Pick up the cutaneous tissue of the scalp and insert the needle under the epicranial aponeurosis parallel to the bone. If the scalp is very tight, this may be difficult, making perpendicular insertion 0.1 to 0.2 cun the only alternative. Because perpendicular needling is not as effective, either choose another point or apply moxibustion or manual techniques to loosen the area.

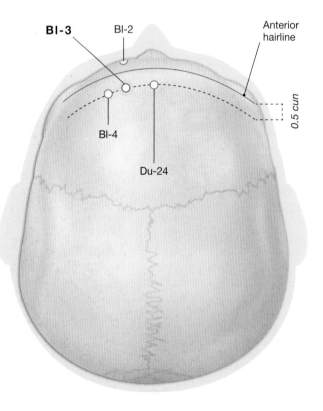

Bl-4   Quchai

曲差

Deviating Turn

1.5 cun lateral to the anterior midline, 0.5 cun within the anterior hairline, one third of the distance between Du-24 to St-8.

Treatment and applications
Similar to Bl-3.

Actions and indications
Bl-4 is primarily used as a *local point, to dispel wind, clear heat and alleviate pain.* It is particularly indicated for *disorders of the nose.*

Indications include headache, fever, sinusitis, rhinitis, nasal congestion, epistaxis, epilepsy, eye disorders and facial paralysis.

Main Areas: Nose. Head.

Main Functions: Dispels wind. Clears heat. Alleviates pain.

Bl-5   Wuchu

五處

Fifth Place

1 cun within the anterior hairline, 0.5 cun posterior to Bl-4. 1.5 cun lateral to Du-23.

Treatment and applications
Similar to Bl-3.

Actions and indications
Although Bl-5 is not a very commonly used point, it can help *clear the head, eyes* and *nose and dispel wind, descend rising yang and clear heat.*

Indications include headache, heavy feeling in the head, dizziness, epilepsy, poor or diminishing eyesight, painful eyes and nasal congestion.

Main Areas: Head. Eyes. Nose.

Main Functions: Dispels wind. Clears heat. Descends yang.

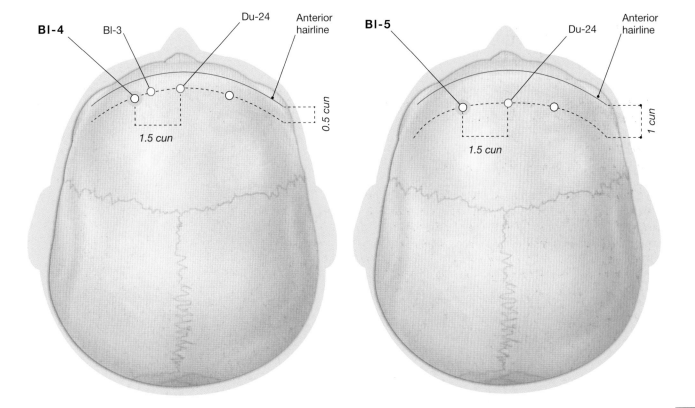

Bl-6 Chengguang 承光

Receiving Light

1.5 cun lateral to the midline, 2.5 cun within the anterior hairline, 1.5 cun posterior to Bl-5.

Treatment and applications
Similar to Bl-3.

Actions and indications
Similar to Bl-4 and Bl-5, Bl-6 also helps to *dispel wind and clear heat from the head* and *benefits the eyes and nose*.

> **Main Areas:** Head. Eyes. Nose.
>
> **Main Functions:** Dispels wind. Clears heat.

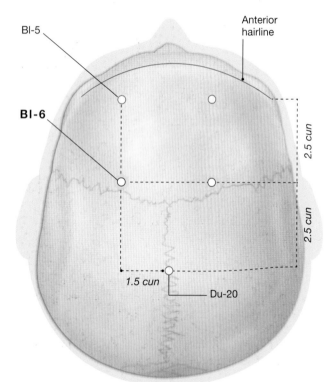

Bl-7 Tongtian 通天

Reaching Heaven

4 cun within the anterior hairline, 1.5 cun lateral to, and 1 cun anterior to Du-20, 1.5 cun posterior to Bl-6.

To aid location, it is at the intersection of the anterior and middle third of the distance between the anterior and posterior hairline.

Treatment and applications
Similar to Bl-3.

Actions and indications
Bl-7 is useful to treat *disorders of the head and nose*. It helps to *dispel wind* and *clear phlegm and heat*.

Indications include headache, dizziness, facial paralysis, loss of sense of smell, nasal congestion, soreness of the nose and epistaxis. For the latter symptoms it is often combined with Du-23.

> **Main Areas:** Head. Nose.
>
> **Main Functions:** Dispels wind. Clears heat.

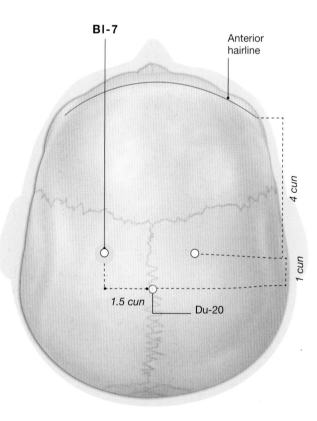

Bl-8 Luoque 絡卻

Declining Connection

5.5 cun within the anterior hairline, 1.5 cun lateral to the midline, 1.5 cun posterior to Bl-7.

To aid location, BL-8 is 1.5 cun lateral and 0.5 cun posterior to Du-20.

Treatment and applications
Similar to Bl-3.

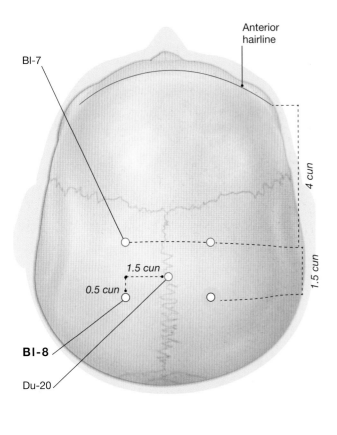

BL-7
Anterior hairline
4 cun
1.5 cun
1.5 cun
0.5 cun
Bl-8
Du-20

Main Areas: Head. Eyes. Nose.

Main Functions: Dispels wind. Clears the eyes.

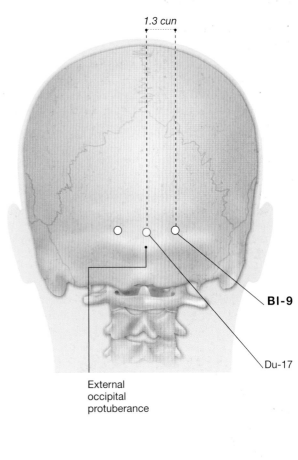

1.3 cun

Bl-9

Du-17

External occipital protuberance

Bl-9 Yuzhen 玉枕

Jade Pillow

1.3 cun lateral to Du-17, in a shallow depression above the superior nuchal line, approximately 2.5 cun within the posterior hairline.

To aid location, Du-17 is in the depression superior to the external occipital protuberance.

Treatment and applications
Similar to Bl-3.

Bl-10 Tianzhu 天柱

Celestial Pillar

Window of Heaven point

On the lateral part of the descending portion of the trapezius muscle, 0.5 cun within the posterior hairline, approximately 1.3 cun lateral to Du-15.

To aid location, Du-15 is directly superior to the spinous process of C2.

Best treatment positions
Needling and manual techniques can be applied with the patient lying down in the prone position, with the head suitably supported in an anatomically shaped cushion or couch. Furthermore, the patient can be lying supine (if there is a lot of tension in the neck, place the head in a slightly extended position).

Unilateral treatment is more effective with the patient lying sideways. Furthermore, this location can be treated with manual techniques and moxa pole therapy with the person sitting up, although needling in this posture can be dangerous.

Needling
• 0.5 to 1 cun perpendicular insertion.

! Do not puncture branches of the occipital artery and vein and deeper, the greater occipital nerve.

!! Do not needle deeply or in an upward direction because the spinal canal and medulla oblongata lies at a depth which may be as little as 2 cm in thin patients.

Manual techniques and shiatsu
Stationary pressure and friction is applicable with the finger and thumb tips. Apply the pressure in a slightly medial direction toward the spine, bilaterally or unilaterally. Squeeze the trapezius and semispinalis capitis muscle bellies by pressing Bl-10 bilaterally, or unilaterally by pressing Bl-10 and Du-15.

Cross-fibre stretching and deep friction of the trapezius and semispinalis capitis muscle is very effective for *chronic pain or stiffness of the neck* and *disorders of the head and sense organs*. Furthermore, the deeper muscles can also be accessed from the Bl-10 and GB-20 sites (the obliquus capitis inferior and superior and the rectus capitis posterior minor and major). Bend the head forward to open the Bl-10 area and stretch these muscles.

! Always apply pressure and stretching to the neck with caution.

Moxibustion
Pole: 5–15 minutes. Direct moxibustion is not recommended.

Guasha
Guasha can be successfully employed across or down the trapezius fibres.

Magnets
Stick-on magnets can be helpful. Use opposite poles on adjacent points such as GB-20, Du-15 and GB-21.

Stimulation sensation
Localised aching and distension, possibly extending down the neck toward the shoulders, or upward, toward the top of the head.

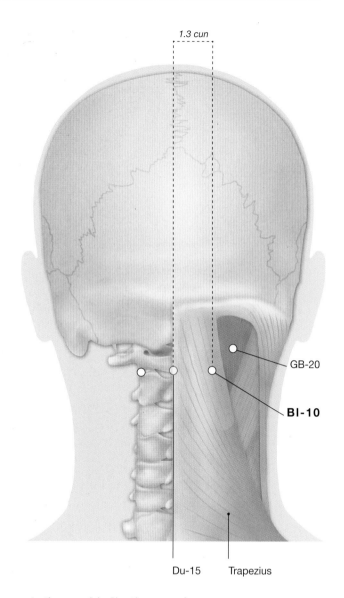

1.3 cun

GB-20

Bl-10

Du-15   Trapezius

Actions and indications
Bl-10 is a *very important point to treat the neck, upper back, head and entire Tai Yang area*. It is primarily used to *dispel wind and cold, regulate qi and Blood circulation,* and *alleviate pain*.

Indications include occipital headache, stiffness of the neck, pain of the body, sore throat, chills and fever, nasal congestion, pain and inflammation of the eyes, excessive lacrimation, blurred vision, epilepsy and dizziness.

Bl-10 helps *calm the mind* and *relax the body*, in common with other adjacent points such as GB-20. Bl-10 also *increases parasympathetic activity.*

Main Areas: Neck. Head. Tai Yang area.

Main Functions: Dispels wind and cold. Regulates qi and Blood. Calms the mind.

The Back Transporting Shu Points
BI-11 to BI-26

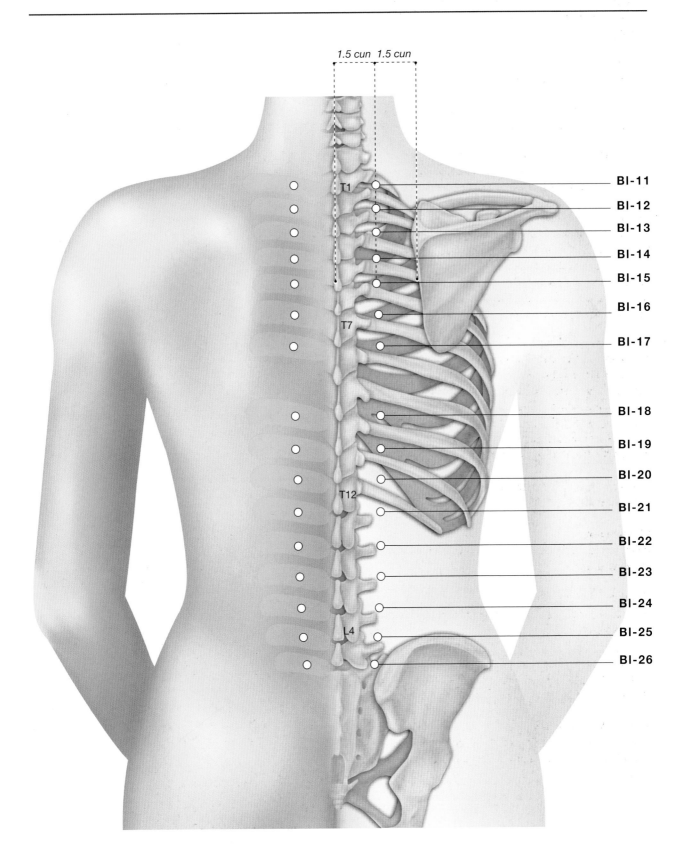

1.5 cun 1.5 cun

T1 — BI-11

BI-12

BI-13

BI-14

BI-15

BI-16

T7 — BI-17

BI-18

BI-19

BI-20

T12 — BI-21

BI-22

BI-23

BI-24

L4 — BI-25

BI-26

Bladder Channel Points of the Back

All the points on the *inner Bladder channel* are located at the highest part of the erector spinae muscle group (longissimus muscle), 1.5 cun lateral to the posterior midline.

To aid location, these points are usually at the top of the paraspinal muscles, in a depression where the fibres divide on pressure.

For the *thoracic points*, the 1.5 cun distance is measured midway between the posterior midline and medial border of the scapula. However, these points are slightly further lateral in the mid-thoracic area, which is often broader. Furthermore, they are usually found over the intercostal spaces, although sometimes they can be more reactive over the ribs.

For the *lower lumbar* and *sacral points*, the 1.5 cun distance is slightly narrower. For the sacral points, the 1.5 cun is measured from the medial border of the posterior superior iliac spine to the posterior midline.

Alternatively or additionally, the inner Bladder channel points may be relocated in the groove running next to the spine, 0.5 cun lateral to the posterior midline (coinciding to the Huatuojiaji points M-BW-35).

The *outer Bladder channel line points* are situated on the iliocostalis muscle, 3 cun lateral to the posterior midline, measured between the medial scapular border and the midline. All the outer Bladder points should be located in the intercostal spaces.

The back varies greatly from person to person, and cases of kyphosis, scoliosis and other variations of the spine must be taken into account.

To treat these points effectively, locate the most reactive sites by superficial and deep pressure palpation. Also, treat sites that are spontaneously tender.

Best treatment positions

A prone position is usually employed to treat points on the back. Use cushion support under the chest and abdomen as necessary. A side-lying posture can also be used to apply manual treatment, and in some cases, needling and other techniques.

Sitting on a stool or an appropriate bodywork chair, or kneeling, are also commonly employed postures for treating Bladder channel points with manual pressure, cupping, moxibustion and guasha. Needling, however, can be dangerous with the patient sitting up.

Furthermore, a 'child's pose' is useful for a variety of manual pressure and stretching techniques (ask the patient to kneel, and then lean the trunk forward; support the trunk with the arms or with cushions).

Needling

In general, the *thoracic points* are needled obliquely 0.4 to 1 cun (or slightly more in some cases) in a medial direction. However, the points on outer Bladder line should be needled slightly more superficially than those on the inner line.

Another common way to needle these points is at an oblique angle to a depth of 0.5 cun in an inferior direction.

Furthermore, points on the inner Bladder line can be needled to a depth of up to 0.5 cun perpendicularly, depending on body type.

!! Points on the back between T1 and L2 should not be needled deeply at a perpendicular angle, or in a lateral oblique direction. This poses a considerable risk of puncturing the lungs and other organs.

! If sharp pain is felt during the inhalation, remove the needles immediately.

The *lumbar points below L2* are needled perpendicularly to a depth of up to 1.5 cun, depending on individual build.

The *sacral points,* however, can be needled (up to 3 cun) deeper.

Manual techniques and shiatsu

Sustained perpendicular pressure and friction techniques are applicable with a variety of different 'tools', depending on the particular features of the area and desired therapeutic results. The thumbs, fingers, elbows, knees and feet can be used effectively.

In general, patients suffering from weakness and deficiency are best treated with gentle sustained finger pressure. Conversely, robust persons require a stronger pressure, which may be applied with the elbows, knees or feet.

Cross-fibre stretching and deep friction of the paraspinal muscles is one of the most important and widely used methods to *reduce tension and invigorate the circulation of qi and Blood.* Applying a combination of friction and sustained pressure onto the muscle spasms is most effective. The surrounding tissues should be noticeably softer after the treatment.

Furthermore, using essential oils with soothing and pain-relieving properties improves the results of the treatment. In addition, various stretching techniques can be employed to open the thoracic and lumbar areas and release tension from these points.

! Only light pressure should be used during pregnancy.

! Occasionally, the patient may feel slightly sore around the points that were treated, usually the following day. This is often unavoidable if the muscles were worked deeply. If this does occur, advise the person to drink a lot of water and do some stretching exercises for a couple of days. Also, having a hot bath may help. However, this reaction probably means that toxins were released into the muscles as a result of the treatment, and were subsequently not adequately flushed out of the tissues.

Next time, apply stretching to flush the muscles after the deep friction, or apply a lighter treatment. Stationary perpendicular pressure poses less risk of injuring the surrounding soft tissues.

!! Avoid strong pressure on the rib cage, especially in the elderly, those suffering from osteoporosis, heart disease or asthma. Ribs can be easily damaged, particularly the lower ribs and floating ribs.

Release sustained pressure slightly during the inhalation when working the lumbar area.

!! Avoid strong pressure on the lumbar area. Only apply the gentlest of pressure to the floating ribs.

Moxibustion
Moxibustion is an extremely important method of treatment for many of these points. Use 3 to 20 cones and indirect moxibustion for 5 to 30 minutes, depending on the specific point and desired result. Furthermore, burning cones on ginger or garlic is widely used on the Back-Shu points. The use of the moxa box on the lumbar area is also extremely beneficial.

Rice-grain moxibustion applied to selected Back-Shu points helps *regulate the qi of the pertaining organ*.

Cupping
Cupping is very useful to treat the Back-Shu points. Use a large or medium cup size. Suction varies from light to strong depending on the desired result.

Empty cupping can be used to *tonify the qi of any of the Zangfu*, separately, or before needling and moxibustion.

Stationary cupping over a particular point helps to *dissipate stagnation and clear heat from the pertaining organ*.

Moving cupping up and down the Bladder channel is *extremely effective to relax the muscles, improve circulation of qi and Blood, dispel stasis, clear heat and calm the body and mind*. Furthermore, it *releases the exterior, clears the Tai Yang, dispels wind and cold and clears interior and exterior heat*.

Needle or *moxa cupping* is also very beneficial in many cases.

! Warn the patient that the area may bruise.

Guasha
Guasha can be effectively applied across the paraspinal muscles in an outward direction, or upward and/or downward, parallel to the spine.

It is particularly useful in the upper back, neck and shoulders to help ease pain and dispel pathogenic factors such as wind and cold.

Magnets
Stick-on magnets and other forms of magnet therapy can be successfully employed to regulate the internal organs and treat spinal disorders. Alternate poles with adjacent and distal points.

For example, for spinal pain and Kidney deficiency, place the north pole on Du-4, the south pole on Bl-23 and the north pole on Kd-3 (or vice-versa). For dyspnoea and coughing, alternate poles between Bl-13, Dingchuan M-BW-1 and LI-4.

Stimulation sensation
The sensation achieved at these points varies depending on the particular point and the condition being treated. In general, it is common to achieve regional aching, soreness, heat or tingling, possibly extending across the back, or reaching the chest and abdomen. In some cases deqi may also extend to the limbs.

Best results seem to be achieved when the sensation reaches the affected organs and areas inside the thorax and abdomen. Furthermore, other reactions such as abdominal rumbling, sighing and changes in the breathing or heart rate and rhythm are indicative of deqi.

Bl-11   Dazhu   大杼
Great Shuttle

Gathering *Hui* point for the Bones
Sea of Blood point
Intersection of the Small Intestine, Sanjiao and Gallbladder on the Bladder channel

1.5 cun lateral to the lower border of the spinous process of T1.

To aid location, if the patient stands up with the arms hanging loosely by the sides, the medial angle of scapula (end of the supraspinal fossa) is approximately level with the spinous process of T3.

Treatment and applications
See pages 166–167.

Needling
• 0.4 to 1 cun oblique medial insertion.
• 0.5 cun oblique inferior insertion.

!! Do not needle deeply or at a different angle. This poses considerable risk of puncturing the lung.

Actions and indications
Bl-11 is the *Gathering Hui point for the Bones* and one of the *three points of the Sea of Blood*. It is useful in the treatment of *disorders of the bones and spine* and has been used to assist the *healing of bone* after fracture and to treat *bone diseases* due to *weakness of Jing and Blood*, including osteoporosis and kyphosis of the spine.

Bl-11 also *effectively releases the exterior, dispels wind and cold, regulates Lung Qi* and *alleviates cough*, in common with Bl-12 and Bl-13. Indications include chills and fever, aversion to cold, absence of sweating, headache, pain of the upper back and shoulders, stiffness and pain of the neck, sore throat, dyspnoea and cough.

Furthermore, Bl-11 is one of the *Eight (bilateral) Points to Clear Heat from the Chest* (together with Bl-12, Lu-1 and St-12) and is therefore considered an *important point to clear heat from the upper jiao.*

> **Main Areas:** Bones. Chest. Lungs.
>
> **Main Functions:** Releases the exterior. Regulates Lung qi and alleviates cough. Nourishes Blood. Benefits the Bones.

Bl-12   Fengmen   風門
Wind Gate

Intersection of the Du Mai on the Bladder

1.5 cun lateral to the lower border of the spinous process of T2.

Treatment and applications
Similar to Bl-11.

Actions and indications
In common with Bl-11 and Bl-13, Bl-12 is widely used in *exterior disorders to clear the Tai Yang area*, particularly at the *initial stage of wind cold invasion*. Additionally, Bl-12 is one of the *Eight (bilateral) Points to Clear Heat from the Chest* (together with Bl-11, Lu-1 and St-12) and is considered important to *clear heat from the upper jiao.*

Indications include chills and fever, aversion to cold, absence of sweating, headache, dizziness, stiffness and pain of the neck, shoulders and back, heaviness of the eyes, sneezing, runny or blocked nose, epistaxis, susceptibility to catching colds, sore throat, high fever, retching, haemoptysis, dyspnoea and cough.

> **Main Areas:** Lungs. Chest. Exterior.
>
> **Main Functions:** Dispels wind and cold. Regulates Lung qi.

Bl-13   Feishu   肺俞
Lung Shu Point

Back *Shu* point of the Lung

1.5 cun lateral to the lower border of the spinous process of T3. In the trapezius, rhomboid, and more deeply, the longissimus muscle.

To aid location, if the patient stands up with the arms hanging loosely by the sides, the medial angle of scapula (end of the supraspinal fossa) is approximately level with the spinous process of T3.

Treatment and applications
Similar to Bl-11.

Actions and indications

Bl-13 is the *Shu point for the Lungs* and is widely employed for both *interior and exterior Lung disorders*. It effectively *dispels wind and releases the exterior, transforms phlegm* and *descends rebellious Lung qi*. It also *tonifies Lung qi, cools and moistens the Lungs* and *nourishes yin*.

Indications include chronic or acute cough, productive or dry cough, chronic or acute respiratory diseases, asthma, fever, thirst, aversion to cold, chronic breathing difficulty, dyspnoea, shortness of breath, chest pain, chronic tiredness, spontaneous sweating, night sweating, low grade fever, steaming bone syndrome, haemoptysis, rhinitis, nasal discharge, nasal congestion, occipital headache and pain at the back of the head and neck.

As a *local point*, it has been successfully employed to treat kyphosis and pain of the upper back. Furthermore, Bl-13 helps *release stuck emotional states*, particularly grief and sadness.

> **Main Areas:** Lungs. Chest. Exterior.
>
> **Main Functions:** Tonifies and regulates Lung qi, Releases the exterior. Nourishes yin.

Bl-14   Jueyinshu

Absolute Yin Shu Point

Back *Shu* point of the Pericardium

1.5 cun lateral to the lower border of the spinous process of T4. In the trapezius, rhomboid, and more deeply, the longissimus muscle.

To aid location, if the patient stands up with the arms hanging loosely by the sides, the medial angle of scapula (end of the supraspinal fossa) is approximately level with the spinous process of T3.

Treatment and applications

Similar to Bl-11.

Actions and indications

Bl-14 is the *Shu point for the Pericardium*. It *regulates Heart* and *Liver qi* and is extensively used to treat thoracic oppression, pain and fullness, palpitations, mental agitation, dyspnoea, coughing, retching and vomiting.

As a *local point,* Bl-14 can be used for pain and stiffness of the upper back.

> **Main Areas:** Chest. Heart.
>
> **Main Functions:** Regulates chest qi. Benefits the Heart and Liver.

Bl-15   Xinshu

Heart Shu Point

Back *Shu* point of the Heart

1.5 cun lateral to the lower border of the spinous process of T5. In the trapezius, rhomboid, and more deeply, the longissimus muscle.

To aid location, if the patient stands up with the arms hanging loosely by the sides, the inferior angle of scapula is approximately level with the spinous process of T7.

Treatment and applications

Similar to Bl-11.

Actions and indications

Bl-15 is the *Shu point for the Heart* and is widely used to *nourish, cool* and *soothe the Heart,* and *calm the mind.* It is also important to *regulate chest qi* and *dispel stasis.*

Indications include palpitations, arrhythmia, tightness, oppression or pain of the chest, angina pectoris, circulation disorders, coughing, dyspnoea, haemoptysis, epistaxis, nasal congestion, pain of the eyes, retching and vomiting, epilepsy, windstroke, hemiplegia, fever, and heat in the palms and soles.

In addition, Bl-15 treats a *wide range of psychosomatic disturbances,* including poor memory, amnesia, depression, insomnia, mental restlessness, anxiety, grief, dream disturbed sleep, nightmares, aphasia, speech disorders, panic attacks, phobias and even madness. As a *local point,* Bl-15 can be used for pain and stiffness of the upper back.

> **Main Areas:** Chest. Heart.
>
> **Main Functions:** Regulates qi and Blood in the chest. Tonifies Heart qi. Calms the mind.

Bl-16 Dushu

督俞

Governor Vessel Shu Point

Back *Shu* point of the Du Mai

1.5 cun lateral to the lower border of the spinous process of T6.

To aid location, if the patient stands up with the arms hanging loosely by the sides, the inferior angle of scapula is approximately level with the spinous process of T7.

Treatment and applications
See pages 166–167.

Needling
• 0.4 to 1 cun oblique medial insertion.
• 0.5 cun oblique inferior insertion.

! In many cases the thoracolumbar fascia is very tight causing needling to be sharp or painful. In such cases, loosen the area first with massage or moxibustion.

!! Do not needle deeply or at a different angle. This poses considerable risk of puncturing the lung.

Actions and indications
Although Bl-16 is the *Shu point for the Du Mai*, it is not as commonly used as the other Back-Transporting Shu points. It can however be employed to help *regulate qi, dispel stasis* and *alleviate pain from the chest, abdomen and back*. Other indications include abdominal pain and distension, thoracic pain, and skin disorders including dryness, scaling and itching of the skin and alopecia.

> **Main Areas:** Chest. Abdomen. Spine. Skin.
>
> **Main Functions:** Regulates qi and Blood in the chest and abdomen. Dispels stasis and pain.

Bl-17 Geshu

膈俞

Diaphragm Shu Point

Back *Shu* point of the Diaphragm Meeting-*Hui* point of Blood

1.5 cun lateral to the lower border of the spinous process of T7.

To aid location, if the patient stands up with the arms hanging loosely by the sides, the inferior angle of scapula is approximately level with the spinous process of T7.

Treatment and applications
Similar to Bl-16.

Moxibustion is the treatment of choice *to nourish the Blood,* whereas needling and manual techniques are more effective *to cool and invigorate Blood.*

Actions and indications
Bl-17 is the *Shu point for the Diaphragm and the Gathering Hui point for Blood*. It is *very important and widely used for many Blood disorders*. Specifically, it is used to *invigorate Blood* and *dispel stasis* as well as to *cool blood* and *arrest bleeding*. Furthermore, it helps *nourish Blood* and is used in many *deficiency conditions*. Bl-17 and Bl-19 are also known as the *Four Flowers* and are indicated for steaming bone syndrome, fevers and to arrest bleeding.

Indications include fever with or without sweating, tidal fever, night sweating, thirst, anaemia, dry eyes, headache, dizziness, asthma, dyspnoea, heart pain, coughing, pain of the whole body including the skin and muscles, amenorrhoea, dysmenorrhoea, dry skin conditions, mental restlessness, depression, insomnia, tightness and oppression of the chest.

Bl-17 also effectively *benefits the diaphragm, harmonises the Stomach and descends rebellious qi*. Indications include abdominal pain and distension, spasm of the diaphragm, hiccup, difficulty swallowing, heartburn, retching, nausea and vomiting.

Bl-17 can also be very effective to treat *pain and stiffness of the spine and mid-upper back.*

> **Main Areas:** Diaphragm. Chest. Abdomen.
>
> **Main Functions:** Nourishes and invigorates Blood. Clears Blood heat. Relaxes the diaphragm. Benefits the skin.

Bl-18 Ganshu　　肝俞

Liver Shu Point

Back *Shu* point of the Liver

1.5 cun lateral to the lower border of the spinous process of T9.

Treatment and applications
Similar to Bl-16.

Actions and indications
Bl-18 is the *Shu point for the Liver* and is very important to *spread Liver qi, invigorate Blood* and *nourish yin and Blood*. Additionally, Bl-18 helps *clear heat and fire from the Liver and sedates interior wind*. It also *benefits the eyes, sinews and muscles*.

Indications include diminishing vision, chronic inflammation, pain or dryness of the eyes, glaucoma, excessive lacrimation, epilepsy, dizziness, hypertension, stiffness, tightness or cramping of the muscles, arthritis, pains in the spine and joints, tightness or pain of the chest and abdomen, shortness of breath, palpitations, hypochondrial pain and distension, jaundice, bitter taste in the mouth, nausea and vomiting, coughing or spitting blood, liver and gallbladder disease, painful palpable masses in the abdomen, enlargement of the liver or spleen, pain of the axilla, breast pain, irritability, insomnia, mental restlessness, mood swings, premenstrual syndrome, infertility, dysmenorrhoea, oligomenorrhoea and amenorrhoea.

> **Main Areas:** Liver. Hypochondrium. Abdomen. Eyes.
>
> **Main Functions:** Spreads Liver qi. Dispels stasis. Nourishes Blood. Clears heat and dampness. Benefits the eyes.

Bl-19 Danshu　　膽俞

Gallbladder Shu Point

Back *Shu* point of the Gallbladder

1.5 cun lateral to the lower border of the spinous process of T10.

Treatment and applications
Similar to Bl-16.

Actions and indications
Bl-19 is the *Shu point for the Gallbladder* and is useful to *clear dampness and heat from the Liver and Gallbladder* and *regulate Liver and Gallbladder qi*. It is useful in disorders of the gallbladder and liver including jaundice, cholecystitis and hepatitis.

Additionally, it can treat disorders of the Shaoyang with symptoms such as alternating chills and fever, sore throat, headache, hypochondrial pain and distension, bitter taste in the mouth, nausea and vomiting.

Furthermore, Bl-19 can be used to tonify the Gallbladder in psycho-emotional disorders such as mental restlessness, anxiety, fright, panic attacks, timidity and indecisiveness.

BL-19 and BL-17 are known as the *Four Flowers* and are indicated for steaming bone disorder, fevers and to arrest bleeding.

As a local point, Bl-19 can be used to treat pain and stiffness of the back.

> **Main Areas:** Gallbladder. Liver. Hypochondrium. Abdomen.
>
> **Main Functions:** Spreads Gallbladder and Liver qi. Dispels stasis. Alleviates pain. Clears dampness and heat. Dispels shaoyang pathogens.

Bl-20 Pishu

脾俞

Spleen Shu Point

Back *Shu* point of the Spleen

1.5 cun lateral to the lower border of the spinous process of T11. See also pages 166–167.

Treatment and applications

See pages 166–167.

Needling

• 0.4 to 1 cun oblique medial insertion.
• 0.5 cun oblique inferior insertion.

! In many cases the thoracolumbar fascia is very tight causing needling to be sharp or painful. In such cases, loosen the area first with massage or moxibustion.

!! Do not needle deeply or at a different angle. This poses considerable risk of puncturing the lung.

Actions and indications

Bl-20 is the *Spleen Shu point* and is important to *tonify and lift Spleen qi*, *boost the middle jiao, nourish Blood* and *resolve dampness*. It has been extensively employed for most symptoms of *Spleen deficiency*, including *qi, yang and Blood deficiency*. Indications include tiredness and weakness of the limbs and body, sweating, flaccidity of the muscles, tendency to gain weight, water retention, swelling, oedema, abdominal distension, loose stools, chronic diarrhoea, undigested food in the stool, poor appetite, indigestion, infertility, oligomenorrhoea and amenorrhoea.

Furthermore, it can treat *urinary and digestive disorders due to damp accumulation*. Indications include diarrhoea, vomiting, jaundice, productive cough due to phlegm damp, dysuria, cystitis, urethritis and leucorrhoea.

As a *local point*, Bl-20 can be useful for pain and stiffness of the back.

Main Areas: Spleen. Stomach. Intestines. Digestive system. Muscles. Entire body.

Main Functions: Boosts Spleen and Stomach qi. Boosts transformation and movement. Clears dampness.

Bl-21 Weishu

胃俞

Stomach Shu Point

Back *Shu* point of the Stomach

1.5 cun lateral to the lower border of the spinous process of T12.

To aid location, the spinous process of T12 is usually visibly smaller than that of L1. To locate T12, it is best to count up from L-5.

Treatment and applications

Similar to Bl-20 and the previous Bladder points.

Actions and indications

Bl-21 is the *Shu point for the Stomach* and is *important to regulate the Stomach, harmonise the middle jiao and descend rebellious qi*. Furthermore, it *boosts Stomach qi and aids in Blood production*.

Indications include epigastric heaviness, distension and pain, heartburn, burping, poor appetite, nausea, vomiting, jaundice, abdominal distension and pain, loose stools and diarrhoea.

Main Areas: Digestive system. Stomach.

Main Functions: Regulates Stomach qi. Benefits the digestion. Descends rebellious qi.

Bl-22 Sanjiaoshu

三焦俞

Sanjiao Shu Point

Back *Shu* point of the Sanjiao

1.5 cun lateral to the lower border of the spinous process of L1.

Treatment and applications

Similar to Bl-20 and the previous Bladder points.

Actions and indications

Bl-22 is the *Shu point for the Sanjiao* and is important to *resolve dampness, open the water passages* and *promote urination*.

Additionally, it *harmonises the middle jiao* and *boosts Spleen qi*. It has been extensively employed to treat water retention, urinary disorders, swelling and oedema of the abdomen, limbs or entire body.

Moxibustion is particularly effective to *tonify and warm the yang qi in the middle and lower jiao*.

> **Main Area:** Urinary system.
>
> **Main Functions:** Resolves dampness. Opens the water passages. Harmonises Sanjiao.

Bl-23   Shenshu   腎俞

Kidney Shu Point

Back *Shu* point of the Kidneys

1.5 cun lateral to the lower border of the spinous process of L2. In the latissimus dorsi, erector spinae and in its deep position, the quadratus lumborum muscle.

To aid location, Bl-23 is approximately level with the thinnest part of the waist.

Treatment and applications
See pages 166–167.

Needling
• 0.5 to 1.5 cun perpendicular insertion.
• 0.5 to 1.5 cun oblique medial insertion.

! In many cases the thoracolumbar fascia is very tight causing needling to be sharp or painful. In such cases, loosen the area first with massage or moxibustion.

!! Do not needle more deeply at a perpendicular angle, or in a superior direction, particularly on the right side. This poses a considerable risk of injuring the kidney.

Actions and indications
Bl-23 is the *Shu point for the Kidney* and is *extremely important for to tonify the Kidneys*. Its primary functions include *nourishing yin, tonifying and warming yang, regulating the water passages, and benefitting the lower jiao, genitourinary system and uterus*.

Bl-23 is also a major point for *many disorders of the spine, lumbar area, lower limbs and bones*. Indications include chronic lumbar pain and weakness, disorders

of the lumbar spine, spasm of the lumbar muscles, difficulty walking, chronic weakness or paralysis of the lower limbs, cold in the lower back, knees and legs and sciatica, pain in the bones, steaming bone syndrome and low grade fever.

Bl-23 has been extensively employed to treat *disorders of the genitourinary system* including frequent urination, renal colic, chronic urinary tract infections, dysuria, haematuria, infertility, amenorrhoea, dysmenorrhoea, oligomenorrhoea, leucorrhoea, diminishing libido, impotence, spermatorrhoea, premature ejaculation and prostatitis.

Other common indications include chronic tiredness, weakness or exhaustion, chronic weak breathing and coughing, spontaneous sweating, night sweating, palpitations, diminishing vision and hearing, chronic diarrhoea, lower abdominal pain and distension, oedema and all chronic disorders in general.

Moxibustion is particularly effective to tonify and warm the *Kidney yang and mobilise the qi in the lower jiao*.

> **Main Areas:** Kidneys. Lumbar area. Abdomen. Genitourinary system. Entire body.
>
> **Main Functions:** Boosts the Kidneys. Tonifies yang and warms the lower jiao. Nourishes yin and cools empty heat. Resolves dampness. Benefits urination. Alleviates pain.

Bl-24   Qihaishu   氣海俞

Sea of Qi Shu Point

Back *Shu* point of the Sea of Qi

1.5 cun lateral to the lower border of the spinous process of L3.

Treatment and applications
Similar to Bl-23.

Actions and indications
Although Bl-24 is the *Shu point for the Sea of Qi*, it is not as commonly used as the other Shu points. It is however effective *to treat regional pain and to strengthen the lumbar area, abdomen and lower limbs*.

Bl-25   Dachangshu   大腸俞
Large Intestine Shu Point

Back *Shu* point of the Large Intestine

1.5 cun lateral to the lower border of the spinous process of L4.

Treatment and applications
Similar to Bl-23.

Actions and indications
Bl-25 is the *Shu point for the Large Intestine* and is very important for many *disorders of the Large Intestine.* Indications include chronic constipation or diarrhoea, undigested food in the stools, abdominal rumbling, abdominal distension and pain.

Furthermore, it *strengthens the lumbar area and lower limbs* and *alleviates pain and sciatica.*

> **Main Areas:** Intestines. Lumbar area.
>
> **Main Functions:** Alleviates constipation and diarrhoea. Regulates qi and alleviates pain.

Bl-26   Guanyuanshu   關元俞

Original Qi Gate Shu Point

Back *Shu* point of the Original Qi Gate

1.5 cun lateral to the lower border of the spinous process of L5.

Treatment and applications
Similar to Bl-23.

Actions and indications
Although Bl-26 is the *Shu point for the Original Qi Gate,* it is not as commonly used as the other Shu points. It is, however, effective *to regulate the lower jiao* and *urinary system, treat pain and stiffness of the lumbo-sacral joint and strengthen the lumbar area and lower limbs.*

> **Main Areas:** Lumbo-sacral joint. Genitourinary system
>
> **Main Functions:** Benefits the urinary system. Clears dampness and heat. Alleviates pain.

Bl-27   Xiaochangshu   小腸俞
Small Intestine Shu Point

Back *Shu* point of the Small Intestine

1.5 cun lateral to the posterior midline, level with the first sacral foramen.

To aid location, it is just medial to the superior border of the posterior superior iliac spine (PSIS), over the sacroiliac joint.

Treatment and applications
See pages 166–167.

Needling
- 0.5 to 1.5 cun perpendicular insertion, slightly laterally between the PSIS and sacrum, toward the sacroiliac joint.

Actions and indications
Bl-27 is the *Shu point for the Small Intestine* and is important for d*isorders of the urinary system and intestines. It clears dampness and heat, harmonises the intestines and Bladder and aids the Small Intestine function of 'separating the pure from the impure'.* Symptoms include dysuria, haematuria, dark or turbid urine, frequent or urgent urination, diarrhoea and lower abdominal pain.

As a *local point,* it can be useful in the treatment of lower back ache, sciatica and *disorders of the sacroiliac joint.*

> **Main Areas:** Small Intestine. Sacroiliac joint. Urinary system.
>
> **Main Functions:** Benefits the urinary system. Clears dampness and heat. Alleviates pain.

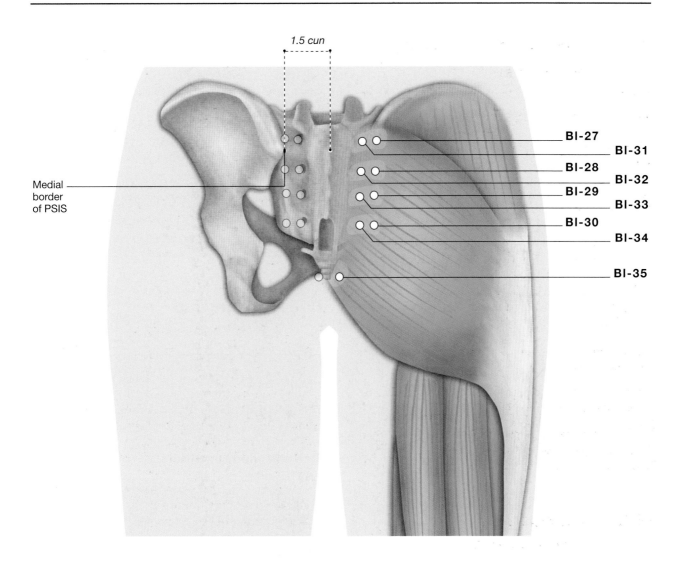

1.5 cun

Medial border of PSIS

BI-27
BI-31
BI-28
BI-32
BI-29
BI-33
BI-30
BI-34
BI-35

BI-28 Pangguangshu 膀胱俞

Bladder Shu Point

Back *Shu* point of the Small Intestine

At the level of the second sacral foramen (Bl-32), 1.5 cun lateral to the posterior midline.

To aid location, it is in the depression between the posterior superior iliac spine (PSIS) and the sacrum.

Treatment and applications
Similar to Bl-27.

Actions and indications
Bl-28 is the *Shu point for the Bladder* and is *important to clear dampness and heat from the lower jiao* and *regulate the Bladder*. Indications include urinary tract infections, dysuria, haematuria, turbid urine, frequent or urgent urination, enuresis, diarrhoea, leucorrhoea, seminal emission, impotence, and pain or inflammation of the genitals.

Furthermore, it *dispels stasis*, *alleviates pain* and *benefits the sacroiliac joint, lumbar region* and *legs*.

> **Main Areas:** Bladder. Sacroiliac joint.
> Urinary system.
>
> **Main Functions:** Regulates the Bladder.
> Benefits the urinary system.
> Clears dampness and heat. Alleviates pain.

Bl-29　Zhonglushu　中膂俞

Middle Spine Shu

At the level of the third sacral foramen, 1.5 cun lateral to the posterior midline.

To aid location, Bl-29 is usually slightly more medial to Bl-28 because the line of the sacral foramina converges slightly towards the midline as it descends.

Treatment and applications
See pages 166–167.

Needling
• 0.5 to 1.5 cun perpendicular insertion.

Actions and indications
Bl-29 is primarily used as a *local point to dispel stasis from the channel and alleviate pain*. It can, however, also help *dissipate cold from the lower jiao* and treat such disorders as weakness and cold of the lower back and legs, diarrhoea, hernia and lower abdominal pain.

> **Main Area:** Sacrum.
>
> **Main Functions:** Regulates qi and Blood. Alleviates pain.

Bl-30　Baihuanshu　白環俞

White Ring Shu Point

At the level of the fourth sacral foramen, 1.5 cun lateral to the posterior midline.

To aid location, Bl-30 is usually slightly more medial to Bl-28 and Bl-29 because the line of the sacral foramina converges slightly towards the midline as it descends.

Treatment and applications
See pages 166–167.

! According to certain classical texts, moxibustion is contraindicated at this location.

Needling
• 0.5 to 1 cun perpendicular insertion.

Actions and indications
Bl-30 is an important point for *disorders of the anal and genital region*. Indications include leucorrhoea, impotence, premature ejaculation, haemorrhoids, diarrhoea, irregular menstruation and amenorrhoea. Furthermore, it is of benefit to the lumbar and sacral area and can help dispel cold and stasis and alleviate pain.

> **Main Areas:** Sacrum. Anus. Genitals.
>
> **Main Functions:** Regulates qi and Blood. Alleviates pain. Benefits the anus.

Bl-31　Shangliao　上髎

Upper Bone-Hole

Over the first sacral foramen, level with Bl-27.

To aid location, it is approximately midway between the posterior superior iliac spine and the posterior midline.

Treatment and applications
See pages 166–167.

Needling
• 0.5 to 1 cun perpendicular insertion.
• 1 to 2.5 cun perpendicular insertion directed slightly medially and inferiorly into the sacral foramen.

Actions and indications
Bl-31 is an important point for *disorders of the sacral, anal and genital area*. Indications include lumbar or sacral pain, irregular menstruation, leucorrhoea, vaginal prolapse, dysmenorrhoea, impotence and difficulty urinating or defecating.

> **Main Areas:** Sacrum. Genitals.
>
> **Main Functions:** Regulates qi and Blood. Alleviates pain.

Bl-32 Ciliao

次髎

Second Bone-Hole

Over the second sacral foramen, level with Bl-28, inferior and slightly medial to Bl-31.

To aid location, Bl-32 is approximately midway between the posterior superior iliac spine and the posterior midline.

Treatment and applications
Similar to Bl-31.

Actions and indications
Bl-32 is also important for *disorders of the sacrum, anal and genital area* and is particularly indicated for *disorders of the uterus and menstruation*.

Symptoms include lumbar or sacral pain, sciatica, numbness and weakness of the lower limbs, irregular menstruation, amenorrhoea, infertility, leucorrhoea, vaginal prolapse, dysmenorrhoea, lower abdominal pain, impotence, difficult urination or defecation.

Furthermore, Bl-32 can be used *during labour for pain relief* and to help the *cervix dilate*.

> **Main Areas:** Sacrum. Uterus. Genitals.
>
> **Main Functions:** Regulates qi and Blood in the lower jiao. Alleviates pain.

Bl-33 Zhongliao

中髎

Middle Bone-Hole

Over the third sacral foramen, level with Bl-29.

To aid location, the line of the sacral foramina converges slightly towards the midline as it descends, placing Bl-33 slightly more medial to Bl-32.

Treatment and applications
Similar to Bl-31 and Bl-32.

Bl-34 Xialiao

下髎

Lower Bone-Hole

Over the fourth sacral foramen, level with Bl-30, inferior and slightly medial to Bl-33.

Treatment and applications
Similar to Bl-31 and Bl-32.

Bl-35 Huiyang

會陽

Meeting of Yang

0.5 cun lateral to the posterior midline, level with the tip of the coccyx.

Treatment and applications
See pages 166–167.

Needling
• 0.5 to 1 cun perpendicular insertion.

Actions and indications
Bl-35 is an *important point for regional disorders* particularly the *coccyx, anus and genitals*. Its primary function is to *clear damp heat, regulate qi in the lower jiao and benefit the anus*. Indications include haemorrhoids, painful defaecation, diarrhoea, coccygeal and sacral pain, impotence, genital pain or itching and dysmenorrhoea.

> **Main Areas:** Coccyx. Anus. Genitals.
>
> **Main Functions:** Regulates qi and Blood. Alleviates pain and swelling.

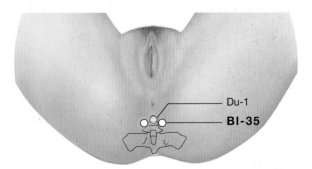

Bl-36 Chengfu

承扶

Support

Bl-37 Yinmen

殷門

Gate of Abundance

At the centre of the transverse gluteal crease, in a sizeable depression, inferior to the gluteus maximus, between the biceps femoris and semitendinosus muscles.

6 cun distal to the transverse gluteal crease (Bl-36), on the line connecting Bl-36 with Bl-40, in the depression between the biceps femoris and semitendinosus muscle.

To aid location, Bl-37 is approximately two hand-widths distal to Bl-36, or one cun proximal to the middle of the line joining Bl-40 to Bl-36.

Best treatment positions
Bl-36 is best treated in a prone position with the knees slightly flexed and the shins supported with cushions.

Needling
• 0.5 to 1.5 cun perpendicular insertion.

! Do not puncture the inferior cluneal nerve, the posterior femoral cutaneous nerve or, more deeply, the sciatic nerve.

Best treatment positions
Similar to Bl-36.

Needling
• 0.5 to 1.5 cun perpendicular insertion.

! Do not puncture the posterior femoral cutaneous nerve, the perforating branch of the deep femoral artery, or more deeply, the tibial nerve and the common peroneal nerve.

Manual techniques and shiatsu
Stationary perpendicular pressure and friction across the attachments of biceps femoris and semitendinosus at the ischial tuberosity are effective techniques. Furthermore, stretching the hamstrings in a lengthwise or cross-fibre direction is very helpful. Use palms, elbows, knees or feet in addition to the thumbs.

An effective self-stretch for this area is performed in the supine position by bringing the one knee toward the chest and pulling it tightly toward the chest with both arms until a stretch is felt in the gluteal area.

Moxibustion
Cones: 3–5. Pole: 5–10 minutes.

Cupping
Stationary and moving cupping can be very effective to treat pain and sciatica.

Guasha
Guasha can be applied distally down the channel or across the muscle fibres.

Actions and indications
Bl-36 in *an important point for disorders of the lower limbs, buttocks and lumbar area* and is widely used to treat sciatica, pain, weakness and atrophy of the legs.

Furthermore, it treats such cases as haemorrhoids, constipation, genital pain and dysuria.

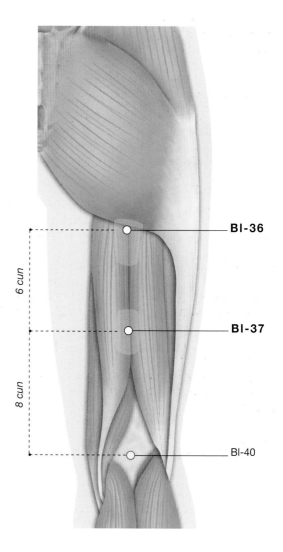

> **Main Areas:** Buttock. Thigh. Lower limb.
>
> **Main Functions:** Regulates qi and Blood. Alleviates pain and sciatica.

Actions and indications

Bl-37 in *an effective point for disorders of the lower limbs,* and is widely used to treat sciatica, pain, weakness and atrophy of the legs.

> **Main Areas:** Thigh. Lower limb.
>
> **Main Functions:** Regulates qi and Blood. Alleviates pain and sciatica.

Bl-38   Fuxi
Superficial Cleft

1 cun above Bl-39 with the knee slightly flexed, on the medial side of the biceps femoris tendon.

To aid location, the patient's knee should be slightly flexed.

Treatment and applications

Similar to Bl-39 although Bl-38 is not a very commonly used point.

> **Main Area:** Knee.
>
> **Main Function:** Regulates qi and Blood.

Bl-39   Weiyang
Outside of the Crease

Uniting Sea-*He* point for the Sanjiao

At the lateral end of the popliteal crease, on the medial side of the biceps femoris tendon (lateral to Bl-40). Locate with the knee flexed.

Best treatment positions

In a prone position with the knees flexed and the shins supported by cushions. However, other positions can also be employed.

Needling

• 0.5 to 1 cun perpendicular insertion.

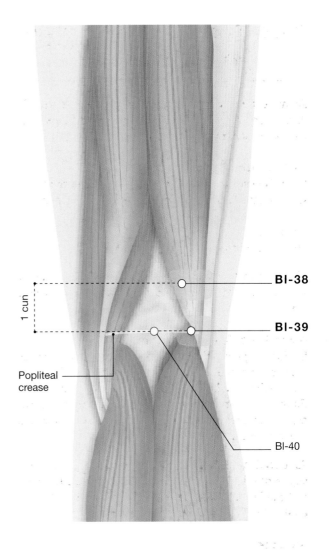

1 cun

Bl-38

Bl-39

Popliteal crease

Bl-40

! Do not puncture the branches of the posterior femoral cutaneous nerve, the common peroneal nerve, or more deeply, the superior lateral genicular artery and vein.

Manual techniques and shiatsu

Stationary pressure and friction across the tendons of biceps femoris is effective. Also, stretching the tendons in a lateral direction can be beneficial.

Moxibustion

Pole: 5–10 minutes, light or light-medium stimulation. Burning cones on Bl-39 is not recommended. However, Rice-grain moxibustion may be applied.

Guasha

Gentle guasha is applicable.

Magnets

Stick-on magnets can also be helpful.

Actions and indications

Bl-39 is the *Lower Uniting Sea-He point of the Sanjiao* and is used to *harmonise the Sanjiao, open the water passages and regulate urination.* Indications include dysuria, urinary retention, incontinence, water retention, swelling and oedema.

Furthermore Bl-39 *regulates qi and Blood* and treats *lower back pain, sciatica* and *disorders of the knee.*

> **Main Areas:** Knee. Lower limbs. Urinary system.
>
> **Main Functions:** Regulates urination and opens the water passages. Alleviates pain.

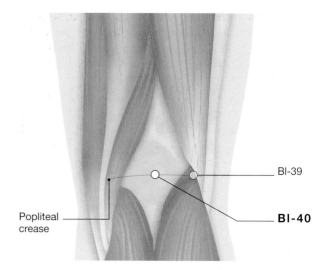

Popliteal crease · Bl-39 · **Bl-40**

Bl-40   Weizhong

Middle of the Crease

委中

Uniting Sea-*He* point of the Bladder
Command point of the Back

At the midpoint of the popliteal crease, midway between the tendons of the biceps femoris and the semitendinosus muscles. Locate with the knee flexed.

To aid location, it is at the site where the pulse of the popliteal artery can be palpated, and usually where it is most sensitive on pressure palpation.

Best treatment positions

This location is best treated in a prone position with the knees flexed and the shins supported by cushions. However, other positions can also be employed.

!! Do not apply any form of treatment to Bl-40 if the possibility of thrombosis has not been ruled out.

Needling

• 0.5 to 1.5 cun perpendicular insertion.

! Do not puncture the femoropopliteal vein or the posterior femoral cutaneous nerve; more deeply, the popliteal vein and artery, and the tibial nerve.

Manual techniques and shiatsu

Perpendicular pressure can be applied carefully to the entire popliteal fossa followed by sustained pressure on Bl-40. Friction to the tendons and insertions of biceps femoris and semitendinosus is also very beneficial.

! Avoid any areas with distended vessels.

Stretching the entire popliteal fossa by extending the knee is very helpful for vascular disorders, poor circulation, water retention and cellulite at the back of the thigh, knee and leg. Also, dorsiflexing the foot while the knee is in extension helps to open this area.

Also, self-acupressure is effective. Place a tennis ball at the back of the knee to apply pressure to the popliteal fossa.

Moxibustion

Cones: 3–5. Pole: 3–10 minutes with light or light-medium stimulation. Rice-grain moxa is also applicable.

Cupping

Medium or light suction can be applied alone or over the needle. Use a small or medium cup size.

Guasha

Guasha can be applied lightly in a distal or cross-fibre direction. Stronger guasha can be applied to the tendons attaching to the medial and lateral aspects of the knee.

Magnets

Stick-on magnets can be effectively employed.

Actions and indications

Bl-40, the *Command point for the back*, is one of the *most important points to treat back problems of both acute and chronic nature.* Combine Bl-40 with local pain points to treat acute back ache, sciatica, weakness of the lower limbs and disorders of the knees. In chronic cases, combine Bl-40 with points such as Bl-23, Bl-52, Kd-3 and Du-4 to strengthen the spine and Kidneys.

Furthermore, Bl-40 is an important point to *clear interior heat and cool the Blood.* Indications include fever, epistaxis, headache, sore throat, epilepsy, loss of consciousness, malaria, night sweating, rashes and other skin disorders, itching, eczema, psoriasis, abdominal pain, diarrhoea and vomiting. It is also mentioned as one of the '*Seven Points for Draining Heat from the Extremities*', together with LI-15, Lu-2 and Du-2.

Bl-40 is also the Uniting Sea-He point of the Bladder and is important in the treatment of *disorders of the urinary system*. Indications include frequent, painful or turbid urination, haematuria, incontinence, water retention, oedema and lower abdominal pain.

Main Areas: Lower back. Knee. Lower limbs.

Main Functions: Regulates qi and Blood. Alleviates pain. Clears heat.

Bl-41 Fufen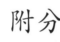

Attached Branch

Intersection of the Small Intestine and Bladder

3 cun lateral to the lower border of the spinous process of T2, just medial to the border of the scapula, lateral to Bl-12. In the trapezius, rhomboideus minor, serratus posterior superior, and in its deep position, the iliocostalis muscle.

Treatment and applications
See pages 166–167.

Needling
• 0.4 to 1 cun transverse oblique medial insertion (toward Bl-12).
• 0.5 cun oblique inferior insertion.

!! Do not needle deeply or at a different angle. This poses considerable risk of puncturing the lung and inducing a pneumothorax.

Actions and indications
Similar to SI-14 and Bl-12.

Main Areas: Shoulder. Upper back. Lungs.

Main Functions: Regulates qi and Blood.

Bl-42 Pohu 魄戶

Door of the Corporeal Soul

---

3 cun lateral to the lower border of the spinous process of T3. Level with Bl-13 and just medial to the medial border of the scapula if the shoulder is relaxed. In the trapezius, rhomboideus major, serratus posterior superior and in its deep position, the iliocostalis muscle.

Treatment and applications
Similar to Bl-41.

Actions and indications
Bl-42 can be *considered as a Back-Transporting Shu point for the Corporeal Soul (Po)*. It is mainly used to treat *psychological disturbances* caused by *disharmony of the Corporeal Soul*, Lungs and Metal Element in general.

Furthermore, it has *similar actions and indications to Bl-13* and, as *a local point*, it can help treat pain of the shoulder, neck and upper back.

Main Areas: Chest. Lungs. Mind.

Main Functions: Regulates Lung qi. Balances the Corporeal Soul.

The Outer Bladder Channel Points
Bl-41 to Bl-54

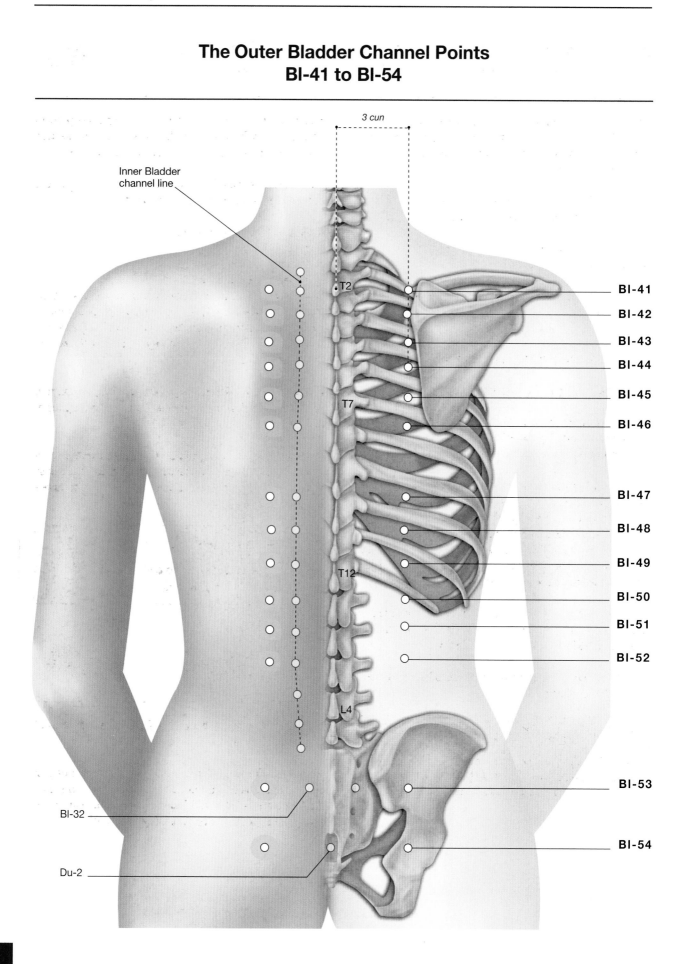

3 cun

Inner Bladder channel line

T2

T7

T12

L4

Bl-32

Du-2

Bl-41
Bl-42
Bl-43
Bl-44
Bl-45
Bl-46
Bl-47
Bl-48
Bl-49
Bl-50
Bl-51
Bl-52

Bl-53

Bl-54

Bl-43   Gaohuangshu   膏肓俞

Vital Region Shu Point

3 cun lateral to the lower border of the spinous process of T4, level with Bl-14. In the trapezius, rhomboideus major, serratus posterior superior and in its deep position, the iliocostalis muscle.

To aid location, Bl-43 is just medial to the medial border of the scapula if the shoulder is relaxed.

Treatment and applications
See pages 166–167.

Many classical texts recommend that only moxibustion is applied to Bl-43.

Needling
• 0.4 to 1 cun transverse oblique medial insertion (toward Bl-14).
• 0.5 cun oblique inferior insertion.

!! Do not needle deeply or at a different angle. This poses considerable risk of puncturing the lung and inducing a pneumothorax.

Actions and indications
Bl-43 is an important point traditionally indicated for any chronic, serious diseases, particularly those affecting the chest, lungs and heart. Its primary functions are to *boost the Lungs, Heart, Kidneys, Spleen and Stomach, resolve phlegm, nourish yin and clear empty heat, tonify yuan qi (Original qi) and calm the mind.*

Symptoms include chronic cough, dry cough, productive cough, haemoptysis, dyspnoea, shortness of breath, emaciation, exhaustion and low grade fever.

As *a local point,* it can help treat pain of the shoulder, neck and upper back.

> **Main Areas:** Chest. Lungs. Heart.
>
> **Main Functions:** Regulates chest qi. Strengthens the Lungs and Heart.

Bl-44   Shentang   神堂

Spirit Hall

3 cun lateral to the lower border of the spinous process of T5, level with Bl-15. In the trapezius, rhomboideus major and in its deep position, the iliocostalis muscle.

To aid location, Bl-44 is just medial to the medial border of the scapula if the shoulder is relaxed.

Treatment and applications
Similar to Bl-43.

Actions and indications
Bl-44 can be *considered as a Shu point for the Mind-Shen* and is used mainly to treat *psychological disorders* relating to disharmony of the Heart and all aspects and levels of consciousness, especially on an *emotional and psycho-spiritual level.*

Indications include anxiety, restlessness, insomnia, dream disturbed sleep, nightmares, depression, epilepsy and even madness.

Furthermore, it helps *regulate qi and Blood in the chest* and is indicated in such cases as dyspnoea, coughing, asthma, thoracic pain, heart pain and pain of the upper back and ribs.

> **Main Areas:** Chest. Heart.
>
> **Main Functions:** Regulates chest qi. Benefits the heart. Balances the mind.

Bl-45   Yixi   譩譆

That Hurts!

3 cun lateral to the lower border of the spinous process of T6, level with Bl-16.

To aid location, apply pressure palpation to the area just medial to the vertebral border of the scapula and locate Bl-45 at the most painful spot (this would cause the patient to cry out 'yi shee' meaning 'that hurts').

Treatment and applications
See pages 166–167.

Needling
- 0.4 to 1 cun transverse oblique medial insertion toward Bl-14.
- 0.5 cun inferior oblique insertion.

!! Do not needle deeply or at a different angle. This poses considerable risk of puncturing the lung.

Actions and indications
Bl-45 is a useful point to *regulate qi and Blood, dispel stasis and alleviate pain*. Furthermore, it *expels wind, clears heat and descends Lung qi*.

Indications include pain and stiffness of the back and shoulder, intercostal neuralgia, rib pain, chest pain, acute and chronic cough, dyspnoea.

> **Main Areas:** Chest. Back.
>
> **Main Functions:** Regulates qi and Blood. Alleviates pain.

Bl-46 Geguan 膈關
Diaphragm Gate

3 cun lateral to the lower border of the spinous process of T7, level with Bl-17.

Treatment and applications
Similar to Bl-45.

Actions and indications
Similar to Bl-17 and other adjacent points.

> **Main Areas:** Diaphragm. Back.
>
> **Main Functions:** Regulates qi and Blood. Alleviates pain.

Bl-47 Hunmen 魂門
Ethereal Soul Gate

3 cun lateral to the lower border of the spinous process of T9, level with Bl-18. In the latissimus dorsi and iliocostalis muscles.

To aid location, the 3 cun line corresponds to a line just medial to the medial border of the scapula if the shoulder is relaxed.

Treatment and applications
Similar to Bl-45.

Actions and indications
Bl-47 can be considered as a *Shu point for the Ethereal Soul (Hun)* and is used mainly to treat *psychological disorders* relating to disharmony of the Ethereal Soul and Liver. Symptoms include irritability, anxiety, dream-disturbed sleep, insomnia, depression, timidity, boredom and lack of inspiration, initiative or goals in life.

Furthermore it helps *spread Liver qi and harmonise the middle jiao*.

Indications include hypochondrial, epigastric and thoracic pain, enlargement of the liver or spleen, hepatitis and diarrhoea.

> **Main Areas:** Hypochondrium. Abdomen. Liver.
>
> **Main Functions:** Regulates qi and Blood. Balances the Ethereal Soul.

Bl-48 Yanggang 陽綱
Yang Headrope

3 cun lateral to the lower border of the spinous process of T10, level with Bl-19. In the latissimus dorsi, serratus posterior inferior, and more deeply, the iliocostalis muscles.

To aid location, the 3 cun line corresponds to a line just medial to the medial border of the scapula if the shoulder is relaxed.

Treatment and applications

Similar to Bl-45.

Actions and indications

Bl-48, can be useful to *harmonise the Gallbladder and Spleen*, *regulate qi* and *clear dampness and heat* from the middle jiao.

Indications include diarrhoea, gastroenteritis, cholecystitis and jaundice. Furthermore, as a local point, it can help treat pain of the back and ribs.

> **Main Areas:** Gallbladder. Spleen. Digestive system.
>
> **Main Functions:** Clears heat and dampness. Regulates qi in the middle jiao.

Bl-49   Yishe

Abode of Thought

3 cun lateral to the lower border of the spinous process of T11, level with Bl-20. In the latissimus dorsi, serratus posterior inferior, and more deeply, the iliocostalis muscle.

To aid location, the 3 cun line corresponds to a line just medial to the medial border of the scapula if the shoulder is relaxed.

Treatment and applications

Similar to Bl-45.

Actions and indications

Bl-49 can be considered as a *Shu point for Thought (Yi)* and is primarily employed in the treatment of *psychological disorders* caused by *disharmony of the Spleen* and the Earth Element in general, particularly in relation to mental processes.

Indications include excessive thinking and worry, poor concentration, diminishing memory and depression.

Furthermore, Bl-49 *harmonises the Spleen and Stomach* and helps *clear dampness and heat*. Indications include abdominal or hypochondrial distension, nausea, vomiting, jaundice, loose stools, diarrhoea, abdominal rumbling and indigestion.

As a *local point,* it can help treat regional pain and stiffness of the back.

> **Main Area:** Spleen.
>
> **Main Functions:** Boosts the Spleen. Improves concentration and thinking.

Bl-50   Weicang

Stomach Granary

3 cun lateral to the lower border of the spinous process of T12, level with Bl-21. In the latissimus dorsi, serratus posterior inferior, and more deeply, the iliocostalis muscle.

Treatment and applications

Similar to Bl-45.

Actions and indications

Bl-50, is a useful point to *harmonise the Stomach and middle jiao and benefit the digestion.* Indications are similar to those of Bl-21.

> **Main Area:** Stomach.
>
> **Main Functions:** Tonifies Stomach qi. Descends rebellious qi.

Bl-51　Huangmen
Vitals Gate

肓門

3 cun lateral to the lower border of the spinous process of the first lumbar vertebra, level with Bl-22. In the latissimus dorsi, serratus posterior inferior, iliocostalis, and in its deep position, the quadratus lumborum muscle.

Treatment and applications
See pages 166–167.

Needling
• 0.5 to 1 cun perpendicular or oblique medial insertion.

!! Do not needle deeply at a perpendicular angle, or in a superior direction, particularly on the right side. This poses considerable risk of injuring the kidney.

Actions and indications
Similar to Bl-22 and other adjacent points.

> **Main Areas:** Abdomen. Epigastrium.
>
> **Main Functions:** Dispels stagnation from the chest and abdomen.

Bl-52　Zhishi
Willpower Room

志室

3 cun lateral to the lower border of the spinous process of L2, level with Bl-23. In the latissimus dorsi, internal abdominal oblique, iliocostalis, and in its deep position, the quadratus lumborum.

To aid location, Bl-52 is approximately level with the thinnest part of the waist.

Treatment and applications
See pages 166–167.

Needling
• 0.5 to 1.5 cun perpendicular insertion.
• 1 to 2 cun oblique medial insertion toward Bl-23.

!! Do not needle deeply, or in a superior direction, particularly on the right side. This poses considerable risk of injuring the kidney.

Actions and indications
Bl-52 can be considered as a *Shu point for the Willpower (Zhi)* and is used to treat *Kidney deficiency and psychological disorders* relating to disharmony of the Kidneys and the willpower.

Furthermore, it helps *regulate urination and strengthen the lumbar area*. Indications are similar to Bl-23.

> **Main Areas:** Kidneys. Lumbar area. Lower jiao.
>
> **Main Functions:** Boosts the Kidneys.

Bl-53　Baohuang
Bladder Vitals

胞肓

3 cun lateral to the lower border of the spinous process of S2, level with Bl-28 and Bl-32. In the gluteus maximus and medius muscles.

To aid location, feel for the most tender spot by palpating laterally from the lower border of the posterior superior iliac spine.

Treatment and applications
Similar to Bl-54, although the latter is more commonly employed.

> **Main Areas:** Sacrum. Buttock.
>
> **Main Functions:** Regulates qi and Blood in the lower jiao. Alleviates pain.

Bl-54   Zhibian

秩邊

Lowermost in Order

On the highest point of the buttock, level with the sacral hiatus, 3 cun lateral to the posterior midline. In the gluteus maximus and medius, and more deeply, the piriformis muscle.

Best treatment positions
Treatment can be applied with the patient lying supine or sideways.

Needling
- 1 to 2.5 cun perpendicular insertion. The needle should enter the piriformis muscle belly during deep insertion.
- 2 to 3 cun oblique insertion toward the anus or perineum.

! Do not puncture branches of the superior cluneal nerve or the inferior gluteal artery, vein and nerve, and in its deep position, the sciatic nerve.

Manual techniques
Perpendicular pressure and friction techniques are applicable with the fingers, knuckles and palms, although often the elbows or knees are most effective, particularly if the recipient is robust.

Moxibustion
Cones: 5–10. Pole: 5–15 minutes.

Cupping
Stationary and moving cupping can be effectively employed. Use a large or medium cup size.

Actions and indications
Bl-54 is a *very effective point for the treatment of pain of the lower back, sacrum and buttocks*, sciatica and *disorders of the lower limbs*. Furthermore, it *regulates qi in the lower jiao* and benefits the *anus* and *genitourinary system*.

Main Areas: Sacrum. Buttock. Anus.

Main Functions: Regulates qi and Blood in the lower jiao. Alleviates pain.

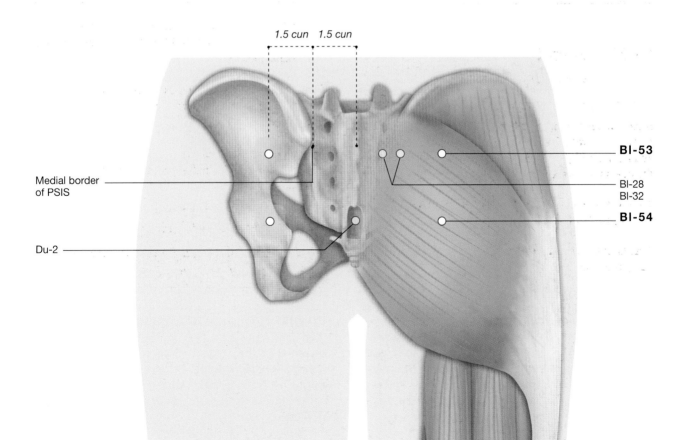

1.5 cun   1.5 cun

Medial border of PSIS

Du-2

Bl-53

Bl-28
Bl-32

Bl-54

Bl-55 Heyang 合陽

Yang Union

2 cun distal to Bl-40, on the line connecting Bl-40 and Bl-57, in the depression between the two heads of the gastrocnemius muscle.

To aid location, Bl-55 is one quarter of the distance between Bl-40 and Bl-57.

Treatment and applications
Similar to Bl-56.

Actions and indications
Bl-55 is a useful point for *disorders of the gynaecological system* and is especially indicated for abnormal uterine bleeding and genital pain. Furthermore, it is effective to *regulate qi and Blood and alleviate pain* of the channel and can be used in similar cases to Bl-56.

Main Areas: Calf. Knee.

Main Functions: Regulates qi and Blood in the lower jiao. Alleviates regional pain.

Bl-56 Chengjin 承筋

Sinew Support

At the centre of the belly of the gastrocnemius muscle, 5 cun distal to Bl-40, midway between Bl-55 and Bl-57.

Needling
• 0.5 to 1 cun perpendicular insertion.

! Do not puncture the small saphenous vein, the medial sural cutaneous nerve or, more deeply, the tibial artery, vein and nerve.

!! According to some classical sources, Bl-56 is contraindicated to needling.

Manual techniques and shiatsu
Pressure must be applied carefully to this area because it is often tight and painful or there may be distended veins. Palm pressure is often most effective. Stretching the gastrocnemius bellies both in a lengthwise and in a cross-fibre direction, helps loosen and relax the calves and improve circulation.

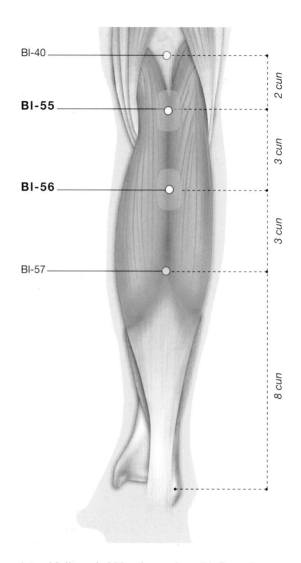

! Avoid distended blood vessels and inflamed areas.

Moxibustion
Cones: 3–5. Pole: 5–15 minutes. Rice-grain moxibustion is also applicable.

!! Do not apply moxibustion over distended vessels.

Guasha
Gentle guasha is applicable distally along the course of the channel toward Bl-57 (between the two heads of the gastrocnemius muscle), or, in a cross-fibre direction.

!! Do not apply guasha on areas with distended veins.

Cupping
Moving cupping over the Bladder channel pathway, as well as the gastrocnemius bellies can be very effective to loosen tight muscles. Use light or medium suction and a medium cup size.

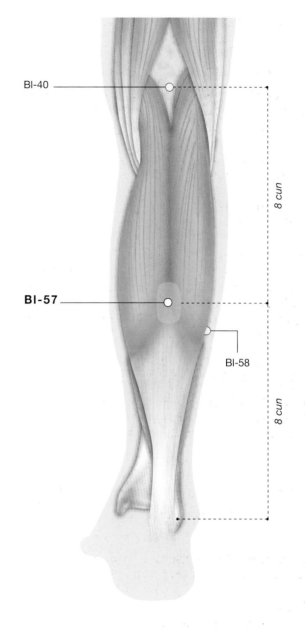

! Do not apply cupping on areas with distended vessels or inflammation.

Stimulation sensation
Regional aching, soreness, numbness or tingling extending distally or proximally along the channel.

Actions and indications
Bl-56 is an *effective local point* to treat pain, cramping, stiffness or weakness of the calf, paralysis, sciatica and lumbar pain.

In common with Bl-57, it is also indicated for *constipation, haemorrhoids and other disorders of the anus*.

Furthermore, it has been traditionally employed to treat a variety of other disorders including, dizziness, headache, epistaxis, axillary swelling and cholera.

> **Main Areas:** Anus. Calf and leg.
>
> **Main Functions:** Regulates qi and Blood. Alleviates pain. Treats haemorrhoids.

Bl-57 Chengshan 承山
Mountain Support

At the centre of the depression below the two bellies of the gastrocnemius muscle, approximately 8 cun inferior to Bl-40, or, midway between Bl-40 and the insertion of the Achilles tendon on the heel.

To aid location, contract the gastrocnemius by asking the patient to press the ball of their foot against the resistance of your hand; then run your finger from the Achilles tendon upwards, along the midline, into the depression.

Treatment and applications
Similar to Bl-56.

Actions and indications
Bl-57 is an *important point for disorders of the channel pathway* and has been extensively used to treat pain, cramping, stiffness or weakness of the calf and leg, paralysis, sciatica and lumbar pain.

In addition, Bl-57 is *important in the treatment of disorders of the anal and genital area* and is especially indicated for haemorrhoids, constipation, rectal prolapse, pain of the perineum or anus and dysmenorrhoea.

> **Main Areas:** Anus. Calf and leg.
>
> **Main Functions:** Regulates qi and Blood. Alleviates pain. Treats haemorrhoids.

Bl-58　Feiyang

Taking Flight

飛揚

Connecting *Luo* point

7 cun proximal to Bl-60, on the posterior border of the fibula, at the lateral margin of the gastrocnemius muscle. Approximately 1 cun distal and lateral to Bl-57.

To aid location, Bl-58 is one cun distal to the midpoint of the line joining Bl-60 with the lateral end of the popliteal crease.

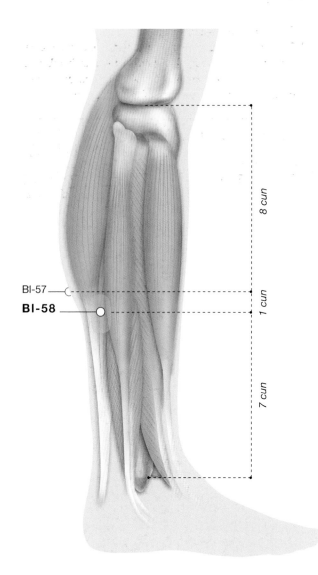

Bl-57

Bl-58

8 cun

1 cun

7 cun

Best treatment positions

This location can be treated with the patient lying down or sitting up.

Needling

• 0.5 to 1 cun perpendicular insertion.

! Do not puncture the lateral sural cutaneous nerve.

Manual techniques and shiatsu

Pressure and friction is applicable with the fingertip or thumb. Palm pressure is also very effective.

Moxibustion

Cones: 3–10. Pole: 5–15 minutes. Rice-grain moxibustion is also applicable.

Guasha

Guasha can be helpful applied across the muscle fibres and downwards along the channel toward Bl-59 and Bl-60.

! Do not apply guasha on areas with distended vessels.

Magnets

Stick-on magnets can be effectively employed at this location.

Stimulation sensation

Regional aching, soreness, numbness or tingling extending distally or proximally along the channel.

Actions and indications

Bl-58 is a useful point to *clear the Tai Yang and dispel wind, dampness and heat.* Furthermore, it *regulates qi and Blood and alleviates pain.*

Indications include pain or cramping of the calf, weakness, stiffness or swelling of the legs, sciatica, lumbar pain, haemorrhoids, chills and fever, headache, dizziness, epilepsy, nasal congestion and epistaxis.

Main Areas: Lower limbs. Anus. Tai yang area. Lower back.

Main Functions: Dispels wind, dampness and heat. Clears the Tai Yang. Regulates qi and Blood. Alleviates pain.

Bl-59   Fuyang

Tarsus Yang

Accumulation Cleft-*Xi* point of the Yang Qiao Mai

3 cun (one hand-width) directly proximal to Bl-60, between the Achilles tendon and the posterior border of the fibula.

Needling
• 0.5 to 1 cun perpendicular insertion.

! Do not puncture the sural nerve and the small saphenous vein, or more deeply, the peroneal artery and veins.

Manual techniques and shiatsu
Pressure and friction is applicable with the fingertip or thumb. Palm pressure is also effective.

Moxibustion
Cones: 3–10. Pole: 5–15 minutes. Rice-grain moxibustion is also applicable.

Guasha
Guasha can be helpful (see Bl-58).

! Do not apply guasha on areas with distended veins.

Magnets
Stick-on magnets can be effectively employed at this location.

Stimulation sensation
Regional aching, soreness, numbness or tingling extending distally along the channel, or upwards along the outer aspect of the leg, possibly reaching the lumbar area. Also, a sensation like a cool breeze may be perceived.

Actions and indications
Bl-59 is a useful point to *dispel wind and dampness and clear the Tai Yang.* Indications include headache, dizziness, nasal congestion, lower backache and pain, atrophy, numbness or swelling of the calf or ankle.

> **Main Areas:** Calf. Head.
>
> **Main Functions:** Dispels wind and damp. Clears the Tai Yang. Alleviates pain.

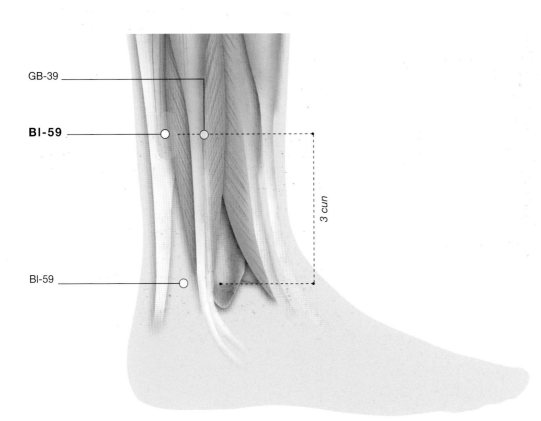

GB-39

Bl-59

3 cun

Bl-59

Bl-60 Kunlun

Kunlun (Mountains)

崑崙

River-*Jing* Fire point of the Bladder channel

At the centre of the large depression formed between the lateral malleolus and the Achilles tendon, level with the tip of the lateral malleolus when the foot is at right angles to the leg. In the triangle-shaped depression posterior to the tendon sheath of peroneus longus and brevis and anterior to the Achilles tendon.

To aid location, Bl-60 is opposite and slightly inferior to Kd-3. Grasp the Achilles tendon between the finger and thumb to locate both points.

Note
The deep position of Bl-60 and Kd-3 is approximately at the same anatomical point, and both needling and acupressure treatment can access it. Additionally, the two superficial points can be joined.

Contraindications
Treatment at this location is not recommended during pregnancy because it can induce abortion or premature labour. However, it may be useful during labour.

Best treatment positions
Bl-60 can be treated with the patient sitting or lying.

Needling
• 0.3 to 5 cun perpendicular insertion.
• 0.5 to 1 cun perpendicular insertion to join with Kd-3.

! Do not puncture the sural nerve (slightly posteriorly), the small saphenous vein and the lateral malleolar artery and vein, or more deeply, the peroneal artery and veins.

If needling to join with Kd-3, ensure the vessels on the medial side are not punctured, particularly the tibial nerve and the posterior tibial artery and vein.

Manual techniques and shiatsu
Stationary pressure and friction techniques are applicable with the tips of the fingers or thumbs. A useful technique is to simultaneously press Bl-60 with the fingers and Kd-3 with the thumb (or vice-versa), so as to grasp and press the flesh between these two points.

Applying perpendicular pressure to the Achilles tendon is very effective, particularly for athletes. Additionally, cross-fibre friction applied to the Achilles tendon (with or without a lubricant) can be very effective to release tension in the lower limbs.

Moreover, careful friction can be applied to the tendons of peroneus longus and brevis at the posterior border of the lateral malleolus.

Moxibustion
Cones: 3–5. Pole: 5–15 minutes. Rice-grain moxibustion is also applicable.

Guasha
Guasha can be applied gently in a distal direction, as well as across the Achilles tendon.

Magnets
Stick-on magnets can be effectively employed. Use opposite poles on Kd-3.

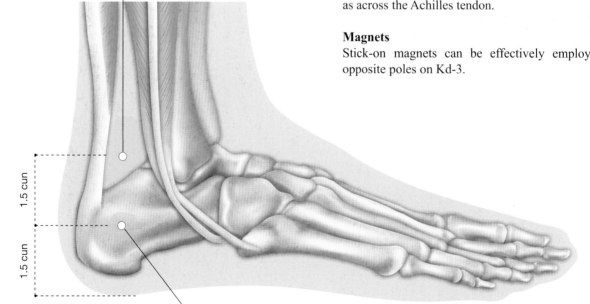

Bl-60

1.5 cun

1.5 cun

Bl-61

Stimulation sensation

Regional aching, soreness, numbness or tingling often extending distally along the channel toward the toes, or upwards along the outer aspect of the leg, possibly reaching the lumbar area. Also, a sensation like a cool breeze may be perceived.

Actions and indications

Bl-60 is a *very dynamic point* and is *very important in the treatment of any blockage along the course of the Bladder channel*, particularly if there is pain. It is widely used to *clear the Tai Yang, treat interior and exterior wind, descend rising yang and clear heat particularly from the head and upper body*. Bl-60 is also used to *strengthen the lumbar area and tonify the Kidneys*.

Indications include headache, stiffness of the neck, heat sensation in the head, inflammation of the eyes, epistaxis, dizziness, hemiplegia, convulsions, chills and fever, acute and chronic lumbar pain, sciatica and pain of the lateral aspect of the leg and heel.

Additionally, Bl-60 has a *powerful effect on the uterus, relieving Blood stasis, alleviating pain and promoting labour*.

Traditionally, Bl-60 has also been used to treat a variety of other symptoms and conditions including infantile epilepsy, malaria, diarrhoea, infertility, toothache, fullness of the chest, dyspnoea and cough.

> **Main Areas:** Tai Yang area. Lower limb. Ankle. Spine and neck. Head. Uterus.
>
> **Main Functions:** Clears the Tai Yang and expels exterior pathogens. Descends rising yang, subdues wind and clears heat. Regulates qi and Blood and dispels stasis from the lower jiao. Promotes labour. Alleviates pain.

Bl-61 Pucan 僕參

Subservient Visitor

Intersection of the Yang Qiao Mai on the Bladder channel

On the lateral aspect of the foot, directly inferior to Bl-60, in a depression on the calcaneus, at the junction of the skin of the plantar and dorsal aspects of the foot.

Best treatment positions

Similar to Bl-62.

Actions and indications

Bl-61 is primarily used as *a local point* for pain, stiffness or swelling.

> **Main Areas:** Ankle. Heel.
>
> **Main Function:** Alleviates pain.

Bl-62   Shenmai

申脈

Extending Vessel

Opening (Master) point of the Yang Qiao Mai
Fifth Ghost point

Directly inferior to the lateral malleolus, between the tendons of peroneus longus and brevis, or posterior to them. Approximately 0.5 cun inferior to the inferior border of the lateral malleolus.

Alternatively, locate Bl-62 slightly more superiorly in the joint space between the talus and calcaneus.

Best treatment positions
Bl-62 can be treated with the patient sitting or lying.

Needling
• 0.3 to 0.4 cun perpendicular insertion between the two tendons.
• 0.3 to 0.5 cun oblique inferior insertion posterior to the tendons.

! Do not puncture the sural nerve or the branches of the lateral malleolar artery.

Manual techniques and shiatsu
Stationary pressure and friction across the tendons is applicable with the tips of the fingers or thumbs.

Moxibustion
Cones: 2–3. Pole: 3–5 minutes.

Guasha
Guasha is effective across the peroneal tendons, and also distally along the course of the channel, toward Bl-63.

Magnets
Stick-on magnets can be effective. Use opposite poles on Bl-62 and SI-3 to treat the Yang Qiao Mai. Combine Bl-62 with SJ-5 for unilateral pain or stiffness due to obstruction of the Yang Qiao Mai.

Stimulation sensation
Regional aching, numbness or tingling, possibly extending distally along the channel toward the toes, or proximally toward the thigh and lower back.

Actions and indications
Bl-62 is the *Opening (Master) point of the Yang Qiao Mai* and is important to *regulate the flow of yang qi, descend rising Yang, clear heat* and *calm the mind*. Furthermore, Bl-62 *clears the Tai Yang area and dissipates exterior wind, cold and heat*.

Indications include headache, stiffness of the neck, redness of the face, dizziness, tinnitus, facial paralysis, windstroke, hemiplegia, convulsions, epilepsy, fever, chills, epistaxis, inflammation and pain of the eyes, palpitations, depression, fright, irritability and insomnia.

Furthermore, Bl-62 *regulates the flow of qi and Blood in the channel pathway and alleviates pain*. Indications include sciatica, cramping, lower back ache and pain, dysmenorrhoea, stiffness or swelling of the ankle.

> **Main Areas:** Head. Lower limb. Ankle.
>
> **Main Functions:** Descends rising yang. Subdues interior wind and clears heat. Clears the head. Calms the mind.

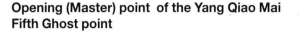

0.5 cun

Bl-62

Bl-63   Jinmen

金門

Golden Gate

**Accumulation Cleft-*Xi* point
Intersection of the Yang Wei Mai on the
Bladder channel**

On the lateral aspect of the foot, inferior and anterior to
Bl-62, in the depression of the cuboid bone, posterior
to the tuberosity of the fifth metatarsal.

To aid location, it is at the site of most tenderness.

Additionally, Bl-63 can be located between the peroneus
brevis tendon and extensor digiti minimi muscle.

Best treatment positions
This location can be treated with the patient lying down
or sitting up in a chair.

Needling
• 0.3 to 0.5 cun perpendicular insertion.

! Do not puncture the small saphenous vein the lateral
dorsal cutaneous nerve, and more deeply, branches of the
lateral malleolar artery.

Manual techniques and shiatsu
Stationary perpendicular pressure and friction is
applicable with the tips of the fingers or thumbs.

Moxibustion
Cones: 3–5. Pole: 5–15 minutes. Rice-grain moxibustion
is also applicable.

Guasha
Guasha can be effectively applied.

Magnets
Use opposite poles on Bl-63 and local pain points.

Stimulation sensation
Regional aching, numbness or tingling, often extending
distally along the channel toward the toes. Deqi may also
be perceived proximally up the channel, toward the lower
back.

Actions and indications
In common with the other Accumulation Xi points, Bl-63
helps *moderate acute conditions and relieve pain*.

Indications include acute pain and cramping along the
course of the Bladder channel, particularly lumbar pain
and sciatica.

Main Areas: Bladder channel. Spine and lumbar
region. Lower limbs.

Main Functions: Regulates qi and Blood.
Alleviates pain.

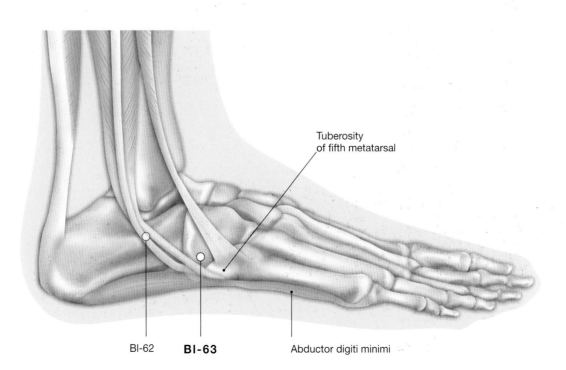

Tuberosity
of fifth metatarsal

Bl-62   **Bl-63**   Abductor digiti minimi

Bl-64   Jinggu

京骨

Capital Bone

Source-*Yuan* point

On the lateral aspect of the foot, in the depression anterior and inferior to the tuberosity of the fifth metatarsal bone, at the junction of the skin of the plantar and dorsal aspects of the foot.

To aid location, apply pressure palpation to the area directly inferior to the tuberosity in order to determine the reactive site that causes a sensation to extend outward from the point.

Some sources place this point directly lateral to the tuberosity of the fifth metatarsal bone, whereas others place it posterior and inferior to it.

Needling
• 0.3 to 0.5 cun perpendicular insertion.

! Do not puncture the small saphenous vein or the lateral dorsal cutaneous nerve.

Manual techniques and shiatsu
Stationary perpendicular pressure and friction is applicable with the tips of the fingers or thumbs.

Moxibustion
Cones: 3–5. Pole: 5–15 minutes.

Guasha
Guasha can be effectively applied.

Stimulation sensation
Regional aching, numbness or tingling, possibly extending distally along the channel toward the fifth toe, or proximally toward the thigh and lower back.

Actions and indications
Although Bl-64 is a Source-Yuan point, it is primarily indicated to *dispel wind* and *clear heat,* especially from the *head and eyes.* It also helps to *calm the mind.*

Indications include headache, stiffness of the neck, chills and fever, heat sensation in the head, epistaxis, pain and inflammation of the eyes, dizziness, fright, epilepsy, palpitations, lower back ache and stiffness or pain along the course of the channel pathway.

Main Areas: Head. Eyes. Bladder channel.

Main Functions: Dispels wind. Clears heat. Calms the mind.

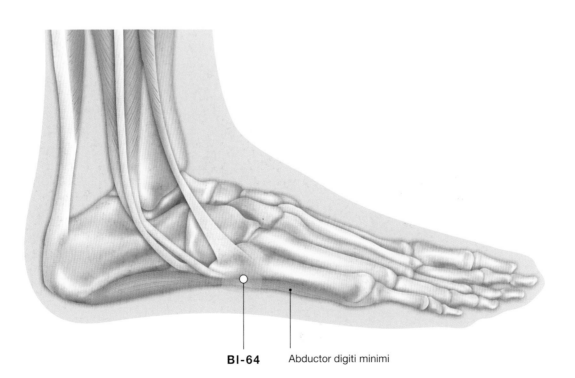

Bl-64   Abductor digiti minimi

BI-65 Shugu   束骨

Restraining Bone

Stream-*Shu*, Wood (Sedation) point

On the lateral aspect of the foot, proximal and slightly inferior to the head of the fifth metatarsal bone, at the junction of the skin of the plantar and dorsal surface.

Treatment and applications
Similar to Bl-64.

Needling
• 0.2 to 0.5 cun perpendicular insertion.

! Do not puncture cutaneous veins of the dorsal network, the lateral dorsal cutaneous nerve or the dorsal metatarsal artery.

> **Main Areas:** Foot. Metatarsal. Head.
>
> **Main Functions:** Dispels wind. Clears heat. Alleviates pain.

BI-66 Zutonggu   足通谷

Foot Valley Passage

Spring-*Ying*, Water (Horary) point

On the lateral aspect of the foot, distal and inferior to the fifth metatarsophalangeal joint, at the junction of the skin of the plantar and dorsal aspects of the foot.

Treatment and applications
Similar to Bl-64.

Needling
• 0.2 to 0.3 cun perpendicular insertion.

! Do not puncture cutaneous veins of the dorsal network, the lateral dorsal cutaneous nerve or the dorsal metatarsal artery.

> **Main Areas:** Foot. Metatarsal. Head.
>
> **Main Functions:** Dispels wind. Clears heat. Alleviates pain.

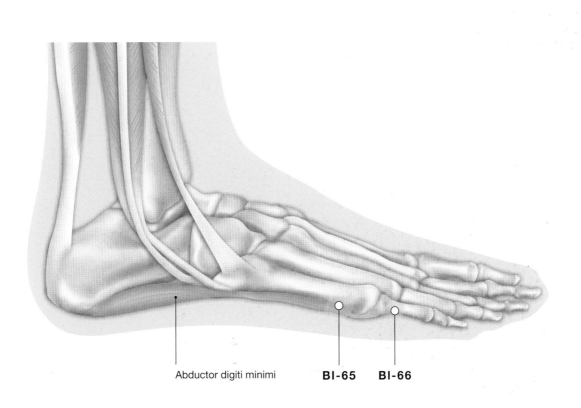

Abductor digiti minimi   **BI-65   BI-66**

Bl-67   Zhiyin

至陰

Reaching Yin

Well-*Jing* Metal (Tonification) point

0.1 cun proximal to the lateral corner of the base of the nail, at the intersection of two lines following the lateral border of the nail and the base of the nail.

!! Contraindicated during pregnancy.

Best treatment positions

Similar to the other Well-Jing points.

Moxibustion

Moxibustion is applied once or twice daily for about 5–10 minutes on each side until the foetus takes position.

!! Discontinue moxibustion as soon as the foetus has turned.

Actions and indications

Bl-67 has a *powerful effect on the uterus* by *activating the Yang Qi of the Bladder and Kidney*. It is therefore contraindicated during pregnancy, except in the case of *breach presentation*, in which event the application of moxibustion is employed to turn the foetus during the seventh and eighth month. It is also used to *induce labour and expedite delivery* of the baby and placenta.

Furthermore, Bl-67 *dispels wind, clears heat and benefits the head and eyes*. Indications include chills and fever, headache, stiff neck, rhinitis and epistaxis.

> **Main Areas:** Uterus. Head.
>
> **Main Functions:** Corrects position of the foetus. Dispels exterior pathogens and clears the Tai Yang.

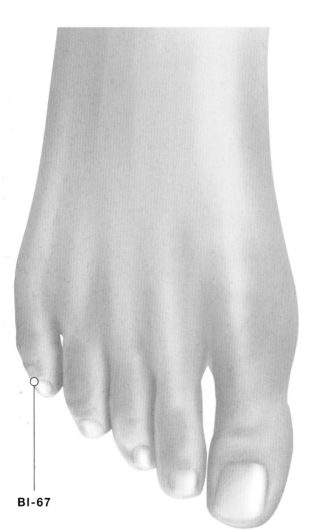

Bl-67

Chapter 17

Points of the

Leg Shao Yin
Kidney Channel

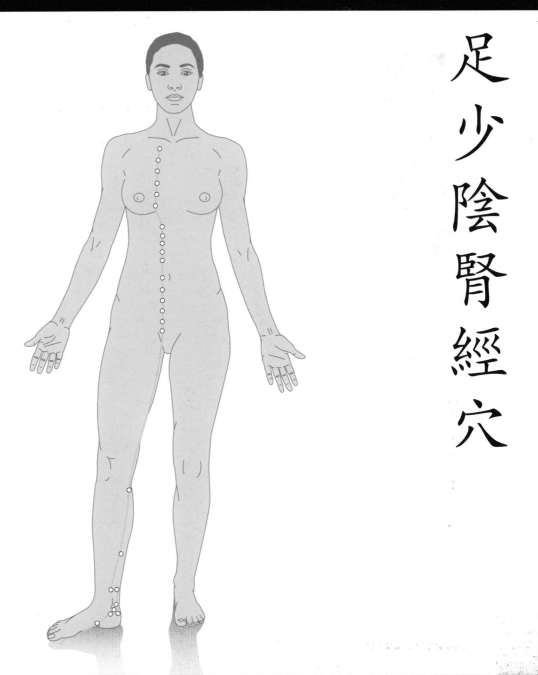

足少陰腎經穴

Kd-1 Yongquan

Bubbling Spring

涌泉

Well-*Jing*, Wood (Sedation) point
One of the nine points for Returning Yang

On the sole of the foot, in the visible depression formed when the foot is plantar flexed, between the second and third metatarsal bones, approximately one third of the distance from the base of the second toe to the heel.

In the second lumbricale muscle, between the tendons of the flexor digitorum brevis and longus attaching to the second and third toes.

Best treatment positions
This location is best treated with the patient lying down prone. However, it can also be treated in other positions.

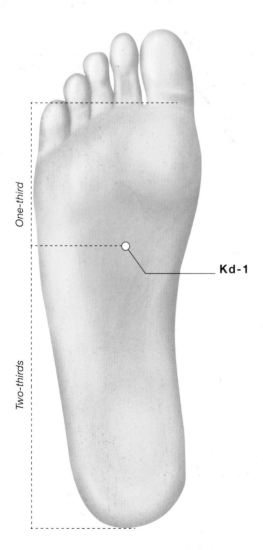

One-third

Two-thirds

Kd-1

Needling
• 0.5 to 1 cun perpendicular insertion.

! This location can be very painful when needled. You may need to use slightly thicker needles if the plantar skin is hard. In general, needling is rarely applied here because it can be so painful.

! Do not puncture the common plantar digital nerve, or more deeply, the plantar metatarsal artery and vein.

Manual techniques and shiatsu
Sustained perpendicular pressure and friction is applicable with the thumbs, elbows, knees or feet.

Regular pressure or massage applied to the sole of the foot with a ball or other specially designed object for this purpose is an effective self-treatment for the disorders mentioned below.

Moxibustion
Cones: 3–5. Pole: 5–15 minutes.

Stimulation sensation
Regional aching, numbness or tingling, extending across the sole of the foot.

Actions and indications
Kd-1 is an important point to *clear heat and fire*, *descend excessive Yang* and *subdue wind (both empty and full)*. It is, however, mostly used in excess conditions, particularly when the upper body is affected. Furthermore, it has a powerful *relaxing and calming effect* on the body and mind.

Indications include headache on the vertex or whole head, dizziness, vertigo, hypertension, insomnia, mental agitation, poor memory, mental confusion, night sweats, sore swollen throat, blurred vision, wind stroke, aversion to cold, cyanosis, hypertension, loss of consciousness, epilepsy, shock, epistaxis, constipation, difficulty urinating, infertility, impotence, sciatica, weakness or paralysis of the lower limbs, lumbar pain, lower abdominal pain, heat in the soles of the feet, pain of the sole of the foot and toes.

Main Areas: Head. Mind. Sole of the foot. Entire body.

Main Functions: Clears fire. Sedates Interior wind. Calms the mind. Resuscitates.

Kd-2 Rangu

Blazing Valley

然谷

Spring-*Ying*, Fire point

On the medial side of the foot, in the depression inferior and slightly anterior to the navicular tuberosity, on the line joining Kd-1 to Kd-3.

To aid location, the navicular tuberosity is the most prominent bony landmark on the medial side of the foot.

Best treatment positions
This location is best treated with the patient lying down supine. However, it can also be treated in other positions.

Needling
• 0.5 to 1 cun perpendicular insertion.

! Do not puncture cutaneous branches of the medial crural nerve, the medial tarsal artery and vein, the plantar digital nerve and deeper, the medial plantar artery and vein.

Manual techniques and shiatsu
Sustained perpendicular pressure and friction is applicable.

Furthermore, this location can be opened by stretching the medial aspect of the foot. Immobilise the heel with one hand, while pressing the medial border of the arch with the other to stretch this area. The foot should be placed with medial side facing upwards (the patient may be lying supine or sideways).

Moxibustion
Cones: 3–5. Pole: 5–15 minutes. Rice-grain moxa is also applicable.

Stimulation sensation
Regional aching, numbness or tingling, possibly extending across the sole of the foot.

Actions and indications
Kd-2 is primarily used to clear *empty fire and heat* due to *Kidney Yin deficiency*. It treats symptoms such as insomnia, restlessness, night sweating, fever, emaciation, pain of the bones and spine which is worse at night, thirst, sore or swollen throat, coughing blood, dry unproductive cough and loss of voice.

Additionally, Kd-2 *regulates menstruation and benefits the uterus*. Indications include uterine prolapse, genital itching, leucorrhoea, infertility, irregular menstruation and excessive menstrual bleeding. It is also used for other *disorders of the lower jiao* including dysuria, haematuria, turbid urination, urethritis, cystitis, prostatitis, impotence and premature ejaculation.

Furthermore, it can be used to *tonify Kidney yang and warm the lower jiao*, particularly if treated with moxibustion.

Main Areas: Kidneys. Spine. Entire body.

Main Functions: Clears empty fire. Nourishes Kidney yin. Benefits the genitourinary system.

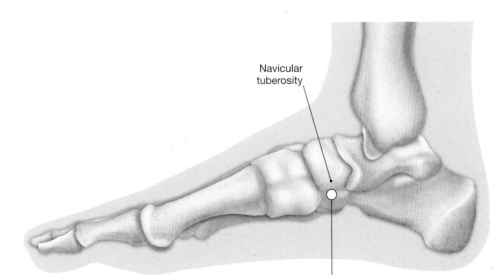

Navicular tuberosity

Kd-2

Kd-3   Taixi

Great Stream

太谿

Stream-Shu Earth point
Source-*Yuan* point
One of the nine points for Returning Yang

In the depression midway between the posterior border of the medial malleolus and the anterior border of the Achilles tendon, level with the prominence of the medial malleolus when the foot is at right angles.

To aid location, Kd-3 is opposite and slightly superior to Bl-60. Grasp the Achilles tendon between the finger and thumb to locate both these points.

Furthermore, it is usually most reactive at the visible centre of the depression, therefore locating it visually may be more helpful (this does not apply in cases of swelling or deformity of the ankle).

Note
The deep position of Kd-3 and Bl-60 is approximately at the same anatomical point, and both needling and acupressure treatment can access it. Additionally, the two superficial points can be joined.

Best treatment positions
Kd-3 is best treated with the patient lying supine. However, it can also be treated in other positions.

Needling
• 0.5 to 1 cun perpendicular insertion toward Bl-60. Palpate for the pulse of the posterior tibial artery and insert the needle posterior to it.

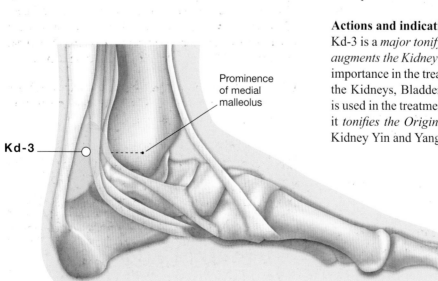

Kd-3

Prominence of medial malleolus

! Do not puncture cutaneous branches of the medial crural nerve, the posterior tibial vein and artery or the tibial nerve, all situated at this exact site. See cautionary note for Bl-60.

Manual techniques and shiatsu
Stationary pressure and friction techniques are applicable with the tips of the fingers or thumbs. Furthermore, Kd-3 can be opened by stretching the foot laterally.

A useful technique is to simultaneously press Bl-60 with the fingers and Kd-3 with the thumb (or vice-versa), so as to grasp and press the flesh between these two points.

For further techniques see Bl-60.

Moxibustion
Cones: 3–6. Pole: 5–15 minutes. Rice-grain moxa is also applicable.

! Do not apply moxibustion on areas of visible capillaries, distended vessels or oedema.

Magnets
Stick-on magnets can be applied to Kd-3 and Bl-60 simultaneously (use opposite poles on Kd-3 and Bl-60). Furthermore, use north pole on Kd-3, south on St-36 and north on Ren-6 to tonify the qi and yang of the whole body; north pole on Kd-3, south on Bl-23 and north on Du-4 for chronic back ache; north pole on Kd-3, south on Sp-6 and north on Ren-4 for dysmenorrhoea, irregular menstruation or infertility.

Stimulation sensation
Numbness, tingling or electricity possibly extending distally toward the sole of the foot, or proximally up the channel. Furthermore, a sensation like a cool breeze is often perceived.

Actions and indications
Kd-3 is a *major tonifying point for the Kidneys* because it *augments the Kidney yin, yang and jing*. It is of particular importance in the treatment of disorders of the lower jiao, the Kidneys, Bladder, reproductive system and spine. It is used in the treatment of *many chronic diseases* because it *tonifies the Original qi* (yuan qi) that stems from the Kidney Yin and Yang.

Indications include exhaustion, diminished hearing and sight, tinnitus, dizziness, hypertension, heat in the five hearts (palms), fever, night sweating, insomnia, dream disturbed sleep, emaciation, thirst, sore throat, infertility, impotence, premature ejaculation, spermatorrhoea, amenorrhoea, irregular menstruation, menopausal syndromes, frequent and abundant urination, dribbling urination, dysuria, dark urine, enuresis, constipation, oedema, swelling of the legs, abdominal pain, chronic lower back ache, coldness and weakness of the lower back, abdomen, knees and legs.

Furthermore, Kd-3 has a *beneficial influence on the Lungs and breathing* and can help the Kidneys in the function of *Grasping qi*. Indications include chronic cough, haemoptysis, epistaxis, chest pain, shallow breathing and asthma due to Kidney and Lung disharmony.

> **Main Areas:** Kidneys. Spine. Entire body.
>
> **Main Functions:** Augments Kidney yin and yang. Tonifies yuan qi. Benefits the genitourinary system. Increases fertility.

Kd-4 Dazhong 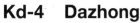 大鐘

Large Bell

Connecting *Luo* point

In a small depression approximately 0.5 cun distal and posterior to Kd-3, at the anterior border of the Achilles tendon.

To aid location, find the midpoint of the line joining Kd-3 to Kd-5 and, from here, move posteriorly to the point just anterior to the Achilles tendon.

! Kd-4 can be tender or sensitive on palpation.

Best treatment positions
This location is best treated with the patient lying down supine. However, other positions can be employed.

Needling
• 0.3 to 0.5 cun perpendicular or oblique anterior insertion.

! Do not puncture cutaneous branches of the medial crural nerve, the posterior tibial vein and artery or the tibial nerve.

Manual techniques and shiatsu
Stationary pressure and friction techniques are applicable with the tips of the fingers or thumbs.

Moxibustion
Cones: 3–5. Pole: 5–10 minutes. Rice-grain moxa is also applicable.

! Do not apply moxibustion on areas of visible capillaries, distended vessels or oedema.

Magnets
Stick-on magnets can be effective. Use north pole on one side and south on the other.

Stimulation sensation
Numbness, tingling or electricity possibly extending toward the sole of the foot, or proximally up the channel.

Actions and indications
Kd-4 is the *connecting point of the Kidney channel* and has been extensively employed to *strengthen the Kidneys* both in the physical and psycho-emotional sense. It is traditionally indicated to increase the *willpower and dispel fear* and has been used to treat such cases as propensity to fright, chronic phobias, psychological insecurity, introverted unconfident behaviour, lack of willpower, sleepiness, anxiety, irritability, fright palpitations, insomnia and other psychological disturbances.

Furthermore, Kd-4 is important to *harmonise the Kidney and Lung* and helps draw down excess causing various respiratory disorders. Symptoms include shallow breathing, asthma, cough, dryness and soreness of the mouth and throat and haemoptysis.

Symptoms relating to *disharmony of the Kidney Connecting (Luo) channel* include lumbar pain, weakness of the lower limbs, pain of the ankle or heel, oppression of the chest, palpitations, heart pain, vomiting, abdominal distension and fullness, dysuria and urinary retention.

Kd-4 also treats other symptoms of *Kidney weakness* including exhaustion, chronic constipation, impotence, infertility and irregular menstruation.

> **Main Areas:** Mind. Kidneys. Lungs.
> **Main Functions:** Reinforces the Kidneys. Strengthens Willpower. Harmonises the Kidney and Lung.

Kd-5 Shuiquan

Water Spring

水泉

Accumulation Cleft-*Xi* point

1 cun inferior to Kd-3, in the depression anterior and superior to the insertion of the Achilles tendon and the calcaneal tuberosity. Locate with the foot at right angles.

Best treatment positions

This location is best treated with the patient lying supine. However, it can also be treated in other positions.

Needling

• 0.3 to 0.5 cun oblique or perpendicular insertion.

Manual techniques and shiatsu

Stationary pressure and friction techniques are applicable with the tips of the fingers or thumbs.

Moxibustion

Cones: 3–5. Pole: 5–10 minutes. Rice-grain moxa is also applicable.

! Do not apply moxibustion to areas of visible capillaries, distended vessels or oedema.

Magnets

Stick-on magnets can be effective.

Stimulation sensation

Numbness, tingling or electricity extending toward the sole of the foot, or proximally up the channel.

Actions and indications

Kd-5 is important to regulate the *flow of qi and Blood in the lower jiao* and *harmonise the Ren and Chong Mai*. It is used to *nourish Blood* as well as to *dispel Blood stasis*.

Indications include abdominal pain, dysmenorrhoea, amenorrhoea, irregular menstruation, infertility, uterine prolapse, frequent urination, dysuria and dribbling.

Furthermore it has been traditionally used to treat *disorders of the eyes*, including nearsightedness and diminishing or unclear vision.

Moxibustion at Kd-5 helps *dispel cold and Blood stasis from the uterus and warm the Kidney yang*.

> **Main Areas:** Lower jiao. Gynaecological and urinary system. Eyes.
>
> **Main Functions:** Dispels Blood stasis. Nourishes Blood. Regulates the Ren and Chong Mai.

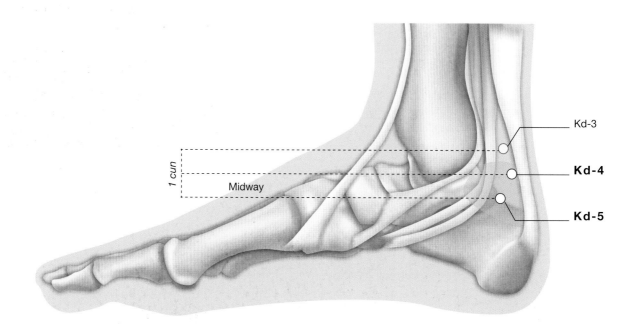

Kd-6   Zhaohai

Shining Sea

照海

Opening (Master) point of the Yin Qiao Mai

In the depression approximately 1 cun below the prominence of the medial malleolus, between the tendons of tibialis posterior and flexor digitorum longus.

To aid location, define the tendons by plantar flexing and inverting the foot.

Alternative location
If the tendons are very stiff and tight, treat Kd-6 in the depression directly below the sustentaculum tali.

Best treatment positions
This location can be treated with the patient lying down or sitting up.

Needling
- 0.3 to 0.5 cun perpendicular insertion in a slightly superior direction. The needle should go between the two tendons. However, if this location is very tight it will be painful, and so needling should be applied below the sustentaculum tali.

! Do not puncture the medial crural cutaneous nerve and more deeply, the posterior tibial artery and vein and the tibial nerve.

Manual techniques and shiatsu
Stationary pressure and friction techniques are applicable with the fingertips or thumbs to the entire area covering the whole of the inner aspect of the calcaneum.

Moxibustion
Cones: 3–5. Pole: 5–10 minutes. Rice-grain moxa is also applicable.

Magnets
Stick-on magnets can be effective. To regulate the Yin Qiao and Ren Mai, use opposite poles on Kd-6 and Lu-7.

Stimulation sensation
Localised aching, numbness, tingling or electricity extending proximally up the channel. Also, a sensation like a cool breeze is often perceived.

Actions and indications
Kd-6 is one of the most important points to *nourish and moisten yin, cool the body and clear empty heat*. Indications include night sweating, heat in the five hearts, low grade fever, chronic thirst, dry mouth, headache, dizziness, palpitations, epilepsy, sore, painful or swollen throat, pharyngitis, exhaustion, hot flushes, menopausal syndromes, dryness and pain of the eyes, photophobia, diminishing vision, tinnitus, soreness of the lower back, pain in the bones and impotence.

Kd-6 is also a significant point for the treatment of *gynaecological complaints* such as infertility, irregular menstruation, amenorrhoea, excessive menstrual bleeding, post partum abdominal pain, excessive lochia, leucorrhoea, uterine prolapse, genital itching and dryness.

Furthermore, Kd-6 helps to *calm the mind in* cases of anxiety, restlessness and insomnia.

Main Areas: Head. Eyes. Ears. Throat. Mind. Lower jiao. Uterus.

Main Functions: Nourishes yin. Cools empty heat. Regulates the Yin Qiao Mai.

Tibialis posterior

Kd-6

Flexor digitorum longus

Sustentaculum tali

1 cun

Kd-7 Fuliu

Returning Flow

復溜

River-*Jing*, Metal (Tonification) point

2 cun proximal to Kd-3, in the depression anterior to the border of the Achilles tendon and inferior to the soleus muscle.

Best treatment positions

This location is best treated with the patient lying down supine. However, it can also be treated in other positions.

Needling

• 0.5 to 1 cun perpendicular insertion.

! Do not puncture the cutaneous branches of the medial crural or saphenous nerve. More deeply and anteriorly, the tibial nerve, artery and vein.

Manual techniques and shiatsu

Stationary pressure and friction techniques are applicable with the fingertips or palms. Furthermore, stretching the Achilles tendon in a posterior direction is beneficial.

Moxibustion

Cones: 3–8. Pole: 5–10 minutes. Rice-grain moxa is also applicable.

Magnets

Stick-on magnets can be effective. For oedema and sweating use opposite poles on Kd-7 and LI-4.

Stimulation sensation

Localised aching, numbness or tingling extending proximally up the channel or distally toward the sole of the foot.

Actions and indications

Kd-7 is *a very important point to tonify Kidney yang* and *promote the body's water metabolism* thus *regulating sweat, urination and movement of interstitial fluids.* It has been extensively used to treat oedema, frequent urination, dribbling urination, anuria, lower back ache, spontaneous, excessive or lack of sweating and lumbar pain.

Furthermore, Kd-7 is important to *clear damp heat* and has been employed to treat such cases as night sweating, tidal fever, urinary tract infections, leucorrhoea, abdominal distension, diarrhoea, haemorrhoids, pus and blood in the stool.

Additionally, Kd-7 treats other symptoms of *Kidney deficiency* including exhaustion, depression, lack of motivation and other psychological disorders.

> **Main Areas:** Water passages. Lower jiao.
>
> **Main Functions:** Regulates sweat and urination. Reduces swelling. Tonifies Kidney yang.

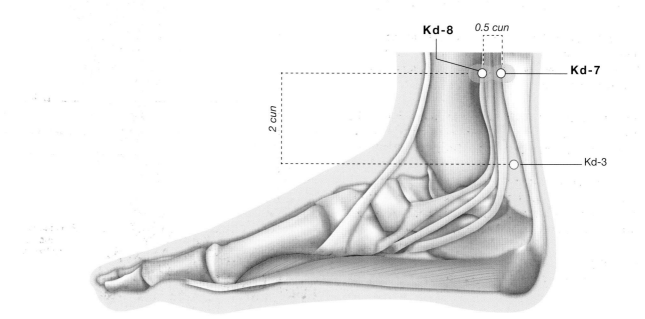

Kd-8 Jiaoxin 交信

Belief Intersection

Accumulation Cleft-*Xi* point of the Yin Qiao Mai
Intersection of the Spleen and Kidney

0.5 cun anterior to Kd-7, posterior to the medial border of the tibia, 2 cun proximal to Kd-3.

Best treatment positions
Similar to Kd-7.

Actions and indications
Kd-8 is a *useful point to harmonise the Ren and Chong Mai* and *regulate menstruation.* Furthermore, it *clears dampness and heat and benefits the lower jiao.*

Indications include irregular or excessive menstrual bleeding, dysmenorrhoea, amenorrhoea, uterine prolapse, genital itching, urinary tract infections, urinary retention, diarrhoea and lumbar pain.

> **Main Area:** Genitourinary system.
>
> **Main Functions:** Regulates menstruation. Clears dampness and heat.

Kd-9 Zhubin 築賓

Guest House

Accumulation Cleft-*Xi* point of the Yin Wei Mai

In the depression below the belly of the gastrocnemius muscle, just anterior to the medial border of the Achilles tendon, approximately 5 cun proximal to Kd-3, on the line joining Kd-3 to Kd-10.

To aid location, it is approximately one third of the distance along the line joining Kd-3 to Kd-10 and approximately 1 cun posterior to Liv-5.

Best treatment positions
Treatment is best applied in a supine position with the knee flexed and the thigh laterally rotated. Use ample cushion support under the thigh, knee and leg.

Needling
• 0.5 to 1.5 cun perpendicular insertion.

! Do not puncture the cutaneous branches of the medial crural or saphenous nerve, or more deeply and anteriorly the tibial nerve, posterior tibial artery and vein.

Manual techniques and shiatsu
Sustained perpendicular pressure can be applied with the fingers and palms. Friction is useful across the soleus and Achilles tendon. Stretching the calf muscles in a posterior direction is also effective.

Moxibustion
Cones: 3–5. Pole: 5–15 minutes. Rice-grain moxa is also effective.

! Direct moxibustion is not recommended at this location in patients with varicosities.

Magnets
Magnets are also effectively employed at this location.

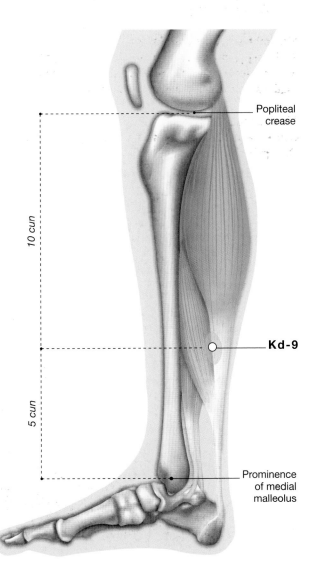

Popliteal crease

10 cun

5 cun

Kd-9

Prominence of medial malleolus

Stimulation sensation
Aching, tingling or numbness locally, or extending proximally along the channel toward the abdomen.

Actions and indications
Kd-9 is primarily indicated to calm the mind, clear the heart and transform phlegm, whilst at the same time, tonifying the Kidney yin and jing.

It has been used to treat psycho-emotional disorders including insomnia, epilepsy, anger, fright and even insanity. Furthermore, it is used in the treatment of other related disorders, including vomiting, oppression of the chest, palpitations, goitre, urinary tract infections, hernia, abdominal pain and swelling.

As a local point, it can be helpful in cases of pain and spasm of the calf muscles.

Main Areas: Heart. Mind. Lower jiao.

Main Functions: Clears and calms the Heart and mind. Regulates qi.

Kd-10 Yingu
Yin Valley

陰谷

Uniting Sea-*He* point of the Kidney channel

At the medial end of the popliteal crease between the tendon of semitendinosus and the lower end of the semimembranosus muscle, located with the knee flexed.

To aid location, it is approximately level with Bl-39 and Bl-40.

Best treatment positions
This location is best treated with the patient lying down prone and the knees slightly flexed (the shins should be supported with cushions). However, it can also be treated with the patient lying supine or sideways.

Needling
• 0.5 to 1.5 cun perpendicular insertion.

! Do not puncture the saphenous vein or nerve just anterior to Kd-10, and more deeply, the medial superior genicular artery and vein.

Moxibustion
Cones: 3–5. Pole: 5–15 minutes. Rice-grain moxa is also effective.

Magnets
Magnets can also be effectively employed.

Stimulation sensation
Localised tingling or numbness extending proximally or distally along the channel and into the knee.

Actions and indications
Kd-10 is an *important point to transform dampness, clear heat, nourish Yin and benefit the lower jiao.*

It has been extensively employed to treat such symptoms as dysuria, haematuria, frequent urination, impotence, chronic leucorrhoea, abnormal uterine bleeding and pain of the lower back and knees.

Main Areas: Lower jiao. Genitourinary system.

Main Functions: Nourishes yin and cools lower jiao heat. Transforms dampness.

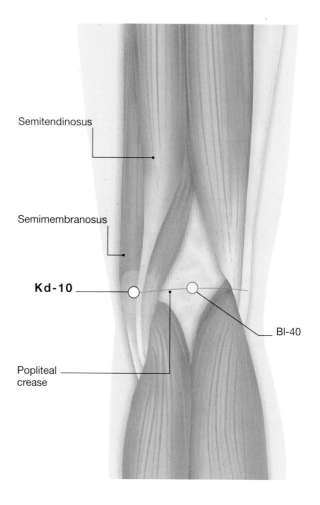

Semitendinosus

Semimembranosus

Kd-10

Bl-40

Popliteal crease

Kd-11 Henggu
Pubic Bone

横骨

Intersection of the Chong Mai and Kidney

On the superior border of the symphysis pubis, 0.5 cun lateral to the anterior midline (Ren-2), 5 cun below the umbilicus.

A number of sources place the points Kd-11 to Kd-17, slightly further lateral at a distance of 1 cun from the anterior midline.

Best treatment positions
This point is best treated with the patient lying in a supine position with the hips flexed and the thighs and knees well supported with cushions.

Needling
• 0.5 to 1 cun perpendicular insertion.

! Do not needle deeply, particularly if the patient is very thin. This poses the risk of puncturing a full bladder.

Manual techniques and shiatsu
Similar to St-30.

Moxibustion
Pole: 5–15 minutes. Direct moxibustion is not easily applicable to this location.

! Do not burn the pubic hair.

Actions and indications
Kd-11 has similar functions to Ren-2 and is primarily used to treat disorders of the genitourinary system, including infertility, genital pain, dysuria, urinary retention, incontinence, prostatitis and impotence.

> **Main Areas:** Bladder. Genitals. Lower jiao.
>
> **Main Functions:** Benefits the lower jiao. Improves sexual function and fertility.

Kd-16 Huangshu
Vital Point

肓俞

Intersection of the Chong Mai and Kidney

At the centre of the abdomen, 0.5 cun lateral to the centre of the umbilicus (Ren-8).

To aid location, it is usually just at the edge of the umbilicus.

Alternative location
A number of sources place Kd-16 1 cun lateral to the anterior midline.

Best treatment positions
Kd-16 is usually treated with the patient lying supine.

Needling
• 0.5 to 1.5 cun perpendicular insertion.

! Do not needle deeply, particularly if the patient is very thin. Do not puncture the peritoneum.

Moxibustion
Cones: 5–15. Pole: 10–20 minutes. Rice-grain moxa is also applicable.

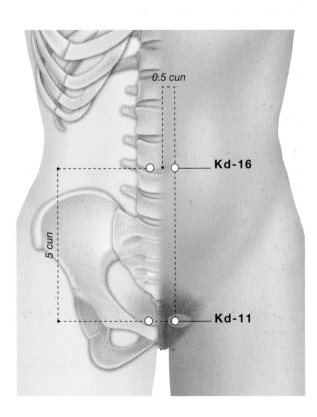

Cupping

Empty or moving cupping is effective applied over the umbilicus, covering Ren-8 and Kd-16.

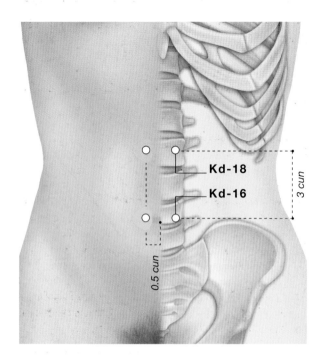

Manual techniques and shiatsu

Sustained perpendicular pressure is applicable with the fingertip or thumb. Pressure can also be applied in a medial direction so that the umbilicus is slightly squeezed. This is more effective in cases where perpendicular pressure is painful. Circular or cross-fibre friction can also be effective to relax the musculature.

Self-acupressure can be applied in a standing or sitting position while bending the trunk forward.

! The umbilicus, and the area immediately around it, is often tender. Great care should be taken to ensure the correct angle and depth of pressure. A sensation of warmth in the whole abdomen should be perceived.

Actions and indications

Similar to Ren-8, St-25 and Sp-15, Kd-16 *warms and regulates qi in the abdomen and intestines* and *helps alleviate pain.* Symptoms include constipation, dry stools, abdominal pain, distension or swelling and vomiting.

> **Main Areas:** Umbilicus. Abdomen. Intestines.
>
> **Main Functions:** Warms the abdomen. Regulates intestinal qi. Alleviates pain.

Kd-18   Shiguan
Stone Gate

石關

Intersection of the Chong Mai and Kidney

3 cun above the umbilicus, 0.5 cun lateral to the anterior midline (Ren-11).

Certain classical sources place Kd-18 1.5 cun lateral to the anterior midline.

Actions and indications

Although Kd-18 is not a very commonly used point, but can be used to *harmonise the Stomach* and treat symptoms such as nausea and vomiting, indigestion, epigastric or abdominal pain and acid reflux.

> **Main Areas:** Epigastrium. Stomach.
>
> **Main Functions:** Harmonises the Stomach. Descends rebellious qi.

Kd-19   Yindu
Yin Metropolis

陰都

Intersection of the Chong Mai and Kidney

4 cun above the umbilicus, 0.5 cun lateral to the anterior midline (Ren-12).

Certain classical sources place Kd-19 1.5 cun lateral to the anterior midline.

Treatment and applications

Similar to Ren-12 and St-21.

> **Main Areas:** Epigastrium. Stomach.
>
> **Main Functions:** Harmonises the Stomach. Descends rebellious qi.

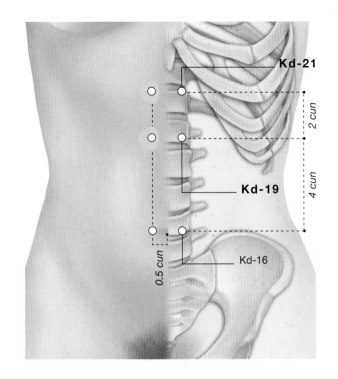

Kd-22 Bulang 步廊

Stepping Upward

In the fifth intercostal space, 2 cun lateral to the anterior midline (Ren-16).

To aid location, the 2 cun line is halfway between the anterior midline and the mid-mammillary line. Kd-22 is three rib spaces below Kd-25.

Best treatment positions
Similar to Kd-25.

Needling
• 0.5 to 1 cun transverse oblique insertion, laterally along the intercostal space.

!! Deep needling may puncture the lung or liver.

Actions and indications
Although Kd-22 is not a very commonly used point, it can be helpful to regulate qi in the chest, dispel stagnation and descend rebellious Lung and Stomach qi.

> **Main Areas:** Chest. Epigastrium.
>
> **Main Functions:** Regulates qi.
> Descends rebellious qi.

Kd-21 Youmen 幽門

Dark Gate

Intersection of the Chong Mai and Kidney

6 cun above the umbilicus, 0.5 cun lateral to the anterior midline (Ren-14).

Treatment and applications
Similar to Ren-14 and St-19.

> **Main Areas:** Epigastrium. Chest.
>
> **Main Functions:** Harmonises the Stomach. Clears Heat.

Kd-25 Shencang 神藏

Spirit Storehouse

In the second intercostal space, 2 cun lateral to the anterior midline (Ren-19).

To aid location, locate the sternal angle, which is level with the second rib; palpate the second rib and drop your finger into the intercostal space below it.

Needling
• 0.3 to 0.4 cun perpendicular insertion.
• 0.5 to 1 cun transverse oblique insertion, laterally along the intercostal space.

!! Deep needling may puncture the lung.

Manual techniques and shiatsu
Ensure the pressure is applied at the correct angle in the intercostal spaces as they are often tight and painful.

! Avoid excessive pressure on the rib cage, particularly if the patient has heart disease, asthma or osteoporosis.

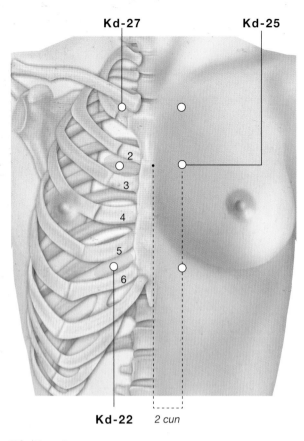

Kd-27   Kd-25

Kd-22   2 cun

Kd-27   Shufu

Shu Mansion

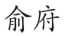

In the depression inferior to the medial end of the clavicle, 2 cun lateral to Ren-21.

Best treatment positions
This location is best treated with the patient lying down supine. However, it can also be treated in other positions.

Needling
- 0.3 to 0.4 cun perpendicular insertion.
- 0.5 to 1 cun transverse oblique insertion, laterally along the inferior border of the clavicle.

!! Deep needling may puncture the lung.

Manual techniques and shiatsu
Perpendicular pressure and friction techniques are applicable with the fingertips or thumbs.

! Avoid strong pressure.

Moxibustion
Cones: 3–5. Pole: 5–10 minutes. Rice-grain moxa is also applicable.

Magnets
Apply opposite poles on the left and right. To treat severe dyspnoea use alternating poles on Kd-25, Lu-1 and Bl-13 (also add LI-4 and other Lung channel points, depending on the case).

Actions and indications
Kd-27 is an important point to treat disorders of the upper thorax and respiratory tract. It is particularly indicated for tightness and constriction of the chest and throat, sore or swollen throat, goitre, cough, dyspnoea and asthma.

It has also been traditionally employed to harmonise the Stomach, descend rebellious qi and treat nausea, vomiting, lack of appetite and abdominal distension.

> **Main Areas:** Chest. Throat.
>
> **Main Functions:** Descends rebellious qi. Regulates qi.

Moxibustion
Cones: 3–5. Pole: 5–10 minutes. Use rice-grain moxa also.

Magnets
Apply opposite poles on the left and right. To treat severe dyspnoea alternate poles on Kd-25, Lu-1 and Bl-13 (also add LI-4 and other Lung points, depending on the case).

Actions and indications
Kd-25 is an important point to treat disorders of the chest and thorax, including rebellious qi. It is particularly indicated for tightness, pain and constriction of the chest, hiccup, palpitations, shortness of breath, chronic weak breathing, dyspnoea, asthma and cough.

Furthermore, Kd-25 harmonises the Kidneys, Lungs and Heart.

> **Main Areas:** Chest. Lungs. Heart.
>
> **Main Functions:** Benefits respiration. Regulates chest qi.

Chapter 18

Points of the

Arm Jue Yin
Pericardium Channel

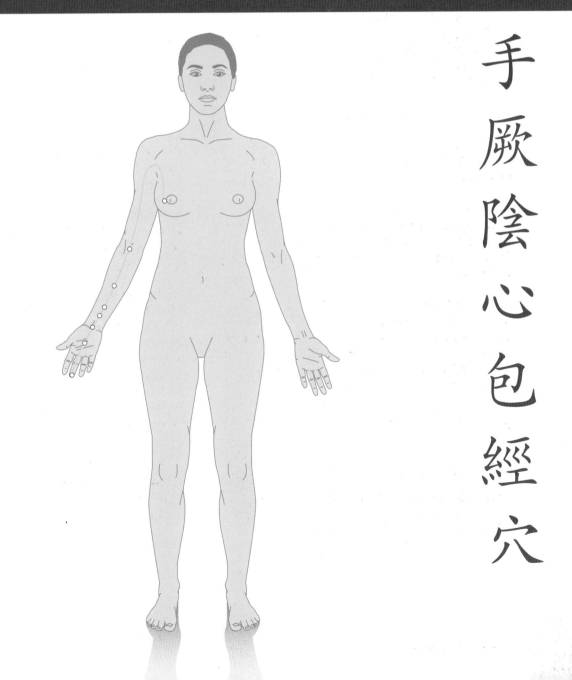

手厥陰心包經穴

P-1   Tianchi

天池

Heavenly Pool

Approximately 1 cun lateral and superior to the nipple, in the fourth intercostal space.

Best treatment positions
P-1 is best treated with the patient in a supine position.

! This location is often very sensitive and treatment should be applied carefully.

Needling
• 0.2 to 0.5 cun oblique supralateral insertion.

! Do not puncture the mammary glands. Also, avoid the thoracoepigastric vein and branches of the lateral thoracic artery and vein, and branches of the anterior thoracic nerve; more deeply, the fourth intercostal artery, vein and nerve.

Moxibustion
Pole: 5–10 minutes. Light stimulation only.

! Direct moxibustion is not recommended.

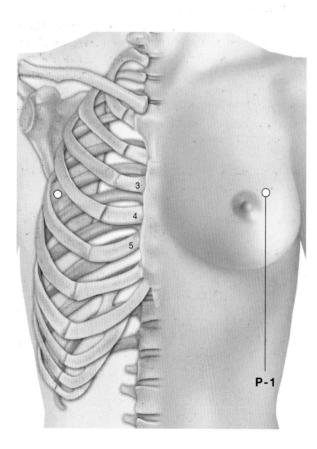

P-1

Manual techniques and shiatsu
Carefully applied stationary perpendicular pressure and friction techniques are applicable to the intercostal space, under the mammary glands. Deep friction of the intercostal muscles can be effective to unbind the chest.

! Do not apply pressure onto the mammary glands and note that they are also present in males. In cases of inflamed glands or painful lumps, do not apply pressure directly to the affected area. Do not apply strong pressure to the ribs.

An effective technique is to support the medial portion of the breast with the palm of one hand, while using the fingertips of the other hand to apply gentle friction and pressure under the glands.

P-1 can't be accessed easily if there is enlargement of the mammary glands. In such cases, work the area supralateral to it.

If there is great swelling or pain of the mammary glands, apply the following technique: in a supine position, with the palm of one hand, press the head of humerus toward the floor, so that the shoulder girdle moves posteriorly to stretch and open P-1 and the surrounding pectoral and breast area.

These techniques can also be applied in a side-lying position.

Stimulation sensation
Localised ache, distension, tingling or numbness spreading into the breast and chest or upward toward the shoulder.

Actions and indications
P-1 is used to treat *disorders of the breasts and chest*, particularly when there is *qi and Blood stagnation* or *phlegm* accumulation. Symptoms include pain, swelling and palpable masses in the breast, insufficient lactation, axillary swelling or nodules, swollen glands, pain and difficulty lifting the arm, intercostal pain, heart pain and fullness of the chest.

It has also be employed to treat coughing, dyspnoea, palpitations, angina pectoris, headaches and blurred vision.

Main Areas: Breast. Chest. Ribs. Heart.

Main Functions: Regulates qi. Dispels stasis and unbinds the chest. Benefits the breast.

P-3   Quze

曲澤

Marsh at the Bend

Uniting Sea-*He*, Water point

On the transverse cubital crease in the depression on the medial (ulnar) side of the tendon of the biceps brachii muscle.

To aid location, flex the elbow to define the biceps brachii tendon.

Best treatment positions
P-3 is best treated with the patient in a supine position with the arm abducted and elbow flexed (the forearm should be supported with cushions).

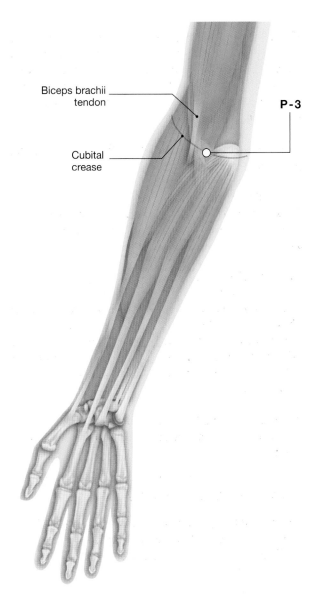

Biceps brachii tendon

P-3

Cubital crease

Needling
• 0.5 to 1 cun perpendicular insertion.
• Prick to bleed.

! Do not puncture the basilic vein and its branches or the branches of the medial antebrachial cutaneous nerve; in its deep position, the brachial artery and vein, and the median nerve.

Moxibustion
Cones: 1–5. Pole: 5–15 minutes. Light stimulation only.

Manual techniques and shiatsu
Stationary pressure and friction techniques are best applied with the fingertips or thumbs. Also apply pressure while simultaneously closing the forearm (flex the elbow) with the other hand.

Open P-3 by stretching the anterior aspect of the elbow: with one palm pressing the upper arm (above the elbow), and the other the forearm (below the elbow); apply pressure for one to five minutes.

Stimulation sensation
Localised ache and distension extending into the elbow. Also, tingling or electricity giving way to numbness is often perceived extending down the forearm toward the fingers.

Actions and indications
P-3 is a powerful point to *clear heat* and *cool Blood, dispel stasis, open the chest, descend rebellious qi* and *harmonise the middle jiao.* Indications include fullness or pain of the chest, palpitations, tachycardia, arrhythmia, dyspnoea, cough, nausea, vomiting, epigastric pain, haemoptysis, skin rashes, insomnia, headache, thirst, excessive menstrual bleeding, convulsions, fevers, heat stroke and febrile diseases.

As a *local point*, P-3 can be used to treat pain, stiffness and impaired mobility of the arm and elbow.

Note: P-3 seems to reflect Bl-40 on the upper limb because it has a similar anatomical location and also shares some of the same functions.

> **Main Areas:** Chest. Heart. Stomach. Elbow.
>
> **Main Functions:** Clears heat. Dispels stasis. Descends rebellious qi.

P-4 Ximen

郄門

Cleft Gate

Accumulation Cleft-*Xi* point

On the anterior aspect of the forearm, 5 cun proximal to the transverse wrist crease, in the depression between the tendons of the palmaris longus and flexor carpi radialis muscles, on the line joining P-7 with P-3.

To aid location, if the palmaris longus is absent, locate P-4 on the ulnar side of the flexor carpi radialis tendon.

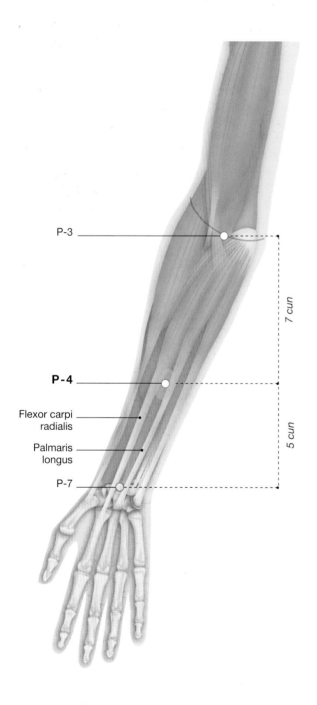

P-3

P-4

Flexor carpi radialis

Palmaris longus

P-7

7 cun

5 cun

Best treatment positions
Similar to P-6. However, both pressure and needling can be applied slightly more deeply.

Moxibustion
Cones: 5–7. Pole: 5–20 minutes.

Cupping
Small or medium sized cups can be effective.

Stimulation sensation
Localised ache, distension, tingling or numbness spreading up the forearm toward the elbow, shoulder and chest. Often an electric sensation is felt radiating down the forearm toward the fingers.

! P-4, P-5 and P-6 can engender particularly strong sensations. Do not overstimulate in cases of qi deficiency or psycho-emotional imbalance.

Actions and indications
P-4 is the Accumulation Xi point of the Pericardium channel and as such, *cools the Blood, dispels stasis* and *alleviates pain.* Furthermore, it *regulates Heart qi* and *calms the mind.*

It is widely employed in such cases as acute or chronic chest or cardiac pain, angina pectoris, arrhythmia, palpitations, vomiting, skin diseases due to heat and Blood stasis, epistaxis, coughing blood, insomnia, fear, fright or depression due to weakness of the heart qi, and pain.

As *a local point,* P-4 is useful in cases of pain, stiffness or hypertonicity of the forearm and impaired mobility of the wrist and fingers.

> **Main Areas:** Heart. Mind. Forearm.
>
> **Main Functions:** Cools Blood. Dispels stasis. Regulates Heart qi. Calms the mind.

P-5   Jianshi

間使

Intermediary Messenger

River-*Jing* Metal point

On the anterior aspect of the forearm, 3 cun proximal to P-7, between the tendons of the palmaris longus and flexor carpi radialis muscle, on the line joining P-7 with P-3.

To aid location, it is one quarter of the distance between the transverse wrist crease at P-7 and the cubital crease at P-3.

If the palmaris longus is absent, locate P-5 on the ulnar side of the flexor carpi radialis tendon.

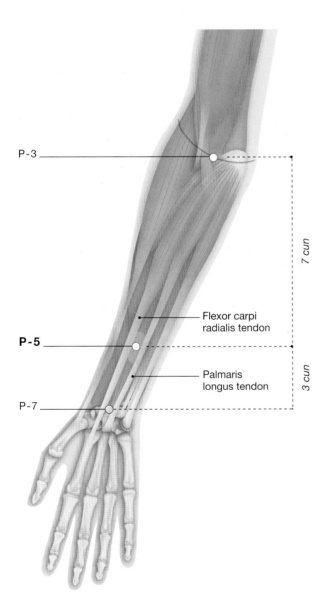

P-3

P-5

P-7

Flexor carpi radialis tendon

Palmaris longus tendon

7 cun

3 cun

Best treatment positions

Similar to P-6. However, both pressure and needling can be applied slightly more deeply here.

Actions and indications

P-5 is a major point to *regulate chest qi, resolve phlegm, clear heat, cool Blood* and *calm the mind*. Similar to other Pericardium points, it also *descends rebellious qi and harmonises the Stomach*.

P-5 is widely used in such cases as chest pain, palpitations, cough, stomach ache, vomiting, malaria, tidal fever, convulsions, epilepsy, insomnia, tongue ulcers, psychosis and hysteria.

P-5 has also been used to *regulate menstruation* in cases of dysmenorrhoea, irregular cycle, retention of the lochia and leucorrhoea.

As *a local point*, P-5 is useful to treat pain and stiffness of the forearm, wrist and fingers.

Main Areas: Chest. Wrist. Heart. Stomach.

Main Functions: Regulates chest qi. Resolves phlegm. Calms the mind. Descends rebellious qi.

P-6   Neiguan

內關

Inner Gate

Connecting *Luo* point
Opening (Master) point of the Yin Wei Mai
Command point for the chest

2 cun proximal to the transverse wrist crease, between the tendons of the palmaris longus and flexor carpi radialis muscle.

To aid location, P-6 is located opposite SJ-5. If the palmaris longus is absent, locate P-6 on the ulnar side of the flexor carpi radialis tendon.

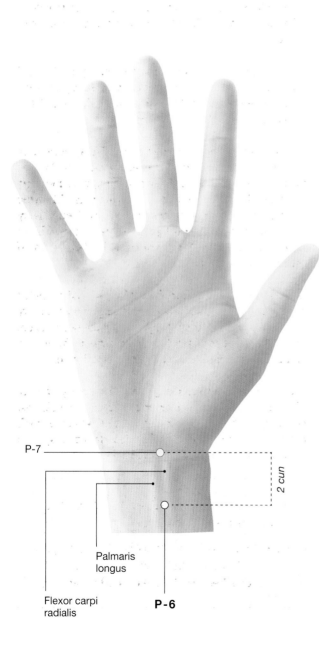

P-7

Palmaris longus

Flexor carpi radialis

P-6

2 cun

Needling
- 0.2 to 0.5 cun perpendicular insertion.
- 1 to 1.5 cun perpendicular insertion to join with SJ-5 on the posterior aspect of the forearm.
- 0.3 to 1.5 cun oblique insertion distally or proximally along the channel, depending on the area to be treated (deqi sensation should vary accordingly).

If the tendons are very tight or if there are visible vessels at the superficial location of P-6, insert the needle on the medial (ulnar) side of the tendon of flexor carpi radialis, so that the tip passes under the tendon to reach P-6.

Note: often, particularly with very 'sensitive', thin or 'tight' patients, deqi is achieved during initial insertion (the tip of the needle reaches only the subcutaneous layer). In this case, further manipulation should not be employed.

In such cases, consider subcutaneous needling only (lift the skin to insert needle transversely). If the patient is very sensitive, pricking the skin lightly with the needle tip is adequate.

! Do not puncture the cutaneous palmar branch of the median nerve or other superficial branches of the medial and lateral antebrachial cutaneous nerves (inspect the skin carefully before inserting the needle because in some cases a cutaneous nerve lies just under the skin at this location). If a strong electric sensation is felt on initial needle insertion at very superficial needling depths (as little as 0.2 cun), it means that the needle tip may be touching a nerve. If the sensation is very strong, remove needle and do not manipulate the needle. Also in many cases, a cutaneous vein lies superficial to this point. Move the vein aside with the finger before needling or choose to needle from the side.

When inserting deeper, do not puncture the median nerve, and deeper still, the anterior antebrachial interosseous nerve.

!! P-6 can be very painful and engender an electric deqi sensation. This means the needle tip may be touching the nerve(s) deep to the point. Do not manipulate strongly.

Manual techniques and shiatsu
Stationary perpendicular pressure applied gently and gradually with the pads or tips of the finger or thumbs is most effective. Connect P-6 to SJ-5 by pressing and squeezing both sides of the forearm simultaneously. Careful friction of the tendons is also applicable.

Furthermore, the P-6 area can be opened by stretching the palm backwards (extension of the wrist).

Moxibustion
Cones: 3–5. Pole: 5–15 minutes. Light stimulation only. Rice-grain moxibustion is also effectively employed.

Magnets
Magnets are also effectively employed. To activate the Yin Wei Mai and Chong Mai, use opposite poles on P-6 and contralateral Sp-4. For diseases of the chest, use opposite poles on Ren-17 and P-6. For carpal tunnel syndrome, use P-6, P-7 and SJ-4 or SJ-5.

Guasha
Effective up and down the channel or lightly across the tendons and muscle fibres.

Stimulation sensation
Regional aching, distension, warmth, tingling and electricity often giving way to numbness and often extending up or down the channel. The sensation can be exceptionally strong and reach the throat and chest area. Often electricity is felt down the forearm toward the fingers.

Deqi at P-6 can cause sighing, coughing or emotional outburst such as sadness, crying or irascibility. Furthermore, the pulse should feel more smooth and regular and the heart rate should decrease.

! P-4, P-5 and P-6 can engender particularly strong sensations. Do not stimulate excessively in cases of qi deficiency or emotional imbalance.

Actions and indications
P-6 *is a very important point* used in a wide variety of conditions. It *regulates the circulation of qi and Blood throughout the three Jiao, dispels stasis of qi, Blood and phlegm, clears heat and has a particularly powerful effect on relaxing the chest*. Furthermore, it has a nourishing effect on the Blood and yin. All these functions are intimately connected to the *Yin Wei Mai* and Pericardium *Luo Connecting channel* which are activated by treatment at P-6.

Indications include pain, fullness and constriction of the chest, cough, plum stone throat, pain or swelling of the throat, goitre, lymphadenopathy, palpitations, arrhythmia, chest or heart pain, dyspnoea, swollen painful throat, phlegm nodules, fever, headache or migraine, hypochondrial and abdominal pain, fever, headache and neck pain.

Needling P-6 has been shown to *relax the coronary arteries* and increase blood supply to the myocardium. It has also been needled for *first aid following or during myocardial infarction*, and has been shown to minimize damage to the myocardium.

P-6 effectively *descends rebellious qi* and *harmonises the Stomach and middle jiao*. It is an extremely important and widely used point in the treatment of epigastric pain, acid reflux, heartburn, hiccup, oesophagitis, gastritis, nausea, vomiting, morning sickness during pregnancy and other digestive disorders.

Furthermore, P-6 is *extremely important to calm the mind* in the treatment of *emotional and psychosomatic complaints* such as insomnia, anxiety, irritability, emotional upset, propensity to crying, mood swings and depression.

It is particularly indicated for women with emotionally related *gynaecological complaints* such as premenstrual syndrome, breast pain, fibrocystic breast disease, mastitis, breast abscess, dysmenorrhoea, irregular menstruation, oligomenorrhoea, infertility and postpartum dizziness or depression.

P-6 also has an *analgesic effect*, and thus it can be used for *post-operative pain* and *pain caused by injury*. Also it can be used in anaesthesia (in conjunction with LI-4, Liv-3 and ear points).

It is also very effective to *open the orifices, resuscitate consciousness* and *clear the mind* in cases of lack of mental concentration, mental exhaustion, poor memory, amnesia, dizziness, vertigo and symptoms following wind stroke. Gentle moxibustion here will effectively warm and revive the Heart yang and is indicated in all conditions of *Heart Yang deficiency leading to Blood stasis or yang collapse*.

It is very important as a *local point* for pain and restricted movement of the forearm, wrist and fingers, particularly if there is hypertonicity and tightness of the wrist flexors due to qi and Blood stasis along the channel pathway. It is particularly indicated for carpal tunnel syndrome.

P-6 has also been traditionally used for a variety of other disorders including tidal fevers, malaria, convulsions, coughing, spitting or vomiting blood, blood in the stool, prolapse of the rectum, jaundice, dysuria, epilepsy, loss of consciousness, coma and even madness.

Main Areas: Chest. Heart. Mind. Stomach. Wrist. Forearm. Neck.

Main Functions: Regulates qi and Blood. Dispels stasis. Relaxes the chest. Calms the mind. Descends rebellious qi. Harmonises the Stomach.

P-7　Daling

大陵

Great Mound

Stream-*Shu* Earth (Sedation) point
Source-*Yuan* point

In the depression in the middle of the transverse wrist crease between the tendons of palmaris longus and flexor carpi radialis. Approximately midway between He-7 and Lu-9.

If the palmaris longus is absent, locate this point on the ulnar side of the flexor carpi radialis tendon.

Needling
• 0.3 to 0.5 cun perpendicular insertion.
• 0.5 to 1 cun oblique distal insertion into the carpal tunnel.

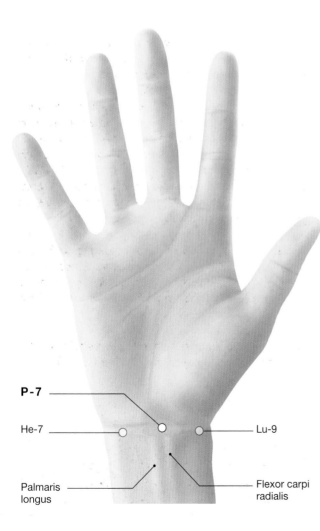

P-7

He-7

Lu-9

Palmaris longus

Flexor carpi radialis

! Superficially, do not puncture the palmar branch of the median nerve or the medial cutaneous antebrachial nerve; more deeply, do not puncture the median nerve.

P-7 can be very painful and engender electric deqi sensation. This means that the needle tip may be touching the median nerve deep to the point. Do not manipulate strongly.

Manual techniques and shiatsu
Extend the wrist slightly to expose the point.

Moxibustion
Cones: 2–4. Pole: 5–10 minutes.

Stimulation sensation
Ache, distension, tingling, electricity or numbness locally and commonly spreading down the channel toward the fingers.

Deqi at P-7 can cause sighing, coughing or emotional outbursts, in common with P-6.

Actions and indications
Although P-7 was traditionally considered to be the Source-Yuan point of the Heart, and have similar functions to He-7, it is not as commonly used as the latter.

It is, however, effective to *regulate qi and Blood, cool the Heart, open the chest and calm the mind.* Furthermore, it *descends rebellious qi and harmonises the Stomach.*

Indications include pain and tightness of the chest, angina pectoris, palpitations, arrhythmia, tachycardia, fever, epigastric pain, nausea, vomiting, gastritis, epilepsy, depression, emotional upset, anxiety and panic attacks.

As a *local point*, it can be effective to treat carpal tunnel syndrome and pain or stiffness of the wrist.

Main Areas: Wrist. Chest. Heart. Stomach.

Main Functions: Regulates qi and Blood. Relaxes the chest. Calms the mind.
Descends rebellious qi.

P-8 Laogong

Palace of Toil

勞宮

Spring-*Ying* Fire (Horary) point
One of the nine points for Returning Yang

At the centre of the palm, in the depression between the second and third metacarpals, on the radial side of the third metacarpal.

To aid location, if the fist is clenched, P-8 is at the point where the tip of the middle finger touches the palm.

Some sources place P-9 on the ulnar side of the third metacarpal, below the tip of the ring finger when the fist is clenched.

Needling
• 0.3 to 0.5 cun perpendicular insertion.

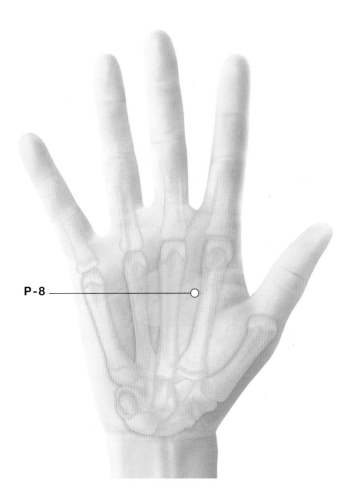

P-8

You may need to use slightly thicker needles if the palmar skin is thick or hard. In practice, needling P-8 is usually employed to treat channel disorders because it is usually very painful.

! Do not puncture the palmar digital artery and nerve.

Manual techniques and shiatsu
Friction and stationary perpendicular pressure may be applied with the thumbs or fingertips. The centre of the palm may also be stretched open to dissipate stagnation and clear heat.

Moxibustion
Cones: 3. Pole: 5–10 minutes.

Stimulation sensation
Ache, distension, tingling, electricity or numbness spreading across the palm toward the fingers.

! Deqi at P-8 can also cause sighing or emotional outbursts, in common with P-6 and P-7.

Actions and indications
P-8 *strongly clears heat and fire from the Heart, subdues wind, restores consciousness and calms the mind.* Furthermore, it *descends rebellious qi.*

It has been employed in a variety of disorders including excessive sweating, fever, loss of consciousness, wind stroke, convulsions, epilepsy, epistaxis, ulceration of the mouth and tongue, glossitis, swelling of the throat, nausea, gastritis, abdominal pain and hardness, halitosis, excessive thirst, blood in the stool, depression, mental agitation, delirium, palpitations, arrhythmia, angina pectoris and chest pain.

P-8 is also *extensively used in qigong* and Eastern bodywork methods as a point to focus and strengthen the qi, which then transmits to the patient during treatment. P-8 can be combined with Kd-1 for mental focus exercises.

As a *local point* P-8 can be used in cases of tendinitis, hypertonicity and injury of the soft tissues of the palm and fingers.

> **Main Areas:** Palm. Chest. Heart. Mind.
>
> **Main Functions:** Clears heat. Restores consciousness. Calms the mind. Descends rebellious qi. Focuses qi in qigong therapy.

P-9　Zhongchong　中衝

Central Surge

Well-*Jing*, Wood (Tonification) point

At the centre of the tip of the middle finger, approximately 0.1 cun distal to the end of the nail.

Alternative location
0.1 cun proximal to the corner of the nail on the radial side of the middle finger, at the intersection of two lines following the radial border of the nail and the base of the nail.

Additionally, it can be treated (by pressure) at both nail points: on the radial and on the ulnar side.

Best treatment positions
This point can be treated easily with the patient sitting or lying. A strong stimulation is most effective if applied regularly until symptoms subside.

Needling
• 0.1 to 0.3 cun perpendicular insertion.

P-9

Manual techniques and shiatsu
Pressure is applied onto the tip of the middle phalanx (flex the distal and middle phalanx). Alternatively, strongly press the points on both sides of the phalanx, level with the base of the nail.

Moxibustion
Cones: 1–2. Pole: 2–5 minutes. Rice-grain moxibustion can also be effectively employed.

First aid for syncope, shock, fainting or coma
If strong pressure with the fingers is not effective, use an object to tap the point (for example a pen or book). If tapping doesn't work, hit the point harder or prick to bleed. Furthermore, rice-grain moxa can be helpful.

Stimulation sensation
Regional distension, ache, tingling or numbness extending up the finger toward the hand. If strong stimulation is applied, deqi should reach the centre of the chest and heart and make the person sigh or breathe more deeply.

! P-9 has a *very powerful sedating effect*, and can cause excessive descent of qi (even to the extent of collapse of qi) if stimulated too strongly on qi-deficient patients. This happens reasonably often following injury to the middle finger (for example, when the finger is trapped in a closing door).

Actions and indications
P-9 has comparable functions to the other Well-Jing points including *clearing heat, sedating interior wind, opening the orifices and restoring consciousness*. It is, however, considered more powerful, and the qi here is seen to be surging rather than still and small like a 'Well'. Anatomically, the middle finger is the strongest of the four fingers and the flesh at the tip is deeper at the corners of the nails than at the other Well-Jing points.

Thus, P-9 is one of the strongest points to *restore consciousness* and *stimulate the Heart* in cases of loss of consciousness, syncope, coma, shock, convulsions, fever and delirium.

Because of its powerful effect as a *Heart tonic,* P-9 is used in *qi gong therapy*, similarly to P-8, to project qi for healing or martial applications.

Main Areas: Heart. Mind.

Main Functions: Restores consciousness. Opens the orifices. Opens the chest.

Chapter 19

Points of the

Arm Shao Yang
Sanjiao (Triple Burner) Channel

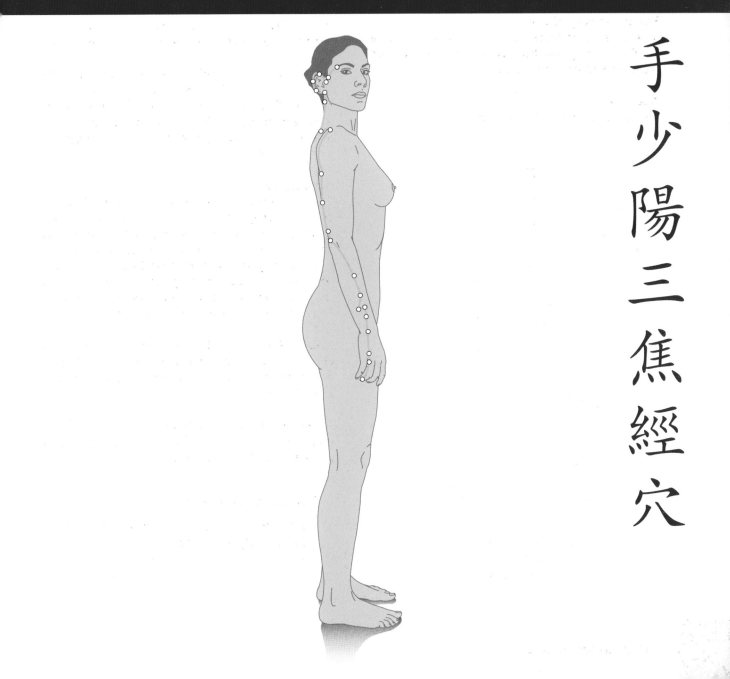

手少陽三焦經穴

SJ-1 Guanchong 關衝
Surge Gate

Well-*Jing*, Metal point

On the ulnar side of the fourth (ring) finger, 0.1 cun proximal to the corner of the nail. At the intersection of two lines following the ulnar border of the nail and the base of the nail.

Best treatment positions
This point can be treated with the patient lying down or sitting up.

Needling
• 0.1 cun perpendicular insertion.

Manual techniques and shiatsu
Friction or sustained pressure may be applied quite strongly with the thumb or fingertip until symptoms subside.

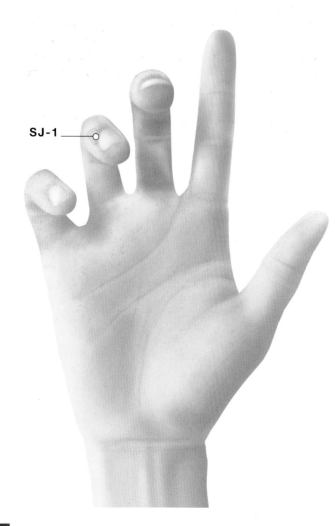

SJ-1

Moxibustion
Cones: 1–3. Pole: 5–10 minutes.

Stimulation sensation
Aching, tingling or pain may be experienced around the point. However, a stronger sensation reaching the chest can be obtained during stimulation of the Well-Jing points.

Actions and indications
SJ-1 is mainly used to *clear exterior heat and wind* causing symptoms such as earache and sore throat. Similarly to other Well-Jing points, SJ-1 will help *restore consciousness* in cases of coma or fainting. Additionally it opens the *Sanjiao sinew channel and treats pain* along the channel pathway.

> **Main Areas:** Mind. Ears. Sanjiao channel.
>
> **Main Functions:** Clears heat. Benefits the ears. Resuscitates consciousness.

SJ-2 Yemen 液門
Fluid Gate

Spring-*Ying*, Water point

0.5 cun proximal to the margin of the web between the fourth and fifth fingers, distal to the metacarpophalangeal joint.

Treatment and applications
Similar to SJ-3. However, SJ-2 is more effective to *clear heat and wind*, whereas SJ-3 can be used to tonify the ears as well.

> **Main Areas:** Mind. Ears. Sanjiao channel.
>
> **Main Functions:** Clears heat. Benefits the ears. Resuscitates consciousness.

SJ-3 Zhongzhu

中渚

Central Islet

Stream-*Shu* Wood (Tonification) point

On the dorsum of the hand, in the depression proximal to the metacarpophalangeal joints between the fourth and fifth metacarpal bones. To aid location, the patient should make a loose fist.

Best treatment positions

This point is best treated with the patient lying supine, with the elbow flexed and the palm facing downward.

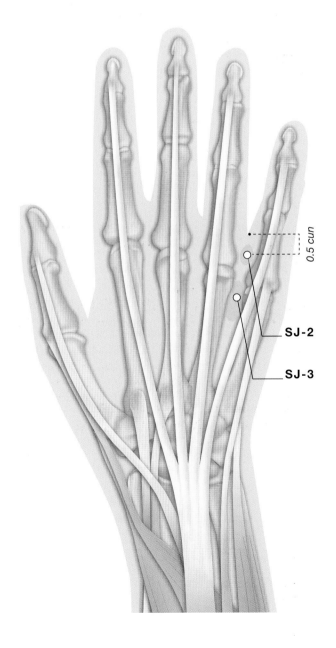

0.5 cun

SJ-2

SJ-3

Needling

• 0.3 to 0.5 cun perpendicular insertion or join to He-8.
• 0.5 to 1.5 cun oblique insertion directed toward the wrist.

! Do not puncture the dorsal digital artery, vein or nerve.

Moxibustion

Cones: 2–3. Pole: 5–10 minutes.

Magnets

Application of a small magnet can be effective.

Manual techniques and shiatsu

Sustained pressure and friction techniques are very effective applied into the channel area between the metacarpal bones and joints.

Stimulation sensation

Local ache, distension, tingling or numbness sometimes extending upward toward the forearm or an electric sensation reaching the fingertips.

Actions and indications

Both SJ-2 and SJ-3 are useful points to *dispel wind, clear heat and fire, regulate qi and Blood* and *dispel stasis,* particularly from the *head* and *ears.* Common indications include ear infections, tinnitus, deafness, inflammation of the eyes and headache.

SJ-2 and SJ-3 can also be used for *regional disorders,* including pain or stiffness of the fingers, elbow and arm.

Main Areas: Metacarpophalangeal joints. Sanjiao channel. Ears.

Main Functions: Clears heat. Benefits the ears. Regulates qi and Blood. Alleviates pain.

SJ-4 Yangchi

陽池

Yang Pool

Source-*Yuan* point

On the dorsum of the wrist between the ulna and carpal bones, in the depression between the tendons of extensor digitorum communis and extensor digiti minimi.

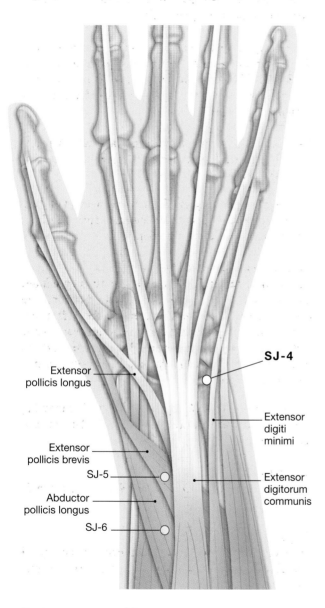

Extensor pollicis longus

Extensor pollicis brevis

SJ-5

Abductor pollicis longus

SJ-6

SJ-4

Extensor digiti minimi

Extensor digitorum communis

Best treatment positions

SJ-4 is best treated with the patient lying in a supine position, with the elbow flexed and the palm facing downward upon the abdomen.

Needling

• 0.3 to 0.5 cun perpendicular insertion between the junction of the triquetral and lunate with the ulna.

• 0.5 to 1 cun transverse insertion radially, under the tendon sheath.

! Do not puncture the cutaneous veins and arteries of the dorsal carpal network, the dorsal branch of the ulnar nerve or the posterior antebrachial cutaneous nerve; more deeply the posterior branch of the anterior interosseous artery and posterior interosseous nerve.

Manual techniques and shiatsu

Sustained perpendicular pressure is best applied into the wrist joint space between the triquetral bone and ulna with the fingertip or thumb. Extending the patient's wrist simultaneously enables a deeper pressure into the joint space. Friction techniques are very effective applied across the fibres of the extensor tendons crossing the wrist. Additionally, stretch and open this point by flexing the wrist and gently mobilising the wrist joint.

Moxibustion

Cones: 3–5. Pole: 5–15 minutes. Rice-grain moxa is also effective.

Magnets

Use opposite poles on SJ-4, SJ-5 and P-7 for disorders of the wrist.

Stimulation sensation

Local ache, distension, tingling or numbness extending into the wrist joint and possibly distally toward the fingers, or proximally along the channel.

Actions and indications

Although SJ-4 is the Yuan Source point of the Sanjiao channel, in clinical practice it is primarily used to treat *regional disorders, particularly of the wrist.* It is particularly effective for pain, restricted movement or swelling of the wrist, hand and arm. Additionally, it *clears exterior and interior heat* and treats *inflammation of the ears, eyes and throat* including tonsillitis, otitis, fever and thirst.

Furthermore, SJ-4 has been *extensively employed to tonify the Yuan qi* and *augment the qi of the entire body*, particularly in Japanese acupuncture traditions.

It is also considered to *reinforce the Penetrating Vessel and Kidney* and improve *fluid transformation*. Indications include chronic tiredness, weakness and exhaustion, wasting syndromes, infertility, amenorrhoea, profuse urination, anuria, fluid retention and oedema.

Main Areas: Wrist. Sanjiao channel. Ears.

Main Functions: Tonifies Yuan qi.
Regulates the Sanjiao.

SJ-5 Waiguan

外關

Outer Gate

Connecting *Luo* point
Opening (Master) point of the Yang Wei Mai

Between the radius and ulna, 2 cun above SJ-4, on the radial edge of the extensor digitorum communis tendon, close to the radial border. Situated in the extensor pollicis brevis muscle.

To aid location, it is approximately 3 finger-widths proximal to the transverse wrist crease.

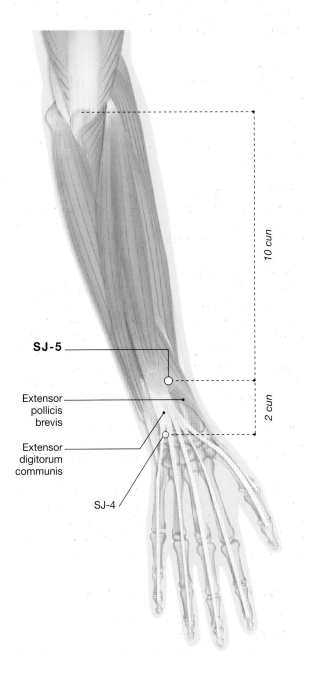

SJ-5

Extensor pollicis brevis

Extensor digitorum communis

SJ-4

10 cun

2 cun

Best treatment positions
SJ-5 is best treated with the patient lying in a supine position, with the elbow flexed and the palm facing downward, so that the radius and ulna are parallel.

Needling
• 0.3 to 1.5 cun perpendicular insertion as far as P-6 on the anterior aspect of the forearm.
• 0.5 to 2 cun oblique insertion distally or proximally along the channel, depending on the area to be treated (sensation should vary accordingly).

Often deqi is achieved during initial insertion with the needle tip reaching only the subcutaneous layer, particularly if there is a lot of tension in this area. It is thus unnecessary to stimulate any further until the sensation disappears.

! Do not puncture the posterior antebrachial cutaneous nerve, or the posterior and anterior interosseous nerves; more deeply the median nerve.

This point can be very painful and engender an electric deqi sensation. This means the needle tip may be touching any of the nerves deep to the point.

Manual techniques and shiatsu
Sustained perpendicular pressure and friction techniques are very effective applied across the fibres of the extensor muscles in the area between the radius and ulna (superficially, the extensor digitorum communis, and more deeply the extensor pollicis longus and the extensor indicis). Additionally, stretch and open this area by flexing the wrist.

Connect SJ-5 to P-6 by pressing and squeezing the anterior and posterior aspects of the forearm simultaneously.

Moxibustion
Cones: 3–5. Pole: 5–15 minutes. Rice-grain moxa is also effective.

Cupping
Small cups with reasonably strong suction can be applied topically and moved up and down the forearm (use ample lubricant).

Guasha
Effective up and down the channel or across the muscle fibres.

Magnets
Magnets are also effectively employed at this location. Use opposite poles on SJ-5, P-6 and GB-41.

Stimulation sensation

A strong aching sensation should be felt deep in the muscles of the forearm radiating up and/or down the arm. Also, electricity giving way to numbness may be perceived downward toward the fingers.

Actions and indications

SJ-5 is one of the *most important and commonly used points*. Its primary functions are to *release the exterior, dispel wind, clear heat, dissipate qi stagnation and smooth the Liver*. Furthermore, it is extensively employed to *descend excessive yang, clear the head, sharpen eyesight and hearing and regulate the Yang Wei Mai.*

Indications include fever with or without chills due to febrile diseases or qi stagnation, upper respiratory tract infections, colds and flu, sore throat, headache, migraine, tinnitus, deafness, pain and inflammation of the ears or eyes, epistaxis, toothache, hypertension, dizziness and hemiplegia.

SJ-5 also successfully treats other manifestations of *Liver qi stagnation* including irritability, mood swings, depression, hypochondrial distension or pain, vomiting, epigastric pain, abdominal distension and pain, and constipation.

SJ-5 is also *important in the treatment of channel disorders* and is indicated in such cases as atrophy, paralysis, stiffness and pain of the arm, wrist, shoulder and neck.

> **Main Areas:** Lungs. Liver. Ears. Head. Eyes. Forearm and wrist. Sanjiao channel.
>
> **Main Functions:** Releases the exterior and dispels wind. Dispels stasis and smooths the Liver. Clears interior and exterior heat. Descends excessive yang. Alleviates pain.

SJ-6 Zhigou

Branch Ditch

支溝

River-*Jing*, Fire (Horary) point

In the depression 3 cun proximal to SJ-4, between the radial side of the extensor digitorum communis muscle and the radius. Situated in the abductor pollicis longus muscle.

To aid location, SJ-6 is approximately one hand-breadth proximal to SJ-4. One quarter of the distance between SJ-4 and the lateral epicondyle of the humerus or the tip of the olecranon process.

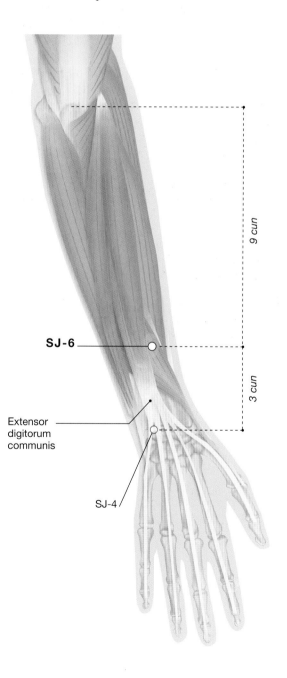

SJ-6

9 cun

3 cun

Extensor digitorum communis

SJ-4

Best treatment positions
Similar to SJ-5.

Actions and indications
SJ-6 is *widely used to clear heat, dissipate stagnation and smooth the flow of qi in all three Jiao,* although it is particularly indicated for *disorders of the chest, sides and abdomen.*

In the Lower Jiao it *purges the Large Intestine* and is commonly used for acute and chronic constipation with abdominal pain. Furthermore, it can be helpful for gynaecological pain.

In the Middle Jiao it *smoothes the flow of Liver qi* and treats symptoms of stagnation including fullness, distension and pain of the epigastrium, abdomen, hypochondrium and chest, nausea and vomiting, oppression and heaviness of the chest.

In the Upper Jiao it unblocks the channel pathway and releases *exterior heat and wind,* treating pain and inflammation of the throat, ear, eye, arm, axilla, and skin; including tinnitus and deafness, headache, redness of the eyes, sudden loss of voice, herpes zoster, intercostal neuralgia, urticaria and other skin diseases.

As a *local point,* SJ-6 can be successfully employed in the treatment of pain, tightness or atrophy of the forearm and wrist.

> **Main Areas:** Chest. Sides. Abdomen.
> Large intestine. Ears. Throat.
>
> **Main Functions:** Clears heat. Dispels stasis.
> Releases the exterior.

SJ-7 Huizong

Convergence and Gathering

Accumulation Cleft-*Xi* point

3 cun proximal to SJ-4, about one finger's breadth to SJ-6, on the radial side of the ulna. In the depression between the extensor digitorum communis muscle and the ulna.

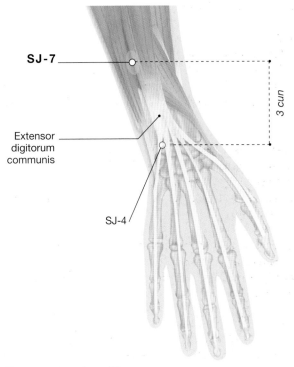

SJ-7

Extensor digitorum communis

SJ-4

3 cun

Best treatment positions
Similar to SJ-5.

Actions and indications
SJ-7 is the Accumulation Xi point of the Sanjiao and is useful to *clear the channel pathway and alleviate pain,* particularly in the shoulder, arm, forearm and wrist. It is also useful for *disorders of the ears* such as tinnitus and deafness.

Furthermore, it has been traditionally used to treat a wide range of other disorders including fevers, dizziness, blurred vision, epilepsy, fright and even madness.

> **Main Areas:** Upper limb. Ears.
>
> **Main Functions:** Dispels stasis and alleviates pain. Clears heat.

SJ-10 Tianjing 天井

Heavenly Well

Sea Uniting *He*, Earth (Sedation) point

On the elbow, in the depression of the olecranon fossa, approximately 1 cun proximal to the tip of the olecranon process when the elbow is flexed.

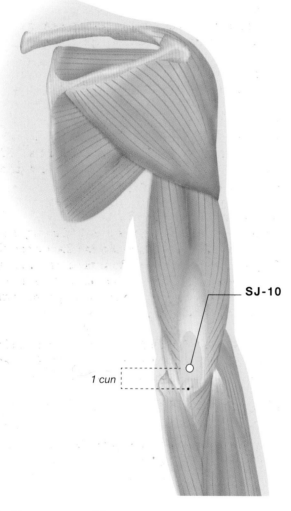

SJ-10

1 cun

Best treatment positions
SJ-10 is best treated with the elbow flexed.

Needling
• 0.5 to 1 cun perpendicular insertion.

Manual techniques and shiatsu
Pressure should be applied perpendicularly to the olecranon fossa, with the elbow flexed. Friction of the triceps tendons is also effective. Pressure and/or friction should be continued up the channel through SJ-11, SJ-12 and SJ-13.

Moxibustion
Cones: 2–3. Pole: 5–15 minutes. Rice-grain moxibustion is also applicable.

Cupping
Use small cups with reasonably strong suction.

Guasha
Effective across triceps brachii fibres and around olecranon process.

Stimulation sensation
A numb aching sensation is often perceived going deep into the elbow and up the arm, toward the shoulder.

Actions and indications
SJ-10 is primarily used to *activate qi and Blood circulation and dispel wind and dampness from the Sanjiao channel.* Symptoms include pain and stiffness of the elbow, arm and shoulder and difficulty in flexing or extending the elbow.

However, it has been traditionally used to *transform phlegm and dissipate stagnation, descend rebellious qi and calm the mind.* Symptoms include nodular swellings in the neck, goitre, productive cough, coughing blood, sore throat, headache, deafness, chest or flank pain, heart pain, chills and fever, malaria, urticaria, epilepsy and even madness.

> **Main Areas:** Elbow. Arm. Sanjiao channel.
>
> **Main Functions:** Regulates qi and Blood. Alleviates pain and swelling.

SJ-14 Jianliao 肩髎

Shoulder Bone Hole

On the posterolateral aspect of the shoulder, in the anterior of the two distinct depressions between the anterior and middle belly of the deltoid muscle. Between the acromion and the greater tubercle of the humerus.

To define the depressions, ask the patient to lift (abduct) the arm. Use resistance if necessary.

To aid location, SJ-I4 is directly posterior to LI-15.

Best treatment positions
SJ-14 is mostly treated with the arm down by the sides of the body, although it can also be needled with the arm abducted (raised).

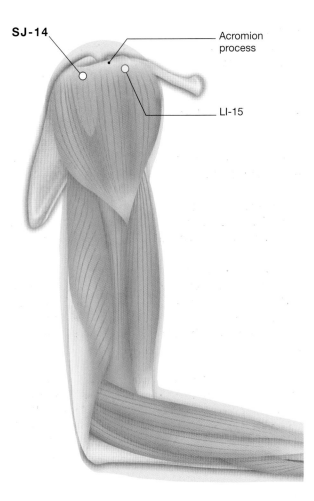

SJ-14

Acromion process

LI-15

Needling

- With the arm down by the side, 0.5 to 1 cun perpendicular insertion. The needle should enter the space between the subacromial bursa and the acromion process.
- With the arm down by the side, 0.5 to 2 cun oblique or transverse insertion distally along the channel, between the anterior and medial fibres of the deltoid.
- With the arm abducted (raised), 1 to 3 cun perpendicular insertion directed toward He-1 at the centre of the axilla.
- With the arm abducted (raised), 0.5 to 2 cun transverse-oblique insertion into the deltoid fibres directed distally down the arm.
- Anterior transverse insertion to join with LI-15.

Manual techniques and shiatsu

Sustained perpendicular pressure and friction techniques may be applied into the space between the acromion process and the tubercle of the humerus with the thumbs or fingertips. Friction distally along the channel between the posterior and middle fibres of the deltoid is also extremely effective. Shiatsu pressure can also be applied to the surrounding area with the forearms or elbows in a side-lying or sitting position.

Moxibustion

Cones: 3–5. Pole: 10–20 minutes. Moxa pole therapy is most effective when applied for 15 to 30 minutes simultaneously to other major points surrounding the shoulder (including LI-15, LI-16, GB-21, SI-12, SI-11 and M-UE-48 Jianqian).

Cupping

Small or medium cups may be used. Curved rim cups are best. Medium to strong suction is effective over needles or separately.

Guasha

Guasha is very effective around the entire shoulder joint, particularly in cases of stiffness and pain.

Magnets

Use opposite poles on SJ-14 and LI-15.

Stimulation sensation

Distension, aching, soreness or electricity extending to the areas being treated (commonly into the shoulder joint, up toward the neck and down the arm toward the elbow, forearm, hand and fingers).

Actions and indications

Similarly to LI-15, SJ-14 is *very useful for many types of shoulder and arm disorders* manifesting along the Sanjiao channel pathway. It effectively *treats weakness, pain and stiffness of the shoulder* particularly if there is difficulty in lifting the arm and moving it backward (abduction and extension).

It is particularly indicated for supraspinatus tendinitis, periarthritis of the shoulder, frozen shoulder and spasticity, atrophy or paralysis of the upper limb.

Main Area: Shoulder.

Main Functions: Regulates qi and Blood. Alleviates pain and stiffness.

SJ-15 Tianliao

天髎

Heavenly Bone Hole

Intersection of the Yang Wei Mai and Gallbladder on the Sanjiao channel

Approximately 1 cun posterior and slightly medial to GB-21, midway between GB-21 and SI-13.

To aid location, it is approximately 1 cun directly posterior to GB-21.

Best treatment positions
Similar to GB-21.

Needling
• 0.3 to 0.5 cun perpendicular insertion.

! Do not puncture cutaneous or deep branches of the suprascapular artery, vein or nerve. Also, the accessory nerve, and more deeply, the transverse cervical artery and vein.

Moxibustion
Cones: 2–3. Pole: 5–10 minutes.

Actions and indications
SJ-15 has *similar functions to GB-21*, albeit not as powerful. It helps *dispel wind and dampness, and moderates pain.* Additionally, it *relaxes the chest and regulates qi.*

It is primarily used *as a local point* in the treatment of pain and stiffness of the shoulder and back, and disorders of the cervical spine.

It has also been traditionally used for a variety of other symptoms including fullness, tightness or pain in the chest, chills and fever, insomnia and mental restlessness.

> **Main Areas:** Shoulder. Chest.
>
> **Main Functions:** Regulates qi and Blood. Alleviates pain and stiffness.

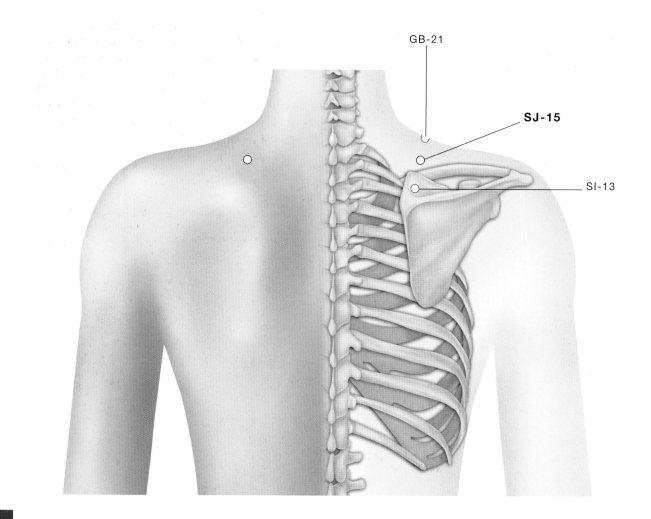

SJ-16 Tianyou

天牖

Window of Heaven

Window of Heaven point

On the posterior border of the sternocleidomastoid muscle, level with the angle of the mandible, posterior and approximately 1 cun inferior to the tip of the mastoid process.

To aid location, it is directly inferior to GB-12, level with SI-17 and Bl-10.

Best treatment positions
Similar to GB-12.

! Great care should be taken when working on the neck to avoid overstimulation or overstretching of this area.

Needling
• 0.3 to 1 cun oblique inferior insertion into the sternocleidomastoid fibres.
• 0.3 to 1 cun perpendicular insertion.

!! Do not insert deeper. Do not puncture branches of the lesser occipital or greater auricular nerve, and in its deep position, the deep cervical artery and vein.

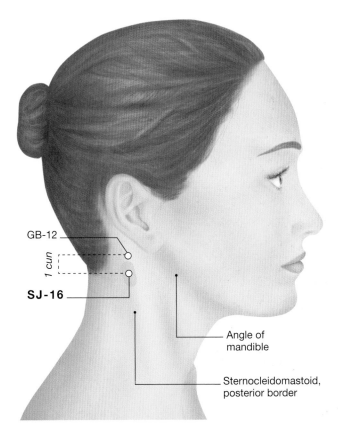

GB-12

1 cun

SJ-16

Angle of mandible

Sternocleidomastoid, posterior border

Manual techniques and shiatsu
It is most effective to apply stationary pressure and friction down the channel toward SJ-15 and to the entire sternocleidomastoid muscle. Also, apply pressure to SJ-17 simultaneously and grasp the sternocleidomastoid muscle belly.

Moxibustion
Pole: 5–15 minutes. Direct moxibustion is not recommended at this location.

! Do not use moxibustion in cases of lymphadenopathy.

Guasha
Guasha can be effectively applied across and down the sternocleidomastoid fibres.

! Warn the patient that bruising may occur.

Stimulation sensation
Localised distension and ache, tingling or numbness extending down the posterior aspect of the neck and along the channel pathway reaching the throat, face and ears.

Actions and indications
SJ-16 is an effective point for *disorders of the ears, neck and entire head*. It *activates qi and Blood circulation* in the channel, *dispels wind, clears heat, transforms dampness and phlegm and reduces swelling*. Indications include pain and inflammation of the ears and eyes, easy lacrimation, impaired hearing, deafness, tinnitus, nasal obstruction, sore throat, headache, dizziness, swelling of the face, phlegm nodules and swollen glands.

SJ-16 also treats *stiffness of the neck* with difficulty rotating and side-flexing the cervical spine.

Furthermore, it has been employed to treat a variety of other disorders including sudden deafness or loss of sight, loss of sense of smell, swelling of the breast, tidal fevers and mental confusion.

Main Areas: Throat and neck. Ears.

Main Functions: Regulates qi and Blood. Alleviates pain. Transforms dampness and reduces swelling. Dispels wind and clears heat.

SJ-17   Yifeng

翳風

Wind Screen

Intersection of the Gallbladder on the Sanjiao channel

Directly behind the ear lobe, at the centre of the deep depression formed between the mastoid process and the mandibular ramus.

To aid location, it is superior to the transverse process of the atlas.

Best treatment positions
This point is best treated with the patient in a supine, sitting or side-lying position.

Needling
• 0.5 to 1 cun perpendicular insertion.
• 1 to 1.5 cun oblique downward medial insertion.

! Do not needle deeper. Do not puncture jugular vein, carotid artery, facial nerve or other nerve branches lying in its deep location.

Manual techniques and shiatsu
Sustained pressure is best applied carefully with the fingers perpendicular to SJ-17. Additionally, pressure can be applied anteriorly onto the mandible and in a posterosuperior direction onto the mastoid process.

! This is a sensitive point, so do not overstimulate. Do not apply strong perpendicular pressure.

Moxibustion
Pole: 5–10 minutes. Direct moxibustion is not recommended.

! Do not apply moxibustion if there is acute inflammation of the ear.

Magnets
Magnets can also be used successfully at this location. Use opposite poles on SJ-16, SI-17 and SJ-3.

Stimulation sensation
Local ache, distension, tingling, numbness, sometimes extending to the throat, tongue, teeth and cheek and into the ear. It is normal that a slight sore feeling of the surrounding area may be felt for a couple of hours after strong stimulation has been applied.

Actions and indications
SJ-17 may be *the most important point for disorders of the ear* due to its powerful action of *clearing the channel pathway*, *dispelling stagnation, alleviating pain*, *clearing heat and dispelling wind of both exterior and interior origin.*

It is effectively used in a wide variety of conditions affecting the ear including tinnitus, diminished hearing, deafness, earache, acute or chronic otitis, itching, discharge and other inflammatory conditions of the ear.

Due to the fact that SJ-17 *subdues internal wind and descends yang from the head*, it may treat stubborn and difficult conditions such as Meniére's disease, dizziness, loss of balance, vertigo, blurred vision, stiffness of the jaw, sore throat, headache, sudden deafness, extreme ear pain or tinnitus with dizziness and nausea due to *Liver yang or phlegm-fire rising upwards*.

SJ-17 is very effective in the treatment of *facial nerve disorders* such as paralysis of the eye, mouth, tongue or submandibular muscles.

> **Main Areas:** Ears. Face. Throat. Neck.
>
> **Main Functions:** Benefits the ear. Alleviates pain. Clears heat. Dispels wind. Treats the facial nerve.

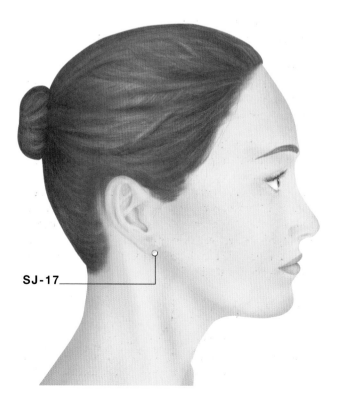

SJ-17

SJ-20   Jiaosun   角孫

Angle Vertex

SJ-21   Ermen   耳門

Ear Gate

Intersection of the Gallbladder and Small Intestine on the Sanjiao channel

In the shallow depression directly above the apex of the ear, just within the hairline.

To aid location, fold the ear forward to locate the apex.

In the depression anterior to the supratragic notch and slightly superior to the condyloid process of the mandible, in line with SI-19 and GB-2.

To aid location, when the patient opens their mouth, the condyloid process of the mandible slides forward to reveal the depression.

Best treatment positions
Similar to GB-2 and SI-19. SJ-21 is often chosen instead of, or in addition to, GB-2 and SI-19 and vice-versa. It is best to palpate these three points in order to ascertain which is most reactive.

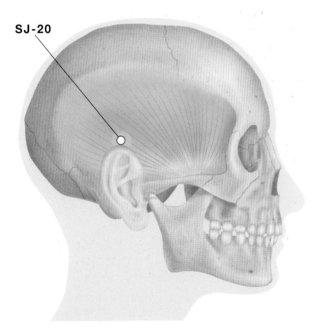

SJ-20

Best treatment positions
Similar to other point of the scalp (see GB-8).

Needling
• 0.3 to 1.5 cun subcutaneous insertion, in the direction of the area being treated, or join to adjacent points, for example GB-8 and GB-5.

Actions and indications
Although SJ-20 is not very commonly used, it can help in the treatment of *regional pain and disorders of the ear and mouth*. Symptoms include earache, tinnitus, discharge from the ear, toothache, bleeding gums, stiffness and dryness of the lips. It has also been traditionally employed in a variety of other cases, including sudden loss of vision, heat rash and stiffness of the neck with difficulty turning the head.

> **Main Areas:** Ear. Mouth.
>
> **Main Functions:** Regulates qi and Blood.
> Alleviates pain and swelling.

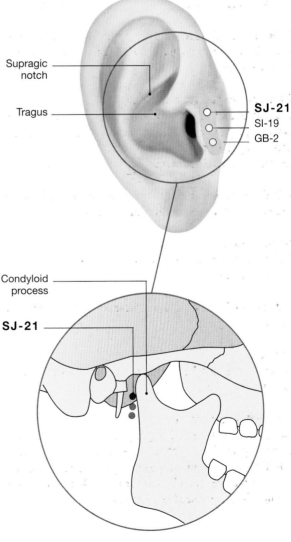

Supragic notch

Tragus

SJ-21
SI-19
GB-2

Condyloid process

SJ-21

Mouth open

Needling

• 0.5 to 1 cun perpendicular needling directed slightly posteriorly. Insert needle with the patient's mouth open. After insertion the patient can close the mouth.
• Join SJ-21, SI-19 and GB-2 by subcutaneous needling.

! Do not puncture the auriculotemporal nerve or the superficial temporal artery and vein, and in its deep position, the facial nerve.

Actions and indications

SJ-21 *is important in the treatment of disorders of the ear* including otitis, tinnitus, deafness and Meniére's disease. It is also effective for other problems of the local area including temporal headache, toothache, facial pain and inflammation of the eyes (see also GB-2, and SI-19).

> **Main Areas:** Ears. Temple. Jaw.
>
> **Main Functions:** Improves hearing. Regulates qi and Blood. Alleviates pain. Clears heat.

Manual techniques and shiatsu
Carefully applied stationary pressure is best with the pads of the fingers or thumbs.

Moxibustion
Contraindicated.

Stimulation sensation
Regional distension or ache, possibly extending to the eye or temporal area.

Actions and indications
SJ-23 is primarily used to *dispel wind, clear heat, alleviate pain* and *benefit the eyes*. Its functions are similar to those of GB-1.

> **Main Areas:** Eyes. Temple.
>
> **Main Functions:** Regulates qi and Blood. Alleviates pain. Dispels wind and clears heat. Clears the eyes.

SJ-23 Sizhukong

Silken Bamboo Hollow

絲竹空

In the depression at the lateral end of the eyebrow.

Best treatment positions
Similar to GB-1.

Needling
• 0.2 to 0.4 cun transverse insertion, posteriorly.

! Do not puncture the temporal branch of the facial nerve, the zygomaticofacial nerve and the superficial temporal artery and vein.

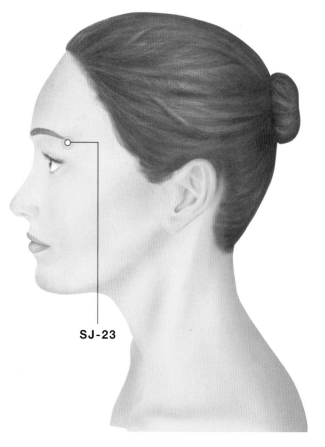

SJ-23

Chapter 20

Points of the

Leg Shao Yang
Gallbladder Channel

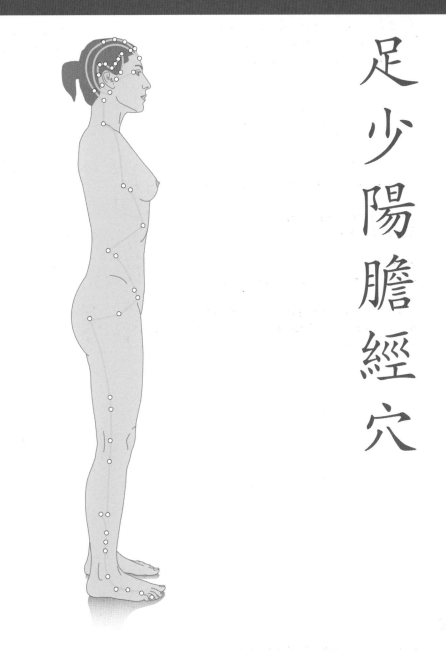

足
少
陽
膽
經
穴

GB-1   Tongziliao
Pupil Crevice

瞳子髎

Intersection of the Sanjiao and Small Intestine on the Gallbladder channel

In the small crevice-like depression, on the lateral margin of the orbit, approximately 0.5 cun lateral to the outer canthus. In the orbicularis oculi muscle.

Palpate the lateral orbital margin gently with the pad of the index finger, to locate the narrow vertical crevice.

Alternatively, treat GB-1 further posteriorly in the temporal fossa, behind the posterior border of the lateral orbital margin. In the temporalis muscle.

Best treatment positions
GB-1 is best treated in a supine position with the patient's head comfortably supported by pillows and the eyes closed. It can also be treated unilaterally lying sideways. Acupressure can also be applied sitting up.

! This is a very delicate and sensitive point. All forms of treatment should be applied carefully.

Needling
• 0.2 to 0.4 cun transverse insertion, posteriorly.
• 0.5 to 1 cun transverse insertion toward Taiyang M-HN-9.

Insert the needle carefully and apply very little manipulation, or none at all. Apply pressure onto the point after removing the needle. During needle retention, the patient should avoid unnecessary blinking.

! Do not puncture branches of the zygomaticoorbital artery and vein; the zygomaticofacial artery, vein and nerve; the temporal branch of the facial nerve; the zygomaticotemporal artery, vein and nerve.

!! This point can bruise easily. If any slight swelling of the skin is observed remove needle immediately and apply pressure, plus a cold compress. See cautionary note and first aid for bruising for St-1.

Moxibustion
Moxibustion is contraindicated at this location.

Manual techniques and shiatsu
Carefully applied stationary pressure is best with the pads of the fingers or thumbs. The pressure can be applied onto the orbital ridge as well as lateral to it.

Stimulation sensation
Local distension or ache should be achieved. It may extend over the eye and toward the ears or temporal area.

Actions and indications
GB-1 is an important point to *clear wind and heat* from the eyes, *promote qi and Blood circulation, alleviate pain* and *benefit vision.*

Indications include pain, redness, swelling, itching and inflammation of the eye, the sclera, the eyelids and the outer canthus, conjunctivitis, pain extending to the ear, trigeminal neuralgia, migraine, facial paralysis, deviation of the eye or cheek, glaucoma, night blindness, short sightedness, cataract and diminishing vision.

> **Main Areas:** Eyes. Outer canthus.
>
> **Main Functions:** Benefits the eyes and improves vision. Dispels wind and heat. Regulates qi and Blood.

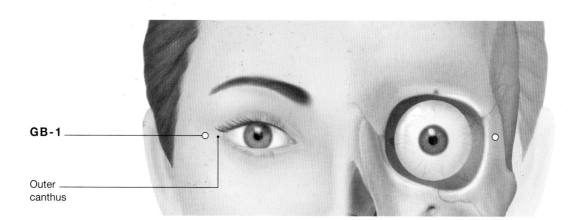

GB-1

Outer
canthus

GB-2   Tinghui

聽會

Hearing Convergence

In the depression anterior to the intertragic notch, directly below SI-19, posterior to the condyloid process of the mandible.

To aid location, when the patient opens their mouth, the condyloid process of the mandible slides forward to reveal the depression.

GB-2 is often chosen instead of, or in addition to, SI-19 and SJ-21, and vice-versa. It is best to palpate these three points in order to ascertain which is most reactive on pressure.

Best treatment positions

This point can be treated in a supine, side-lying or sitting position, depending on the desired results and treatment methods applied. In cases where one side is only affected, it is best treated in a side-lying position.

! This is a sensitive point and care should be taken in all forms of treatment.

Needling

- 0.5 to 1 cun perpendicular needling directed slightly posteriorly. Insert the needle with the patient's mouth open. After insertion, the patient can close the mouth.
- Join SJ-21, SI-19 and GB-2 by subcutaneous needling.

! Do not puncture the auriculotemporal nerve, the great auricular nerve, the superficial temporal artery and vein and the facial nerve.

Manual techniques and shiatsu

For unilateral problems, apply simultaneous finger pressure to GB-2 and other surrounding points, such as SJ-17, SI-19 and SJ-21. Joining some or all of these points with qi projection techniques is most effective.

For bilateral complaints apply sustained perpendicular pressure to both sides. The patient can allow the jaw muscles to relax during the treatment so that the mouth will be slightly open.

! Administer pressure very gradually, particularly if there is pain and inflammation. Excessive pressure can exacerbate pain.

Moxibustion

Pole: 2 to 10 minutes. Light or medium stimulation only. Direct moxibustion is not recommended at this site.

! Do not overheat this area. Do not apply moxibustion if there is acute inflammation of the ear.

Magnets

Stick-on magnets can be very effective for pain and other disorders of the ears. Alternate poles on GB-2, SI-19 and SJ-21 or other adjacent points.

Stimulation sensation

Local distension, ache or tingling radiating to the inside of the ear and possibly extending anteriorly and superiorly into the temporomandibular joint, cheek, eye and temporal area is often achieved.

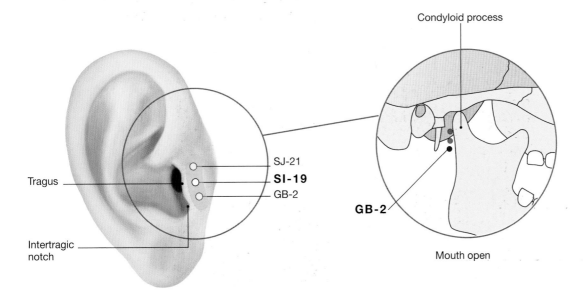

Condyloid process

SJ-21
SI-19
GB-2

Tragus

Intertragic notch

GB-2

Mouth open

! Treatment at GB-2 can occasionally bring about a tinnitus-like buzzing in the ears or the sound of water moving. This is due to an increase in blood circulation or other reaction in the inner ear as a result of the treatment. It could, however, mean that the needle is touching the artery, or that excessive heat from moxibustion has been applied.

Actions and indications

GB-2 is an important point to *improve hearing* and treat a *variety of ear disorders*. It effectively *dispels wind and clears heat, promotes qi and Blood circulation, dispels stagnation, relieves swelling* and *alleviates pain*. Indications include *acute or chronic inflammatory conditions of the ear*, itching, pain, swelling or discharge from the ear, diminished hearing, tinnitus, deafness, deviation of the eye or mouth, facial paralysis, facial pain, trigeminal neuralgia, migraine, headache, toothache, temporomandibular syndrome and stiffness or injury of the jaw.

Furthermore, treatment applied to GB-2 is effective for other *disorders of the face and head* including temporal headache, toothache and inflammation of the eyes (see also SJ-21 and SI-19).

Main Area: Ears.

Main Functions: Dispels wind and heat. Regulates qi and Blood. Alleviates pain. Improves hearing.

GB-3 Shangguan 上關

Above the Arch

Intersection of the Sanjiao and Stomach on the Gallbladder channel

In the depression above the superior border of the zygomatic arch, directly above St-7.

Contraindications

According to classical texts, needling GB-3 is contraindicated. This may be due to the observation that puncturing vessels at this location can cause internal bleeding and lead to deafness or even death.

Best treatment positions

This location can be treated supine, side-lying or sitting.

! This is a sensitive point and care should be taken in all forms of treatment.

Needling
• 0.2 to 0.4 cun perpendicular insertion.

!! Do not needle deeper. Do not puncture branches of the superficial temporal artery and vein, the auriculotemporal nerve and the branches of the facial nerve; more deeply, the zygomatico-orbital artery and vein and the middle temporal artery and vein. Deeper still, the deep temporal artery, vein and nerve.

Moxibustion
Direct moxibustion should not be applied to this location. Pole: 3–5 minutes. Light stimulation only.

Magnets
Small stick-on magnets can be effective for channel disorders. However, because of the numerous blood vessels found at this location, the application of magnets may also be beneficial in circulation and vessel disorders due to their anticoagulant effect.

Manual techniques and shiatsu
Sustained perpendicular pressure and gentle friction is applicable.

Stimulation sensation
Local distension, ache or tingling extending to the ear, eye, temporomandibular joint and sides of head. Similarly to GB-2, treatment here can, on occasion, bring about a tinnitus-like buzzing in the ears (see also GB-2).

Actions and indications
Although GB-3 is not very commonly used, it can be remarkably effective to *promote qi and Blood circulation, dissipate stasis* and *alleviate pain from the jaw, temporomandibular joint, sides of the face* and *ears*. Furthermore it helps *dispel wind and clear heat*. Indications include earache, acute or chronic inflammatory conditions of the ear, tinnitus, deafness, facial paralysis and pain, trigeminal neuralgia, facial paralysis, migraine, toothache, stiffness of the jaw, temporomandibular joint syndrome, headache, parotitis and swelling of the side of the face.

Main Areas: Temple. Jaw. Ears.

Main Functions: Regulates qi and Blood. Alleviates pain. Clears heat. Improves hearing.

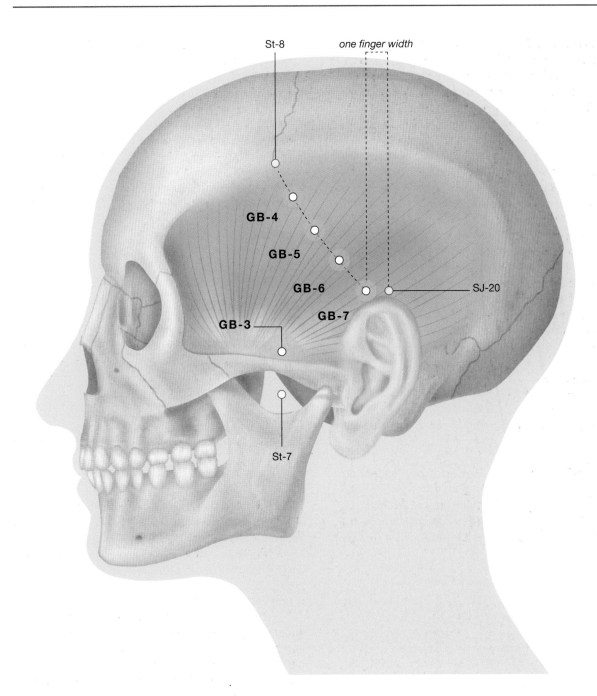

St-8

one finger width

GB-4

GB-5

GB-6

GB-7

GB-3

SJ-20

St-7

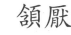

GB-4 Hanyan

頜厭

Forehead Fullness

Intersection of the Sanjiao and Stomach on the Gallbladder channel

In a shallow depression within the temporal hairline, below St-8, one quarter of the distance between St-8 and GB-7.

To aid location, it is just superior to a bulge in the flesh, appearing when the jaw is closed tight.

Needling

• 0.3 to 1.5 cun subcutaneous insertion, in the direction of the area being treated. Join with adjacent points.

Pick up the cutaneous tissue of the scalp (pinch the scalp) and insert the needle subcutaneously, under the epicranial aponeurosis parallel to the bone. If the scalp is very tight, this may be difficult; therefore needle perpendicularly 0.1 to 0.2 cun.

However, because perpendicular needling is not as effective, consider applying moxibustion or massage to loosen the area or choose another technique.

Manual techniques and shiatsu

Friction or sustained pressure may be applied carefully with the tips of the thumbs or fingers. This location can be extremely sensitive in certain cases, particularly if there is a lot of tension of the epicranial tissues. In such cases, it may be best to apply friction, trying to loosen the scalp over the bone in circles. Also stretching the scalp in various directions to loosen the subcutaneous connective tissue is very effective (use the fingers or palms).

! GB-4 and surrounding scalp points can be extremely sensitive or painful on pressure, particularly if the person has a lot of stress. Ensure that the therapeutic pressure starts off gently and increases gradually to avoid aggravating the condition.

Moxibustion
Pole: 3–10 minutes. Direct moxibustion is not recommended at this location.

Guasha
Gently applied guasha can be effective.

! Strong stimulation can exacerbate pain conditions.

Actions and indications
GB-4 is used mainly as a *local point* in the treatment of headache and pain on the lateral aspect of the face and temple. Indications include migraine, trigeminal neuralgia, toothache, earache, tinnitus and pain or inflammation of the eyes, particularly at the lateral aspect.

Traditionally it has been used in such cases as dizziness, convulsions, epilepsy and stiffness of the neck.

Main Areas: Temple. Jaw. Ears.

Main Functions: Regulates qi and Blood. Alleviates pain.

GB-5 Xuanlu
Suspended Skull

Intersection of the Sanjiao, Stomach and Large Intestine on the Gallbladder channel

In a shallow depression within the temporal hairline, below GB-4 and midway between St-8 and GB-7.

Treatment and applications
Similar to GB-4.

GB-6 Xuanli
Suspended Tuft

Intersection of the Sanjiao, Stomach and Large Intestine on the Gallbladder channel

In a shallow depression within the temporal hairline, midway between GB-5 and GB-7 (one quarter of the distance between GB-7 and St-8).

Treatment and applications
Similar to GB-4.

GB-7 Qubin
Temporal Hairline Curve

Intersection of the Bladder on the Gallbladder channel

On the temple, approximately one finger's breadth anterior to SJ-20, level with the apex of the auricle.

To aid location, the shallow depression is easier to ascertain if the patient opens and closes the jaw.

Treatment and applications
Similar to SJ-20 and GB-4.

GB-7 is indicated for swelling and pain of the cheek and submandibular area, stiffness and pain of the jaw and neck, toothache, trigeminal neuralgia and migraine.

Needling
• 0.3 to 1.5 cun subcutaneous insertion, in the direction of the area being treated or join with adjacent points, for example GB-8, SJ-20 and GB-6. See needling note for GB-4.

Main Areas: Temple. Ear. Cheek.

Main Functions: Regulates qi and Blood. Alleviates pain.

GB-8 Shuaigu 率谷
Leading Valley

Intersection of the Bladder on the Gallbladder channel

In the shallow depression superior to the apex of the auricle, approximately 1.5 cun within the hairline and 1 cun directly above SJ-20.

Treatment and applications
Similar to GB-4 and SJ-20.

Needling
• 0.3 to 1.5 cun subcutaneous insertion in the direction of the area being treated, or join to adjacent points.

Actions and indications
Similar to GB-7 and SJ-20. GB-8 is primarily employed to treat *regional pain and disorders of the ear and temple*. It has however, been traditionally used to treat nausea, vomiting, headache and symptoms of alcohol poisoning.

> **Main Areas:** Temple. Ear. Brain.
>
> **Main Functions:** Regulates qi and Blood. Alleviates pain.

GB-9 Tianchong 天衝
Heavenly Surge

Intersection of the Bladder on the Gallbladder channel

In the shallow depression approximately 0.5 cun posterior to GB-8.

Best treatment positions
Similar to GB-7 and GB-4.

Actions and indications
Similar to GB-8. Furthermore, it has been employed to treat *psychological disturbances*, anxiety, agitation, panic attacks, fright and shock, epilepsy and even madness.

> **Main Areas:** Head. Brain. Mind. Ear.
>
> **Main Functions:** Regulates qi. Calms mind.

GB-12 Wangu 完骨
Mastoid Process

Intersection of the Bladder on the Gallbladder channel

In the small depression posterior and inferior to the tip of the mastoid process. Superficially situated in the sternocleidomastoid muscle and more deeply in the splenius capitis and longissimus capitis muscles.

Best treatment positions
With the patient in a prone position and the head suitably supported in an anatomically shaped cushion or couch. However, sitting up can also be employed for the application of manual pressure techniques (acupuncture at this location is not recommended in a sitting position). Ensure the cervical spine is straight. Side-lying is very effective for unilateral treatment and is the position of choice.

Furthermore, manual pressure treatment can be effectively applied with the patient lying down supine. In certain cases, needling can also be applied with the patient supine.

Needling
• 0.3 to 1 cun oblique inferior insertion into the sternocleidomastoid fibres.

! Do not puncture the greater auricular or lesser occipital nerves or the posterior auricular artery and vein.

• 0.3 to 0.5 cun perpendicular insertion under the tip of the mastoid process, pointing anteromedially (the needle tip should be directed toward the space between the mastoid process and the transverse process of the atlas).

!! Do not insert deeper. Do not puncture branches of the lesser occipital or greater auricular nerves, the posterior auricular artery, vein and nerve. More deeply, the occipital artery and vein, and branches of the facial nerve. Posteromedially, in its deep position, the vertebral artery and vein.

Moxibustion
Pole: 5–15 minutes. Direct moxibustion is rarely applied to this location.

! Do not burn the hair.

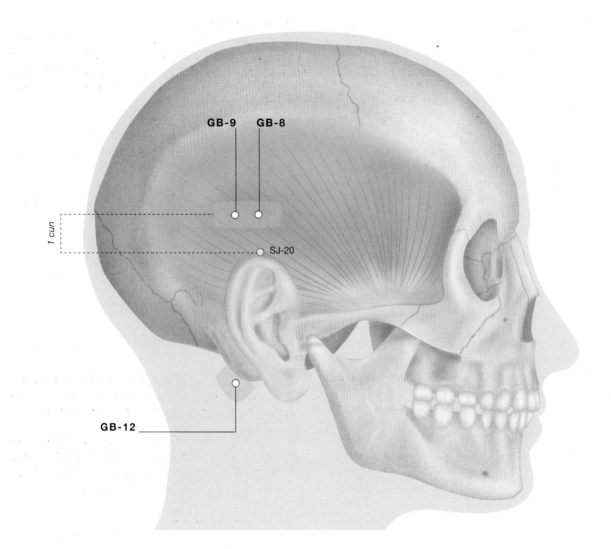

Guasha

Guasha is effective applied surrounding the mastoid process and down the sternocleidomastoid fibres.

! Warn the patient that bruising can occur.

Manual techniques and shiatsu

Similar to GB-20. It is most effective to apply stationary pressure and friction to the entire mastoid process and surrounding soft tissue attachments. Also, friction of the sternocleidomastoid muscle is beneficial.

Actions and indications

The functions of GB-12 are closely related to those of adjacent points at the base of the cranium, particularly Du-15, Bl-10, GB-20 and Anmian N-HN-54. All these points tend to *strongly relax the patient* by *balancing the nervous system* and *regulating the ascending and descending of qi* from the head. They are thus all useful in cases of *excessive rising yang* or deficiency of the Marrow causing *disorders of the brain and sense organs*.

Note that Anmian N-HN-54, located next to GB-12, has been named the *Peaceful Sleep,* reflecting the relaxing properties of the acu-points in this area. However, GB-12 is primarily used as *a local point* to treat regional disorders, particularly pain, stiffness and swelling.

Indications include pain or stiffness of the neck or jaw, earache, painful swelling of the throat, cheeks and submandibular area, lymphadenopathy, toothache and facial paralysis.

Additionally, it has been employed to treat *interior symptoms of Gallbladder imbalance* such as headache, insomnia and sensations of heat.

> **Main Areas:** Ears. Back and sides of the head.
>
> **Main Functions:** Relaxes the body and calms the mind. Dissipates stasis. Alleviates pain.

GB-13   Benshen   本神

Spirit Root

Intersection of the Yang Wei Mai on the Gallbladder channel

In the shallow depression, 0.5 cun within the anterior hairline, approximately two-thirds of the distance between Du-24 and St-8. Directly above the outer canthus.

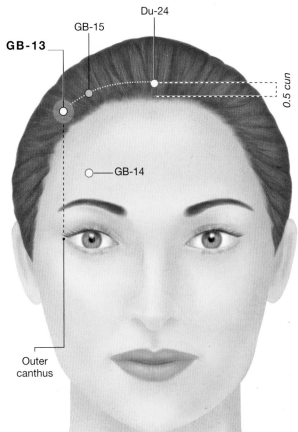

Best treatment positions
Treatment is best applied in a supine position. However, side-lying or sitting up can also be employed.

Needling
• 0.3 to 1 cun transverse insertion posteriorly, or in other directions depending on the desired result. Join with adjacent points such as St-8 or GB-15.

Manual techniques and shiatsu
Friction or sustained pressure may be applied with the pads of the thumbs or fingers.

Moxibustion
Pole: 2–5 minutes. Light stimulation only.

Actions and indications
GB-13 is primarily used as a *local point in the treatment of pain* and headache. Furthermore, it has been employed to treat eye disorders, stiffness of the neck, dizziness, epilepsy and psychological or emotional restlessness, agitation or anxiety.

> **Main Areas:** Head. Mind.
>
> **Main Functions:** Regulates qi and Blood. Alleviates pain. Calms the mind.

GB-14   Yangbai   陽白

Yang Bright

Intersection of the Stomach, Large Intestine, Sanjiao and Yang Wei Mai on the Gallbladder

On the forehead, in a shallow depression approximately 1 cun above the midpoint of the eyebrow, one-third of the distance from the eyebrow to the anterior hairline.

To aid location, the small pulse of the supraorbital artery should be perceived on gentle palpation with the pad of the finger. The midpoint of the eyebrow is level with the pupil when the gaze is fixed straight ahead.

Best treatment positions
Treatment is best applied in a supine position. However, sitting up can also be employed.

Needling
• 0.3 to 1 cun subcutaneous insertion in an inferior direction toward Yuyao M-HN-6. Pick up the skin to insert the needle subcutaneously, parallel to the bone.

! Apply pressure to the point after removing the needle. Do not puncture the supraorbital artery, vein or nerve.

Moxibustion
Pole: 1–3 minutes, light stimulation only. Use a moxa boat over GB-14 and surrounding area to relax the forehead and bring colour to a pale face.

! Do not overheat this location.

!! Direct moxibustion is contraindicated.

Manual techniques and shiatsu
Gentle sustained pressure or stronger friction techniques may be applied effectively with the tips of the thumbs or fingers.

Stimulation sensation
Local distension, ache, tingling or pulling sensation extending out across the forehead and down toward the eyelid.

Actions and indications
GB-14 is very important and widely used to *relax the forehead, calm the mind* and *brighten the eyes*. It *dispels wind* and *clears heat, regulates qi and Blood, dissipates stasis* and *alleviates pain*. Furthermore, it is an important beauty point, used to smoothe the forehead and brighten the eyes.

Symptoms include headache, dizziness, pain of the forehead, itching, pain or inflammation of the eyes, excessive lacrimation, diminishing vision, deviation of the eye or mouth and paralysis, twitching or spasm of the eyelids.

Main Areas: Forehead. Eyes. Supraorbital area.

Main Functions: Calms the mind. Dispels wind and heat. Dispels stasis. Alleviates pain.

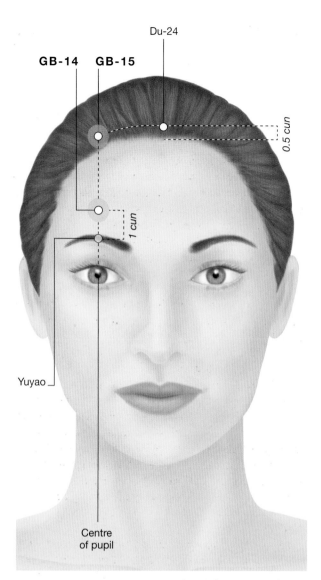

GB-15   Toulinqi   頭臨泣

Head Governor of Tears

Intersection of the Bladder and the Yang Wei Mai on the Gallbladder channel

In the shallow depression 0.5 cun within the anterior hairline, directly above GB-14, midway between Du-24 and St-8.

Needling
• 0.3 to 1.5 cun subcutaneous insertion, in a posterior or lateral direction.

Moxibustion
Cones: 3. Pole: 3–5 minutes.

Manual techniques and shiatsu
Perpendicular pressure and friction is applicable with the tips of the fingers and thumbs. See also GB-4.

Stimulation sensation
Local ache, tingling or electric sensation extending outward around the location.

Actions and indications
Although GB-15 is not a very commonly used point, it has been used to treat such cases as headache, vertigo, dizziness, epilepsy, convulsions, coma, nasal obstruction and inflammation of the eyes.

Main Areas: Head. Forehead.

Main Functions: Dissipates fullness. Regulates qi and Blood.

GB-20   Fengchi

風池

Wind Pool

Intersection of the Sanjiao, Yang Wei and Yang Qiao Mai on the Gallbladder channel

At the centre of the sizeable depression directly below the occipital bone, within the posterior hairline. This depression is formed between the trapezius (medially), the sternocleidomastoid (laterally) and the splenius capitis (inferiorly). Situated superficially in the semispinalis capitis and in its deep position in the rectus capitis posterior major and the obliquus capitis superior on its lateral side.

To aid location, it is approximately midway between Du-16 and the tip of the mastoid process. See also Bl-10.

Best treatment positions
GB-20 is often treated with the patient in a prone position with the head suitably supported in an anatomically shaped cushion or couch. For unilateral disorders, use a side position. Furthermore, manual techniques and moxa pole therapy can be applied with the patient sitting up, although needling should not. Additionally, manual treatment can be applied with the patient in a supine position. Needling can also be applied in supine.

Needling
• 0.5 to 1.2 cun perpendicular insertion into the space between the occiput and the transverse process of C1, directed toward the opposite corner of the mouth.

!! In certain albeit rare cases, needling this location can cause symptoms of needle shock, due to sympathetic nerve stimulation. Symptoms include pallor, sweating, nausea, dizziness and possibly fainting (see also stimulation sensation note below).

GB-20 is usually needled reasonably deeply in order to induce adequate deqi. The needle should be inserted at the level of the space between the occipital bone and transverse process of the atlas. It should go through the semispinalis capitis and reach a depth of 2–4 cm close to the obliquus capitis and posterior rectus capitis muscles.

!! Do not needle deeper or at another angle. Do not puncture veins of the suboccipital network and branches of the lesser and greater occipital nerve and the occipital artery and vein. More deeply, branches of the suboccipital nerve, and deeper still, the vertebral artery and vein and the medulla oblongata.

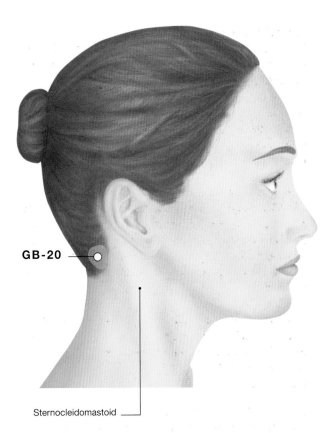

GB-20

Sternocleidomastoid

Manual techniques and shiatsu
Perpendicular pressure and friction techniques, with or without lubricants, can be applied to this location. Sustained perpendicular pressure is most effective applied with the fingertips in a supine position (bilaterally), without a cushion under the head. Curl the tips of the fingers under the occipital bone and apply the pressure whilst allowing the patient's head to extend slightly (the chin should appear to lift during pressure application). Also, sitting up can be employed (the practitioner must support the patient's head so that the neck muscles can be as relaxed as possible).

Stretching the head in an anterior and opposite direction effectively opens the GB-20 area.

! Great care should be taken when working on the neck in order to avoid overstimulation of the area and overstretching of a nerve. This is particularly important in the elderly and patients with vascular disease, hypertension, arthritis and other disorders of the cervical spine.

Moxibustion
Pole: 5–15 minutes. Warm the channel between GB-20 and GB-21 in order to expel cold. Although 3–5 cones can be used, direct moxibustion is not easily applied to this location.

! Do not burn hair.

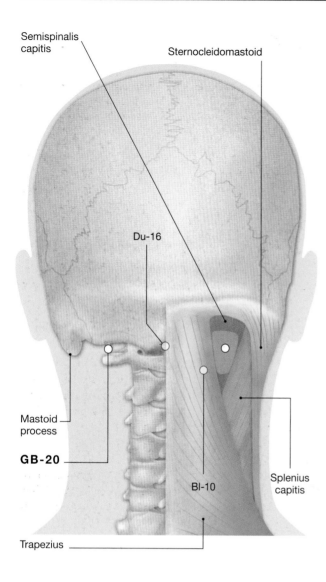

Semispinalis capitis

Sternocleidomastoid

Du-16

Mastoid process

GB-20

BI-10

Splenius capitis

Trapezius

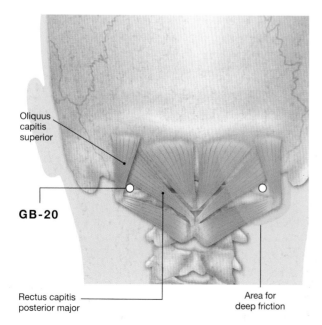

Oliquus capitis superior

GB-20

Rectus capitis posterior major

Area for deep friction

Cupping
Small cups with medium or light suction can be very effective.

Guasha
Guasha is effectively applied across the trapezius and down the semispinalis and splenius capitis fibres.

Magnets
Stick-on magnets can also be very effective at this location. For pain and stiffness of the neck, headache, dizziness, tinnitus and other symptoms of rising yang, place the south poles on GB-20 and the north poles on GB-21 bilaterally or vice-versa (see also GB-21).

Stimulation sensation
Localised ache, tingling and distension, extending into the head, vertex, temple, ears, eyes or downward across the posterior aspect of the neck and along the channel pathway, depending on the condition being treated.

! In some instances, tiredness, dizziness and nausea may occur as a result of excessive sympathetic stimulation of the cervical nerves, indicating that the treatment employed was too strong for the recipient.

!! In certain rare cases, clinical signs of shock may present (sinking or collapse of qi). These include pallor, cold sweat, vomiting, loss of consciousness (fainting), tachycardia and decrease in blood pressure. Although this can occur from wrongly applied pressure or stretching to the suboccipital region, it is more commonly seen as a reaction to needling.

Actions and indications
Gb-20 is a very important point because it *effectively descends pathological qi* from the head whilst at the same time *raising clear qi* and *nourishing the Sea of Marrow*. It is possibly the most powerful point of the region and has been extensively employed to *clear heat, descend rising yang, sedate interior wind* and treat symptoms of *wind stroke*. Furthermore, it is indicated for initial invasion of *exterior pathogenic factors at the Tai Yang stage*.

GB-20 has a marked effect on the head and brain and is important to *calm the mind* and *relax the body*. It is also widely used for *disorders of the sense organs*, and is especially indicated to *brighten the eyes* and *improve vision and hearing*. It also *dynamically activates qi and Blood circulation* in the channel and is important to treat pain, stiffness, spasticity, atrophy and paralysis.

It has been extensively used in a *wide variety of disorders* including headache, migraine, pain and stiffness of the neck, shoulder and back, difficulty flexing the neck and turning or bending the head forward, degenerative disorders of the cervical spine, postural hypotension, pain and inflammation of the eyes, tired eyes, excessive lacrimation, diminishing vision, earache, tinnitus, impaired hearing, disorders of the inner ear, Meniére's disease, facial paralysis, disorders of the jaw, temporomandibular syndrome, swelling and tumours of the neck, tidal fever, chills and fever, blocked nose, sinusitis, epistaxis, dizziness, vertigo, aphasia, hypertension, transient ischaemic attack, hemiplegia and other symptoms following wind stroke, epilepsy, convulsions, spasticity, tiredness, heavy feeling in the head, mental exhaustion, diminishing mental functions, amnesia, difficulty concentrating, poor memory, depression, premenstrual syndrome, insomnia, mental restlessness, irritability and mood swings.

> **Main Areas:** Head. Occiput. Neck. Eyes. Ears. Brain. Mind. Muscles. Entire body.
>
> **Main Functions:** Relaxes. Descends rising yang. Benefits the Sea of Marrow.

GB-21 Jianjing   肩井
Shoulder Well

Intersection of the Stomach, Sanjiao and Yang Wei Mai on the Gallbladder channel

On the top of the shoulder, midway between the spinous process of C7 and the tip of the acromion. On the highest point of the trapezius, where the muscle fibres separate on pressure palpation, directly posterior to St-12. GB-21 is usually at the site of most tenderness.

To aid location, if the therapist places the base of each palm on the scapular spine with the thumbs touching the spinous process of C7 and the fingers resting on the upper portion of the trapezius, GB-21 lies below the tip of the middle finger if it is flexed slightly.

Contraindications
Do not treat GB-21 during pregnancy or in cases of severe deficiency or sinking qi with manifestations such as excessive uterine bleeding, prolapse, diarrhoea, tiredness, dizziness, palpitations and very low blood pressure.

Best treatment positions
GB-21 can be treated in most positions. For unilateral complaints use side-lying, for bilateral complaints choose supine or sitting. Prone may also be used in certain cases.

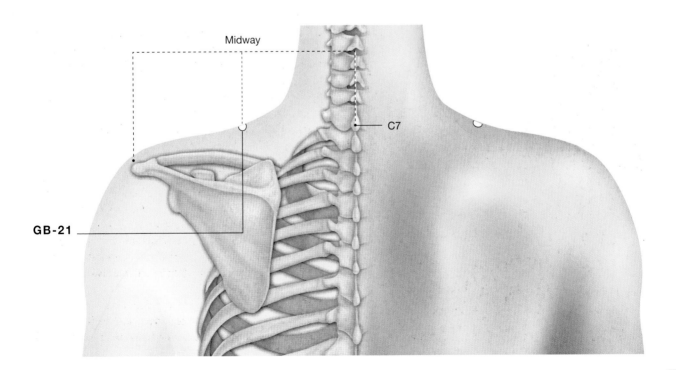

Midway

C7

GB-21

Another thing to take into account is that it can be easier to effectively stimulate GB-21 by manual techniques, because correct needling at this location can be dangerous and requires great skill. Furthermore, deqi is easier to induce by manual pressure techniques.

! GB-21 descends the qi very strongly (this is particularly true if the patient is sitting up during treatment). Accordingly, only light stimulation should be applied in debilitated or qi and Blood deficient patients.

GB-21 is commonly chosen to descend rising yang causing such manifestations as inflamed eyes, headache and hypertension. This means that although the physiological effects of qi descent are a desired part of the treatment, careful assessment of the patient's ability to regulate qi is necessary to avoid undesirable reactions. If it is the first treatment, only apply light stimulation.

Also, according to some classical sources, it is recommended that St-36 should be needled in the same treatment as GB-21 to ensure that the qi is not depleted.

Needling
• 0.5 to 1.5 cun posterior oblique insertion into the trapezius muscle fibres.

With the left hand, pick up and squeeze as much of the muscle as possible, pulling it up from the underlying tissues, while inserting the needle in a posterior direction with the right hand.

• 0.3 to 0.5 cun perpendicular insertion.

! Do not puncture the cutaneous or deep branches of the suprascapular artery, vein or nerve. More deeply, the accessory nerve, and deeper still, the transverse cervical artery and vein.

!! Do not needle deeper. Deeper needling, particularly in thin recipients holds considerable risk of puncturing the lung apex and causing pneumothorax. Never leave a patient unattended with needles in a sitting position.

Manual techniques and shiatsu
Sustained pressure, friction, kneading and stretching the trapezius muscle are all very effective techniques and can be applied with the fingers, thumbs, palms, forearms and elbows. The patient may be sitting up or lying down.

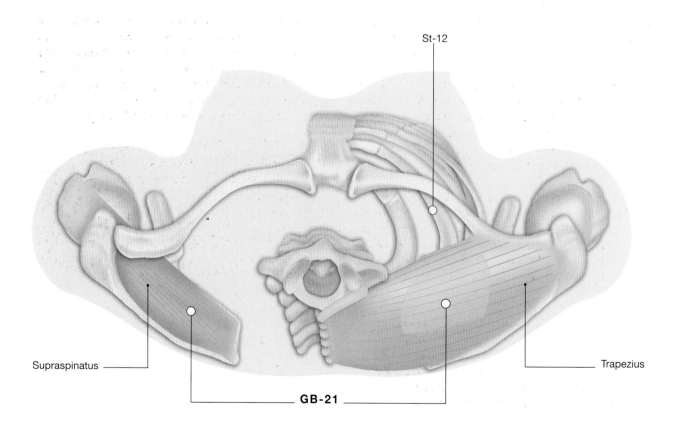

St-12

Supraspinatus

GB-21

Trapezius

! Do not apply perpendicular pressure to GB-21 with the patient sitting up if there is degeneration or pain of the spine. A supine or side-lying posture is preferred.

! Strong stimulation on the accessory nerve can cause central neurological reactions (see cautionary note in the stimulation sensation section).

Moxibustion
Cones: 3–10. Pole: 10–30 minutes.

Cupping
Stationary or moving cupping is very effective. Use small or medium cups with reasonably strong suction.

! Strong cupping around GB-21 will cause bruising that may, in certain cases, last for more than a week.

Guasha
Guasha is effectively applied down the trapezius toward the acromion, or in a cross-fibre direction.

Magnets
Stick-on magnets can be very effective. Place north poles on GB-21 bilaterally and south pole on Du-14, or vice-versa to treat pain and stiffness of the neck. Also, add south poles to GB-20 to make this treatment stronger.

Stimulation sensation
Local ache, distension, tingling, numbness or electricity, radiating toward the shoulder and back, downward into the chest, or up the neck to the head, ears and eyes.

! In some cases, light headedness or dizziness may occur as a result of the treatment. This means that the treatment employed was too strong for the recipient. This situation can occur both from needling and excessive pressure or stretching of a nerve (particularly the accessory nerve). See also cautionary note for GB-20.

Actions and indications
GB-21 is one of the *most commonly used* and *dynamic points* in the body and has been extensively employed in a wide variety of cases. It is one of the *strongest points to activate qi and Blood circulation* and *dispel stasis.* Importantly, it also powerfully *descends qi* and *clears heat.*

It is extensively used to *treat pain* and *calm the mind* as well *clear the head* and *open the sense organs.* Indications include headache, migraine, sinusitis, facial paralysis, temporomandibular syndrome, pain and inflammation of the eyes, earache, tinnitus, deafness, hypertension, tidal fevers, amnesia, depression and insomnia.

GB-21 is probably the *strongest point of the region* and has been extensively used in the treatment of *disorders of the neck, shoulder and head.* Indications include pain and stiffness of the neck, shoulder and back, difficulty in turning the head, disorders of the cervical spine, swelling, phlegm nodules or tumours of the neck, goitre, spasm of the trapezius, frozen shoulder, difficulty lifting the arm, periarthritis and paralysis of the upper limb.

Moreover, it effectively *dispels wind and cold* and is important to *open and relax the chest* and *alleviate dyspnoea and cough.* Indications include pain and tightness of the chest, shortness of breath, asthma, respiratory diseases, chills and fever, headache and sore or swollen throat.

GB-21 also descends the qi dynamically through to the lower jiao making it very effective for *gynaecological disorders* and *inducing labour* for which it is extensively employed. Indications include amenorrhoea, dysmenorrhoea, abnormal uterine bleeding, prolonged labour, difficult delivery, retention of the placenta, uterine bleeding following miscarriage or delivery, swelling and pain of the breasts, mastitis and difficult lactation.

GB-21 is also used to *sedate interior wind* and treat such cases as dizziness, vertigo, Meniére's disease, epilepsy, windstroke, hemiplegia and other neurological disorders.

Diagnostically, spontaneous tenderness at GB-21, and the area posterior to it (including SJ-15 and SI-12) may indicate referred pain from stomach disease on the left side and from the liver or gallbladder on the right. Moreover, chronic stiffness and tightness of the trapezius muscle surrounding GB-21, indicate long-standing Liver qi stagnation, interior cold or Blood deficiency.

> **Main Areas:** Neck. Shoulder. Upper back. Lungs. Chest. Breasts. Uterus. Head. Mind. Temple. Face. Eyes. Ears. Nose.
>
> **Main Functions:** Strongly descends qi. Dispels stasis. Clears the chest. Induces menstruation and labour.

GB-22   Yuanye

Armpit Source

淵腋

Approximately 3 cun below the centre of the axilla, on the mid-axillary line. In the fifth intercostal space, approximately level with the nipple.

To aid location, GB-22 is one hand-width inferior to the axilla, or one quarter of the distance between He-1 and GB-26.

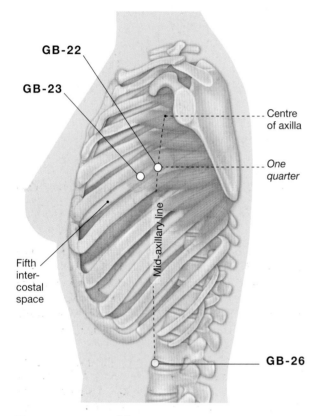

- GB-22
- GB-23
- Centre of axilla
- One quarter
- Mid-axillary line
- Fifth inter-costal space
- GB-26

Best treatment positions

This location is best treated in a side-lying or supine position. Manual techniques can also be applied sitting up.

! GB-22 and GB-23 are often tender on palpation.

Needling

• 0.3 to 0.8 cun oblique insertion along the intercostal space toward GB-23.

! Do not puncture the cutaneous branches of the fifth intercostal nerve, the thoracoepigastric vein or the long thoracic nerve. Anteriorly, the lateral thoracic artery and vein. Also, do not puncture the lymph nodes.

!! Deep needling poses considerable risk of puncturing the lung and causing a pneumothorax.

Moxibustion

Pole: 5–10 minutes, light stimulation only. Direct moxibustion is contraindicated.

Cupping

Gentle cupping can be of benefit in certain cases.

Manual techniques and shiatsu

Gentle pressure can be applied with the fingertips, but also with the palms to a slightly wider area. Friction to the intercostal space is also very effective.

! Do not press distended lymph nodes. Do not apply strong pressure to the thoracic cage.

Actions and indications

GB-22 and GB-23 are not very commonly used, although treatment at these sites can be very effective for *regional pain, stiffness* and *swelling*. It is useful in such cases as intercostal neuralgia, herpes zoster swellings, masses and nodules, excessive sweating, and disorders of the axilla, mammary glands and shoulder. Additionally, it helps *open and relax the chest* and hypochondrial area and regulate qi in the Liver and Gallbladder and throughout the three jiao.

Main Areas: Axilla. Breast. Ribs.

Main Functions: Regulates qi. Dissipates stasis and accumulation.

GB-23   Zhejin

Sinew Seat

輒筋

Intersection of the Bladder on the Gallbladder channel

1 cun anterior and slightly inferior to GB-22, in the fifth intercostal space, approximately level with the nipple.

Treatment and applications

See GB-22.

According to the *Great Compendium*, this is the Alarm-Mu point of the Gallbladder.

Due to its location closer to the breast, GB-23 may be more effective to treat *disorders of this area*. It is also traditionally indicated to descend rebellious qi and clear stagnation causing symptoms such as heartburn, vomiting, hiccup, cough, excessive salivation, jaundice, insomnia and depression.

GB-24　Riyue

日月

Sun and Moon

Alarm *Mu* point for the Gallbladder
Intersection of the Bladder and Yang Wei Mai
on the Gallbladder channel

Below the breast, in the seventh intercostal space, inferior and slightly lateral to Liv-14.

To aid location, GB-24 is in the most medial palpable depression of the seventh intercostal space. It is often described as located on the mid-mamillary line. In practice, however, it is apparent that the shape of the costal cartilages varies in a large percentage of the population, placing this point slightly further lateral on most people.

Best treatment positions
This point is best treated with the patient lying supine.

! This location is usually sensitive or tender on palpation.

Needling
• 0.3 to 1 cun oblique or transverse insertion, laterally along the intercostal space.

!! Deep needling poses considerable risk of puncturing the lung and causing a pneumothorax.

Moxibustion
Cones: 3–5. Pole: 5–20 minutes.

Cupping
Cupping with small cups can be very effective.

Guasha
Apply guasha to the intercostal space and gently across the costal cartilages to release stuck qi.

Magnets
Stick-on magnets are effective for gallbladder disorders, including cholelithiasis. Use south pole on GB-24 and north pole on Dannangxue M-LE-23, or vice-versa.

Manual techniques and shiatsu
Perpendicular pressure is applicable with the fingertips. Also, deep friction of the intercostal space can be very useful to help release stuck qi and regulate the Gallbladder. Massage any spasms in the intercostal muscles until they soften.

! Only apply very light pressure to the ribs.

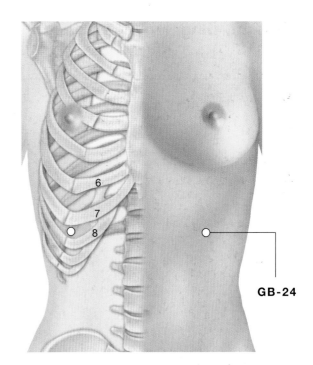

GB-24

Stimulation sensation
Local ache, distension, tingling or numbness extending into the thoracic wall, hypochondrium and abdomen.

Actions and indications
GB-24 *particularly on the right side*, is an important point for *disorders of the Gallbladder*. It regulates Liver and Gallbladder qi and is very important to *transform dampness* and *clear heat* from these organs. It also effectively *descends rebellious qi*, *harmonises the middle jiao* and benefits the hypochondrial area and ribs.

Indications include nausea, vomiting, epigastric pain, heartburn, gastric ulceration, eructation, hiccup, diarrhoea, abdominal rumbling, gastroenteritis, abdominal distension, hypochondrial pain and distension, jaundice, cholecystitis, acute or chronic hepatitis, pain and tightness of the chest, breast pain, mastitis, pain of the ribs, intercostal neuralgia and shingles.

GB-24 has also been traditionally employed to treat *psychosomatic disorders* including frequent sighing, depression, propensity to sadness, indecisiveness and lack of courage.

Furthermore, spontaneous pain at GB-24 on the right side is a *diagnostic indication of gallbladder disorders*.

Main Areas: Hypochondrium. Ribs. Gallbladder. Chest. Epigastrium. Abdomen.

Main Functions: Spreads Gallbladder qi. Alleviates pain. Dispels dampness and heat.

GB-25   Jingmen

Capital Gate

京門

Alarm *Mu* point of the Kidney

On the lower back, at the free end of the twelfth rib.

To aid location, it is usually tender on light palpation because it is a very sensitive location.

Alternative location
At the inferior border of the free end of the twelfth rib.

Best treatment positions
This location is best treated with the patient in a prone or side position. However, manual techniques can also be applied with the patient sitting up.

Needling
• 0.3 to 1 cun oblique or transverse insertion, medially along lower border of twelfth rib.
• 0.3 to 0.5 cun perpendicular insertion.

!! Do not needle deeply. Do not puncture the peritoneum. Deep needling may puncture the colon, liver, spleen or kidney.

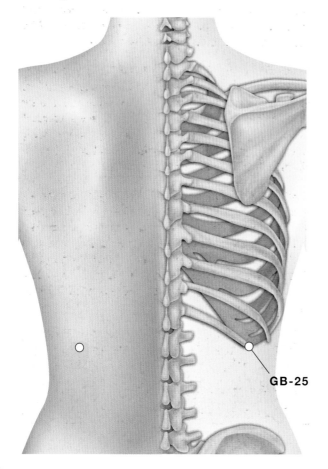

GB-25

Manual techniques and shiatsu
Gently applied sustained perpendicular pressure can be applied with the fingertips onto the tip of the twelfth rib, and directly below it.

! Only apply very gentle pressure to the false ribs. This location is very sensitive and can be very painful if pressed carelessly.

Moxibustion
Cones: 3–10. Pole: 10–30 minutes.

Cupping
Cupping with medium or light suction or empty cupping can be very beneficial for kidney disorders and lumbar pain. Use a medium or large cup size.

Guasha
Gently applied guasha is applicable.

Magnets
Stick-on magnets are helpful for kidney disorders. Apply south pole to GB-25 and north to Bl-23 for lumbar pain and kidney disorders including colic and haematuria.

Stimulation sensation
Local ache, distension, tingling or numbness radiating across the lumbar area, possibly extending toward the groin or into the kidneys.

Actions and indications
Although GB-25 is not as commonly used as other Alarm-Mu points, it can be effective to *tonify the Kidneys* and *strengthen the lumbar area*, *dispel dampness* from the lower jiao and *open the water passages* as well as *regulate the intestines*. It also *activates qi and Blood circulation* and *alleviates pain*.

Indications include acute or chronic lumbar pain, renal colic, frequent urination, dysuria, haematuria, lumbar pain, cold lower back, hip pain, abdominal rumbling, diarrhoea, vomiting, intercostal neuralgia, hypochondrial or abdominal distension and pain.

Spontaneous pain at this location on one or both sides may be a *diagnostic indication* of kidney disease.

Main Areas: Kidneys. Lumbar area. Flank.

Main Functions: Benefits the Kidneys. Transforms dampness and heat. Regulates qi and blood. Alleviates pain.

GB-26   Daimai

Girdle Vessel

帶脈

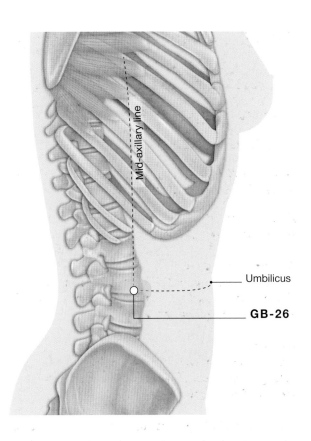

Umbilicus

GB-26

Mid-axillary line

Intersection of the Dai Mai and Gallbladder

On the lateral aspect of the abdomen, level with the umbilicus, below the free end of the eleventh rib, approximately on the mid-axillary line.

Best treatment positions
This location is best treated with the patient in a supine or side-lying position. However, prone or sitting up may also be employed.

Needling
• 0.5 to 1 cun perpendicular insertion.

!! Do not needle deeply. Do not puncture the peritoneum. Deep needling may puncture the colon, liver, spleen or kidney.

Moxibustion
Cones: 3–5. Pole: 10–20 minutes. Rice-grain moxa is also useful.

Magnets
Small stick-on magnets can be effective. For weight loss and harmonising or tonifying the abdomen, alternate north and south poles on points level with the umbilicus including GB-26, Sp-15, St-25, Ren-8, Bl-23 and Du-4.

Manual techniques and shiatsu
It is generally not so easy to stimulate this location by pressure and massage because of the soft nature of the underlying tissues. However, it can be effective to press both sides simultaneously (this is not so easy to achieve on overweight patients) or one side only in a side-lying position.

An effective shiatsu technique is to open this area by stretching the space between the pelvis and rib cage. This is achieved either in a side-lying position (grasp the iliac crest and stretch the pelvis down toward the feet, or apply crossed arm diagonal stretch with one palm resting on the pelvis and the other on the lower ribs), or, in a sitting position (side flex the torso toward the opposite side, while stabilising the pelvis).

! Only apply very light pressure to the floating ribs.

Stimulation sensation
Local distension, dull ache or tingling spreading across the abdomen and lower back, or down toward the hip on the side that is being treated.

Actions and indications
GB-26 is an important point to *activate qi and Blood circulation* in the lower jiao and *regulate the Dai Mai* (Girdle Vessel), from which it takes its name.

It is useful to *clear dampness and heat from the abdomen, harmonise the lower jiao* and *regulate menstruation*. Indications include pain, distension, swelling or flaccidity of the abdomen, lumbus and girdle area, lower abdominal pain in women, irregular menstruation, amenorrhoea, chronic leucorrhoea, blood-stained discharge, hernia, diarrhoea and abdominal rumbling.

Treatment at GB-26 is useful in *weight loss* programmes because it helps *tonify the intestines* and *strengthen the abdominal wall*, helping to lose inches around the waist. In such cases it is most effective to combine treatment with embedding needles or stick-on magnets. Furthermore, self-moxibustion, applied daily for a few minutes, is helpful to tonify the Kidneys and Spleen in such cases.

Main Areas: Abdomen. Sides. Lumbar area. Uterus. Girdle Vessel.

Main Functions: Clears dampness and heat. Benefits the lower jiao. Regulates menstruation.

GB-27 Wushu 五樞

Fifth Pivot

Intersection of the Dai Mai on the Gallbladder channel

On the lower abdomen in the depression just medial to the tip of the ASIS.

To aid location, it is approximately level with Ren-4 and St-28, 3 cun below the umbilicus.

Best treatment positions
GB-27 and GB-28 are usually treated with the patient lying down supine. However, however lying sideways may also be employed.

Choose between GB-27 and GB-28, depending on which is most reactive on pressure palpation.

! These points can be sensitive on palpation.

Needling
• 0.5 to 1.5 cun perpendicular insertion.
• 1 to 2 cun oblique inferior insertion toward GB-28 and Zigong (M-CA-18).

!! Do not needle deeply. Do not puncture the peritoneum.

Manual techniques and shiatsu
Pressure and friction techniques are applicable with the fingers and thumbs. However, the palms are usually more effective.

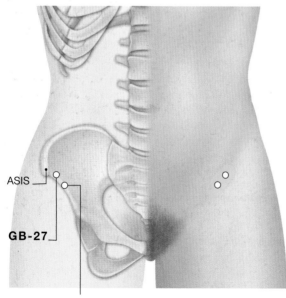

ASIS

GB-27

GB-28

An effective shiatsu technique is to open GB-27 and GB-28 by stretching the ASIS in a posterior direction (curl the fingers over the medial border of the ASIS). The recipient should be lying down supine or sideways.

Moxibustion
Cones: 5–10. Pole: 10–20 minutes. Rice-grain moxa is also applicable.

Cupping
Gentle or medium suction can be effective.

Stimulation sensation
Local distension, ache or tingling spreading across the lower abdomen, maybe extending to the loin.

Actions and indications
GB-27 and GB-28 can both be very effective to treat symptoms such as pain and distension of the lower abdomen, hardness of the abdomen, acute abdominal pain, peritonitis, chronic appendicitis, testicular or hernia pain, testicular torsion, renal colic pain, hip pain, chronic constipation or diarrhoea, irritable bowel, irregular menstruation, prolapse of the uterus and leucorrhoea.

These points help *activate qi and Blood circulation in the Dai Mai* and *dispel stasis from the lower abdomen.*

GB-27 is generally considered more important for men's complaints, whereas GB-28 is more for women.

Main Areas: Lower abdomen. Uterus. Intestines. Testicles.

Main Function: Regulates the lower jiao.

GB-28 Weidao 維道

Linking Path

Intersection of the Dai Mai on the Gallbladder channel

On the lower abdomen in the depression just medial to the inferior border of the ASIS, 0.5 cun inferior and slightly medial to GB-27.

Treatment and applications
See GB-27.

GB-29   Juliao   居髎

Squatting Bone Hole

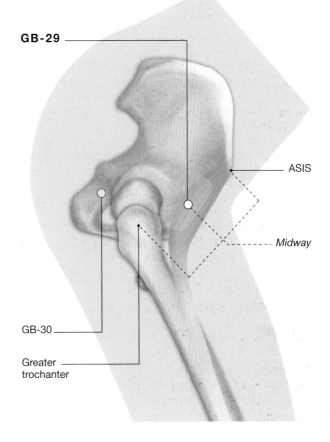

GB-29

ASIS

Midway

GB-30

Greater
trochanter

Intersection of the Yang Qiao Mai on the Gallbladder channel

Superior to the hip joint, at the centre of the large depression formed when the hip joint is flexed. Midway between the anterior superior iliac spine and the protuberance of the greater trochanter.

GB-29 is situated in the tensor fasciae latae muscle superficially, and more deeply, in the gluteus medius and minimus muscles. In its deep position lie the rectus femoris attachments.

Best treatment positions
GB-29 is treated in a side-lying position, with the hip flexed and the thigh and leg well supported by cushions. Ensure the thigh is adequately supported, so that the knee is at the same level as the hip (thigh parallel to the floor). Changing the angle of hip flexion slightly may help to find the most reactive location on pressure palpation.

Needling
• 1.0 to 3.0 cun perpendicular insertion.

! Do not puncture the cutaneous branch of the superficial circumflex iliac artery or vein or the lateral femoral cutaneous nerve. More deeply, the ascending branches of the lateral circumflex femoral artery and vein and branches of the superior gluteal artery, vein and nerve.

Manual techniques and shiatsu
Stationary perpendicular pressure applied with the thumbs, forearms, elbows or even knees can be very effective. Friction techniques are also very useful applied to the deeper muscle layers.

Moxibustion
Cones: 5–10. Pole: 10–30 minutes.

Cupping
Medium or strong suction is applicable on its own or over needles.

Guasha
Guasha is very effective across the fibres of tensor fasciae latae.

Stimulation sensation
Aching, distension, tingling or electricity locally, extending into and across the sides of the hip joint and possibly down the channel pathway toward the feet.

Actions and indications
GB-29 is an extremely powerful and widely used point for many *disorders of the hip joint*. It *dispels wind, cold and dampness, regulates qi and blood and dissipates stasis.*

It is probably the most important point for *pain at the lateral and anterior aspects of the hip and thigh* and helps restore mobility, even in chronic cases.

Main Areas: Hip. Thigh.

Main Functions: Alleviates pain.
Dispels stasis. Restores mobility to the hip.

GB-30 Huantiao

環跳

Jumping Circle

Intersection of the Bladder and Gallbladder
One of the nine points for Returning Yang
Heavenly Star point

In the large depression behind the hip joint, one third of the distance between the prominence of the greater trochanter and the sacral hiatus. Locate with the thigh flexed. Superficially, in the gluteus maximus muscle and more deeply, between the inferior margin of the piriformis and superior margin of the internal obturator. In its deep position in the gemellus superior muscle.

To aid location, place the palm on the thigh with the fingers facing toward the knee, and stroke upward following the femur until the fingers slide over the greater trochanter, directly into the large depression of GB-30. Apply pressure palpation to determine the reactive points that cause a radiating sensation in both the superficial and deep tissue layers.

Alternatively, locate the epicentre of GB-30 and then find four, eight or twelve points around it in a circle. Determine which is most reactive on pressure palpation.

Best treatment positions
GB-30 is best treated in a side-lying position with the hip and knee flexed. Use adequate cushion support under the thigh and leg (3–6 pillows). The knee should be at the same level as the hip and the thigh parallel to the floor.

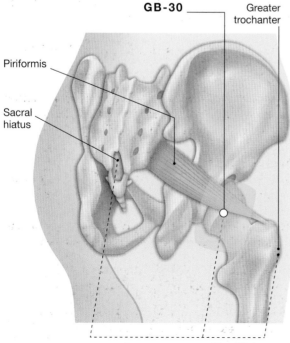

GB-30

Greater trochanter

Piriformis

Sacral hiatus

One third

Changing the angle of hip flexion slightly helps to locate the most reactive location on pressure palpation. Treat GB-30 bilaterally (with the patient prone) to regulate qi, dispel cold and tonify the lower jiao.

Needling
• 1 to 3 cun perpendicular or slightly oblique insertion.

! Do not puncture the cutaneous branches of the superior cluneal nerve. Deeper, the inferior gluteal nerve, artery and vein. In its deep position, the sciatic nerve.

Manual techniques and shiatsu
Strong pressure can be applied (use the elbows, knees and feet as well as the hands). Friction to the deep lateral rotator muscles of the hip, particularly the piriformis, is very effective for sciatic pain.

Moxibustion
Cones: 5–15. Pole: 10–30 minutes.

Cupping
Medium or strong suction is applicable on its own or over needles. Use a large cup size. Moving the cup in a circular motion around this location is also beneficial.

Guasha
Guasha can be applied quite strongly distally along the channel pathway or across the muscle fibres.

Magnets
Use of stick-on and other magnets can be very helpful at GB-30 and adjacent points. For hip disorders and sciatica, alternate poles between GB-30, GB-29 and GB-34 or Bl-60 plus other points of the lumbar or sacral area.

Stimulation sensation
Deqi at GB-30 should bring on a relieving sensation and soreness or aching extending to the affected areas. If strong pressure or deep needling is used, electricity is perceived extending down the legs toward the feet. Also, deqi may extend toward the sacrum and lower back.

Actions and indications
GB-30 is a very *dynamic point*, widely used for *many disorders of the hip*, thigh, entire lower limb, gluteal and lower back areas. It effectively *strengthens the hips, pelvic area* and *lower jiao, tonifies Yang qi and dissipates cold*. It is particularly indicated for sciatica, pain of the hips, lower back, knees and legs, stiffness, restricted movement or atrophy of the lower limbs, hemiplegia and genital or gynaecological pain.

> **Main Areas:** Thigh. Entire lower limb.
>
> **Main Functions:** Dispels wind. Cold and damp. Regulates qi and Blood. Alleviates pain.

GB-31   Fengshi

風市

Wind Market

On the midline of the lateral aspect of the thigh, 7 cun proximal to the popliteal crease, at the posterior border of the iliotibial tract. In the vastus lateralis muscle.

To aid location, ask the patient to stand with the arms hanging relaxed by the sides. Find GB-31 at the point where the tip of the middle finger touches the thigh.

Best treatment positions
This point is best treated with the patient lying down sideways or supine; however, prone can also be employed.

! Do not apply guasha, cupping or strong pressure to areas of visible capillaries, varicosities or cellulite.

Needling
• 0.5 to 1.5 cun perpendicular insertion.
• 1 to 2 cun transverse insertion distally or proximally.

! Do not puncture branches of the lateral femoral cutaneous nerve, and deeper, the muscular branch of the femoral nerve and the descending branch of the lateral circumflex femoral artery.

Moxibustion
Cones: 3–5. Pole: 5–15 minutes. Use the moxa pole to warm the entire iliotibial tract and lateral knee area.

Cupping
Use a medium or large cup size and medium-light or medium-strong suction. Also, move the cup up and down the entire length of the iliotibial tract (apply adequate lubricant). This technique is very effective in cases of pain and stiffness and also helps reduce swelling and cellulite.

Guasha
Guasha is effective across the iliotibial tract or along the channel pathway.

! Although effective, wrongly applied guasha can be extremely painful at this location.

Manual techniques and shiatsu
Stationary pressure is mainly applicable with the fingers, thumbs and palms. However, because this location is often painful, friction techniques may be more effective. Applying cross-fibre friction to the iliotibial tract is also very beneficial.

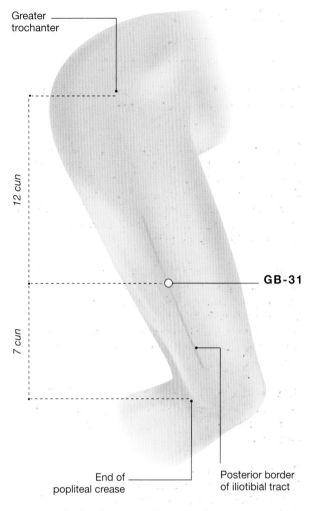

Greater trochanter

12 cun

7 cun

GB-31

End of popliteal crease

Posterior border of iliotibial tract

Another highly effective technique is to apply cross-fibre stretching to the iliotibial tract by moving it in an anterior and posterior direction. Apply this method along the length of the thigh down to the knee.

! Avoid very strong pressure as it can often be painful.

Stimulation sensation
Distension, dull aching, tingling or a mild electric sensation, extends out around the point and proximally and/or distally along the channel pathway.

Actions and indications
GB-31 is a useful point in cases of *weakness, pain, sciatica, atrophy* and *paralysis of the lower limbs*.

It has also been employed to *expel wind* causing swelling or itching of the skin on the legs or the whole body.

Main Areas: Thigh. Entire lower limb.

Main Functions: Dispels wind and dampness. Regulates qi. Alleviates pain.

GB-32　Zhongdu　中瀆
Ditch Centre

5 cun proximal to the popliteal crease, in the depression between the tendon of biceps femoris and the posterior border of the iliotibial tract, posterior to the shaft of the femur.

Note: Select GB-33 instead of GB-32 if it is more tender on pressure palpation.

Best treatment positions
Similar to GB-31.

Actions and indications
Similar to GB-31, *it dispels wind, dampness and cold, stimulates the circulation of qi and Blood in the channel and alleviates pain.*

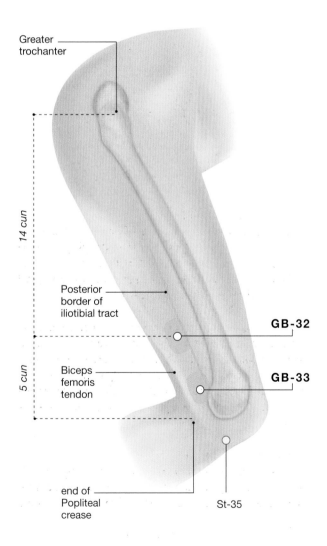

Greater trochanter

14 cun

Posterior border of iliotibial tract

GB-32

5 cun

Biceps femoris tendon

GB-33

end of Popliteal crease

St-35

GB-33　Xiyangguan　膝陽關
Yang Knee Gate

At the centre of the large depression formed between the tendon of biceps femoris and the posterior border of the iliotibial tract, directly superior the lateral condyle of the femur. In the short head of biceps femoris muscle. Locate and treat with the knee flexed at an angle of 90 degrees.

To aid location, GB-33 is directly lateral to St-35, when the knee is flexed and approximately 3 cun proximal to GB-34.

Best treatment positions
See GB-31.

Needling
• 0.5 to 1 cun perpendicular insertion, directed slightly posteriorly.

! Do not puncture the lateral femoral cutaneous nerve, the common peroneal nerve, and more deeply, the lateral superior genicular artery and vein.

Moxibustion
Cones: 3–7. Pole: 5–15 minutes.

! According to certain traditional medical texts, this location is contraindicated for moxibustion.

Actions and indications
Similar to the previous two points, GB-33 *dissipates wind, dampness and cold, regulates qi and Blood in the channel* and *alleviates pain.*

It is an *important local point* for disorders of the lateral aspect of the knee and is particularly indicated for tightness and shortening of the soft tissues in this area.

Main Areas: Knee. Lateral thigh.

Main Functions: Dissipates wind and cold.
Dispels stasis of qi and Blood.

GB-34 Yanglingquan 陽陵泉
Yang Mound Spring

**Uniting Sea-*He*, Earth point of the Gallbladder
Gathering *Hui* point of the sinews
Heavenly Star point**

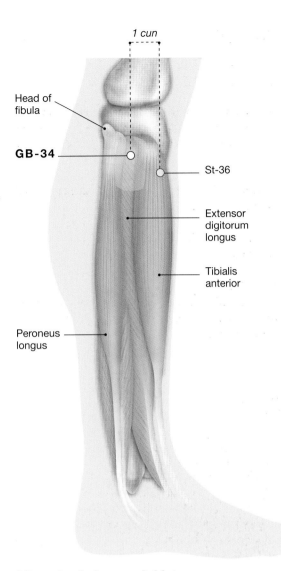

In the palpable depression anterior and inferior to the head of the fibula. Approximately 1 cun lateral and superior to St-36. At the anterior border of the peroneus longus muscle, in the extensor digitorum longus muscle. Locate with the knee flexed.

To aid location, place your fingertip on the prominence of the head of fibula and slide it anteriorly and inferiorly until it slips into the depression.

Best treatment positions
This point is best treated with the patient in a side-lying or a supine position with the knee flexed and well supported with cushions. However, treatment can also be applied in other positions.

Needling
• 0.5 to 1.5 cun perpendicular insertion.
• 2 to 3 cun, through the interosseous membrane behind the tibia, to join with Sp-9.

! Do not puncture the superficial or deep branches of the peroneal nerve, branches of the lateral sural cutaneous nerve or the circumflex peroneal artery. Deeper and in a slightly anterior direction, the anterior tibial artery and veins. Deeper still the peroneal artery and veins.

Moxibustion
Cones: 3–7. Pole: 5–20 minutes. Rice-grain moxa is also applicable.

Cupping
Medium or strong cupping with small cups can be very effective. Apply a cup over the head of fibula. Also, sliding the cup up and down along the lateral aspect of the leg, anterior and posterior to the fibula, as well as moving the cup around the head of fibula, is very effective.

Guasha
Guasha can be very effective, both down the channel pathway (down the centre of fibular shaft and down its posterior and anterior borders) and in a cross-fibre direction, particularly across the head and upper part of the shaft of the fibula (peroneus longus muscle).

Manual techniques and shiatsu
Perpendicular pressure can be applied quite strongly to this location, and is most effective in a side-lying or supine position with the knee flexed to 120–90 degrees. Friction techniques are effectively applied to the surrounding soft tissue attachments on the head and shaft of fibula.

Deep friction of the Gallbladder channel, anterior to the shaft of the fibula, all the way down to the external malleolus, on the peroneus longus and brevis and extensor digitorum longus muscles and underlying fascia is very effective. The same can be applied on the posterior aspect of the fibula to work through all the points from GB-34 to GB-39.

Actions and indications
GB-34 is one of the ten most commonly used points with a wide range of applications. It is one of the most significant locations to *regulate qi throughout the entire*

body, relieve stagnation and smooth the Gallbladder and Liver thus alleviating pain of both exterior and interior origin. GB-34 is also important to *clear dampness and heat from the Liver and Gallbladder.*

Common indications include hypertension, headaches, hypochondrial distension and pain, jaundice, cholecystitis, cholelithiasis, bitter taste, chills and fever due to shaoyang disharmony, nausea, vomiting, abdominal distension and pain, diarrhoea, constipation, intercostal neuralgia, breast pain or swelling, dysmenorrhoea, premenstrual syndrome, irritability and depression.

GB-34 is also extremely important to benefit the *joints and sinews* and has a special effect on the *sides of the body, rib cage* and *breasts*. It is very important in the treatment of *musculo-skeletal disorders* affecting any part of the body, including tendinitis, arthritis, cramps, spasm, tic, stiffness, contraction, shortening and weakness or atrophy of the soft tissues. It is widely used to treat disorders of the neck, shoulder, arm, knee or hip, arthritis, lumbar or thoracic pain, sciatica and hemiplegia.

GB-34 is also useful as a general treatment to *strengthen and relax the musculo-skeletal system* in athletes and other professionals who place great demands on the body.

> **Main Areas:** Sinews (muscles, tendons, ligaments and other soft tissues). Joints. Flank. Hypochondrium. Gallbladder. Chest.
>
> **Main Functions:** Regulates qi. Dissipates stagnation. Alleviates pain. Benefits the sinews. Regulates the Gallbladder and Liver.

GB-35   Yangjiao

Yang Intersection

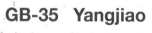

Accumulation Cleft-*Xi* point of the Yang Wei Mai

In the depression at the posterior border of the fibula, 7 cun proximal to the prominence of the lateral malleolus, level with GB-36, St-39 and Bl-58.

Best treatment positions
Similar to GB-34. Treatment is best applied with the knee in a flexed position.

Needling
• 0.5 to 1.5 cun perpendicular insertion.

! Do not puncture the cutaneous branches of the lateral sural nerve. In its deep position, the tibial nerve, artery and veins.

Actions and indications
Although GB-35 is the Accumulation Xi point for the Yang Wei, it is not very commonly used for interior disorders, because GB-34 and other points are considered more effective. It is, however, useful to treat pain at the lateral aspect of the lower leg, ankle and knee.

Nevertheless, it has been traditionally employed to treat *disorders of the Gallbladder and Yang Wei Mai*. Symptoms include chills and fever, dyspnoea, sore throat, swelling of the face, palpitations, fright, anxiety, depression and irritability.

> **Main Area:** Leg.
>
> **Main Functions:** Regulates qi. Dissipates stagnation. Alleviates pain. Benefits the Yang Wei Mai.

GB-36   Waiqiu

Outer Hill

外丘

Accumulation Cleft-*Xi* point

On the anterior border of the fibula, 7 cun proximal to the prominence of the lateral malleolus, level with and anterior to GB-35 and Bl-58, posterior to St-39.

Best treatment positions
Similar to GB-34. Treatment is best applied with the knee in a flexed position.

Needling
• 0.5 to 1.5 cun perpendicular insertion.

! Do not puncture the cutaneous branches of lateral sural nerve or the superficial peroneal nerve. More deeply, and in a slightly anterior direction, the anterior tibial artery and veins and deep peroneal nerve. Deeper still, the peroneal artery and veins.

Actions and indications

Although GB-36 is the Accumulation point of the Gallbladder, it is not as commonly used as other points for interior disorders. It can, however, be useful in the treatment of pain or swelling at the lateral aspect of the leg or ankle.

Traditionally it has been used for *clearing heat and expelling poisons*. Indications include irritability, depression, febrile diseases and fullness of the abdomen and chest.

> **Main Area:** Leg.
>
> **Main Functions:** Alleviates pain.
> Clears the Gallbladder.

GB-37   Guangming   光明
Bright Light

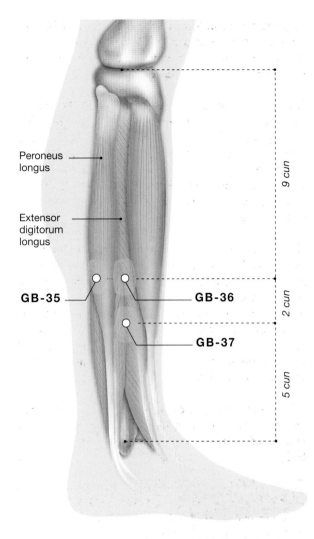

Connecting *Luo* point

In the depression between the peroneus longus and brevis and the extensor digitorum longus muscles, at the anterior border of the fibula, 5 cun proximal to the prominence of the lateral malleolus.

Best treatment positions
Similar to GB-36 and GB-34. Treatment is best applied with the knee flexed.

Needling
• 0.5 to 1.5 cun perpendicular insertion.

! Do not puncture the cutaneous branches of lateral sural nerve or the superficial peroneal nerve. Deeper, and slightly anteriorly, the anterior tibial artery and veins and deep peroneal nerve. Deeper still, the peroneal artery and veins.

Actions and indications
GB-37 is an important location for treating *disorders of the eyes*. Indications include pain, itching, inflammation, swelling and redness of the eyes, excessive lacrimation, migraine, glaucoma, keratitis, night blindness and failing vision.

It can also be effectively employed as *a local point* in the treatment of pain, stiffness or atrophy of the leg, similarly to GB-34, GB-35 and GB-36.

Additionally, it has been traditionally used to treat *interior Gallbladder* and *Liver disorders*. Symptoms include distension, fullness or pain of the hypochondrial area and chest, pain or swelling of the breast, headache, grinding of the teeth, depression and irritability.

> **Main Area:** Eyes.
>
> **Main Functions:** Benefits eyesight.
> Regulates the Gallbladder.

GB-38   Yangfu

Yang Assistance

陽輔

River-*Jing*, Fire (Sedation) point

In the depression 1 cun below GB-37, 4 cun proximal to the prominence of the lateral malleolus, on the anterior border of the fibula.

To aid location, it is one quarter of the distance between the lateral malleolus and the popliteal crease.

Best treatment positions
Similar to GB-37. Treatment is best applied with the knee in a flexed position.

Needling
Similar to GB-37.

Actions and indications
Although GB-38 is the Gallbladder sedation point and is thus useful in *excess conditions to sedate qi*, it is not as commonly used for interior conditions as other points.

GB-38 has been traditionally employed to *clear heat from the Gallbladder*, but in practice it is rarely used for this purpose. It can, however, be effective to treat pain of the lateral aspect of the leg.

> **Main Area:** Gallbladder fu and channel.
>
> **Main Functions:** Clears heat. Regulates qi.

GB-39   Xuanzhong (Juegu)

Suspended Bell (Severed Bone)

Gathering *Hui* point for the Marrow

In the depression 3 cun (one hand-width) proximal to the prominence of the lateral malleolus, between the posterior border of the fibula and the tendon of the peroneus brevis muscle.

GB-39 can also be located in the small space between the tendons of peroneus longus and brevis. In cases of extreme tightness of the peroneal muscles, or difficulty in inducing deqi at the above locations, treat it on the anterior border of the fibula, inferior to GB-38.

Best treatment positions
See GB-34. It is generally best to treat all Gallbladder points of the leg with the knee in a (slightly) flexed position.

Needling
• 0.5 to 1.5 cun perpendicular insertion.

Actions and indications
GB-39 is an important point to *benefit the sinews and bones and to strengthen the skeletal system*. Its primary functions are to *dispel wind and dampness* from the channel and *clear heat from the bones and Marrow*. It is widely used to treat *disorders of the musculo-skeletal system*, particularly weakness and chronic conditions, especially in the elderly.

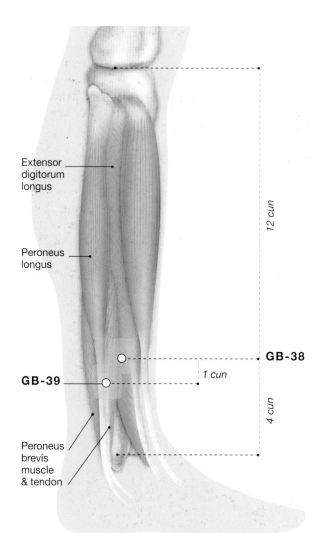

Extensor digitorum longus

Peroneus longus

12 cun

GB-38

1 cun

GB-39

4 cun

Peroneus brevis muscle & tendon

It is indicated for disorders of the joints, spine and neck, although classical texts emphasise the latter. These include osteoporosis, arthritis, spinal diseases, ankylosis, pain, swelling, stiffness of the joints, pain or heat in the bones, difficulty walking, sciatica, atrophy or paralysis of the lower limbs and hemiplegia.

Additionally, GB-39 can treat other disorders of the Marrow such as chronic tiredness, dizziness, reduced concentration, diminishing mental faculties in the elderly, headache, chronic inflammatory diseases and fever.

Furthermore, it *clears heat from the Gallbladder* and can be used to treat various manifestations of Gallbladder disharmony, including hypochondrial pain and distension, fullness of the chest, coughing, swelling of the axilla, anxiety and irritability.

Main Areas: Neck. Spine. Joints. Bones. Marrow. Sinews.

Main Functions: Benefits the Marrow. Sinews and bones. Clears heat. Regulates the Gallbladder channel.

GB-40 Qiuxu

丘墟

Mound

Source-*Yuan* point

At the centre of the sizeable depression, anterior and inferior to the lateral malleolus. Lateral to the tendon of peroneus tertius and distal to the inferior peroneal retinaculum, situated in the extensor digitorum brevis muscle.

To aid location, it is at the intersection of two lines following the anterior and the inferior border of the lateral malleolus.

Best treatment positions
GB-40 can be treated with the patient lying down in a supine or side position. However, sitting up in a chair can also be employed.

Needling
• 0.5 to 1.5 cun perpendicular insertion.

! Do not puncture the **small saphenous vein** or the dorsal cutaneous branch of the superficial peroneal nerve. More deeply, muscular branches of the deep peroneal nerve and the lateral tarsal artery. In a slightly posterior direction, the anterior lateral malleolar artery.

Manual techniques and shiatsu
Stationary pressure is best applied with the tips of the fingers or thumb to the exact location. However, gentle friction over the extensor retinaculum and underlying muscles (extensor digitorum and hallucis brevis) is also extremely effective for stiffness and pain of the ankle.

! GB-40 can be tender or painful on pressure palpation.

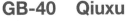

Anterior border of lateral malleolus

GB-40

Peroneus tertius

Inferior border of lateral malleolus

Moxibustion

Cones: 3–5. Pole: 5–20 minutes. Light or medium stimulation.

Guasha

Gently applied, guasha can be effective.

Stimulation sensation

A distending numbness, dull aching, tingling or electric sensation spreading out around the point and downward toward the metatarsals and toes is often achieved.

Actions and indications

GB-40 is the Source-Yuan point for the Gallbladder and is used to treat both *deficiency and excess disorders*. Its main functions are to *clear dampness and heat from the Gallbladder, promote qi and Blood circulation and alleviate pain.* Symptoms include hypochondrial distension and pain, and heartburn.

Furthermore, it is an important point for psychological disorders and is beneficial in cases of depression, mental irritability and inability to make decisions or act with courage.

As a local point, GB-40 can be useful in the treatment of injury and other disorders of the ankle and foot. Symptoms include pain, swelling, stiffness and cramping.

> **Main Areas:** Ankle. Foot. Gallbladder. Mind. Emotions.
>
> **Main Functions:** Regulates qi. Clears dampness and heat.

GB-41   Zulinqi   足臨泣

Foot Governor of Tears

Opening (Master) point of the Dai Mai
Stream-*Shu*, Wood (Horary) point

In the depression distal to the junction of the fourth and fifth metatarsal bones between the tendons of the extensor digitorum longus of the little toe and peroneus tertius.

To aid location, lift the patient's little toe to define the extensor digitorum longus tendon. Also, GB-41 may be located one hand-width distal to GB-40.

Best treatment positions

A supine or sitting position is best.

Manual techniques and shiatsu

Pressure must be applied carefully with the fingertips to ensure reaching the epicentre of the point inside the crevice between the two metatarsal bones.

! GB-41 is often painful on light pressure.

Needling

• 0.3 to 0.5 cun perpendicular insertion.

! Do not puncture veins or nerves of the dorsal cutaneous network. More deeply, the dorsal metatarsal artery.

Moxibustion

Cones: 2–3. Pole: 3–10 minutes.

Guasha

Gently applied, guasha can be effective.

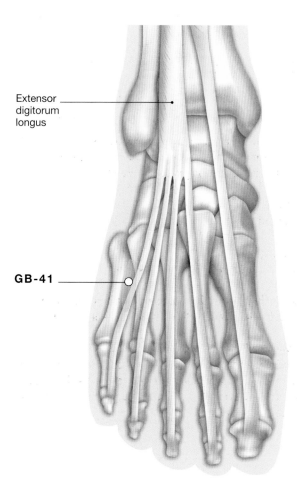

Extensor digitorum longus

GB-41

Actions and indications

GB-41 is the opening point of the Dai Mai (Girdle Vessel) and treats a wide variety of disorders. Its main functions are to *smooth Liver qi, clear damp heat, transform phlegm, open the chest and sides, benefit the breasts, clear the head and eyes and regulate the lower jiao.*

Indications include abdominal, hip and lower back pain, dysmenorrhoea, leucorrhoea, pain and distension of the hypochondrium, breasts and axilla, lumps and nodules, tightness of the chest, headache, migraine, dizziness and disorders of the eyes and ears.

Furthermore it has been employed to *regulate menstruation*, and is *beneficial during pregnancy* for pain of the lower back or hips.

As a *local point*, GB-41 is useful for disorders of the foot and toes. Moreover, it can be treated to *release tension along the entire course* of the Gallbladder channel.

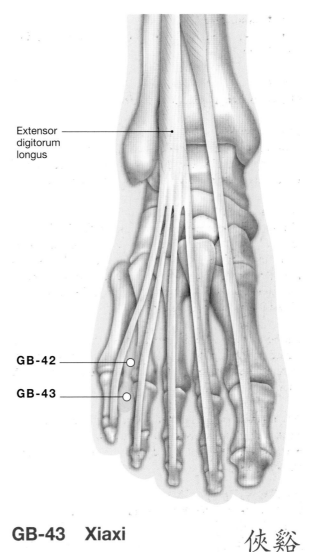

Extensor digitorum longus

GB-42

GB-43

> **Main Areas:** Foot. Breast. Flanks. Girdle Vessel. Gallbladder. Head. Eyes. Mind.
>
> **Main Functions:** Regulates qi. Clears dampness and heat.

GB-42   Diwuhui   地五會

Earth Fivefold Convergence

In the depression proximal to the heads of the fourth and fifth metatarsal bones, medial to the tendon of the extensor digitorum longus of the little toe.

Best treatment positions
Similar to GB-41.

Needling
• 0.3 to 0.4 cun perpendicular insertion.

! Do not puncture veins or nerves of the dorsal cutaneous network. More deeply, the dorsal metatarsal artery.

Actions and indications
GB-42 can be used in cases of local problems of the foot, including pain, swelling and tendinitis. In clinical practice however, this point is very seldom used for interior complaints.

GB-43   Xiaxi   俠谿

Narrow Stream

Spring-*Ying*, Water (Tonification) point

On the dorsum of the foot, between the fourth and fifth toes, proximal to the margin of the web, level with the fourth metatarsophalangeal joint.

Furthermore, GB-43 is also one of the M-LE-8 Bafeng points.

Best treatment positions
Similar to GB-41.

Needling
• 0.3 to 0.5 cun oblique insertion between the fourth and fifth metatarsophalangeal joints.

Actions and indications

GB-43 is a useful point to *clear interior heat and descend rising yang from the head, ears and eyes.* Indications include fever, dizziness, hypertension, red painful, swollen, eyes, headache, migraine and tinnitus.

As *a local point* it can be employed in the treatment of pain, swelling and inflammation of the dorsum of the foot and the fourth and fifth toes.

Furthermore, according to the *Five Phase* model, GB-43 is *a tonification point and has been used to strengthen the Gallbladder and Liver,* although it is seldom used for this purpose.

Main Areas: Gallbladder. Head. Eyes. Mind.

Main Functions: Clears heat. Descends yang. Clears the head. Ears and eyes.

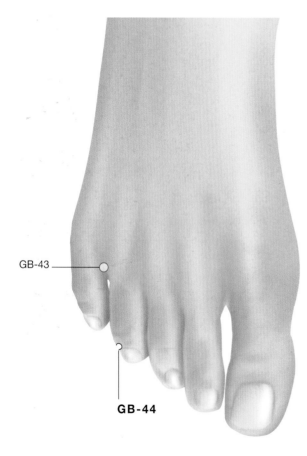

GB-43

GB-44

GB-44 Zuqiaoyin   足竅陰

Foot Opening to Yin

Well-*Jing*, Metal point

On the lateral side of the fourth toe, about 0.1 cun proximal to the corner of the nail. At the intersection of two lines following the lateral border and the base of the nail.

Best treatment positions

This location can be treated easily with the patient sitting or lying.

A strong stimulation is most effective if applied regularly until symptoms subside.

Needling
• 0.1 cun perpendicular insertion.

Manual techniques and shiatsu

Friction or sustained pressure may be applied with the tip of the finger or thumb. For optimum results, the stimulation should be reasonably strong.

Moxibustion

Cones: 3. Pole: 3–5 minutes.

Actions and indications

In common with the other Well-Jing points, GB-44 *restores consciousness, drains heat* and *clears the head and brain.*

Additionally, GB-44 *benefits the eyes, the chest and sides of the body.*

Main Areas: Gallbladder channel. Head. Eyes. Mind.

Main Functions: Restores consciousness. Clears the head and brain. Benefits the eyes.

Chapter 21

Points of the

Leg Jue Yin
Liver Channel

足厥陰肝經穴

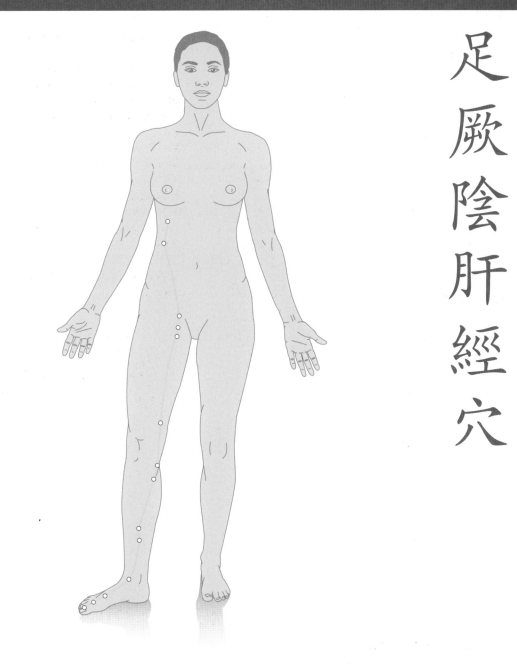

Liv-1 Dadun
Big Mound

大敦

Well-*Jing*, Wood (Horary) point

On the dorsum of the big toe, midway along the line connecting the lateral corner of the base of the nail and the centre of the interphalangeal crease.

Alternative location
Similarly to the other Well-Jing points, locate Liv-1 0.1 cun proximal to the lateral corner of the base of the nail.

Best treatment positions
Similar to the other Well-Jing points, although Liv-1 seems to cover a slightly larger area.

Needling
· Needling may be applied slightly deeper than other Well-Jing points, up to 0.3 cun perpendicularly.

Manual techniques and shiatsu
Friction and sustained perpendicular pressure can be applied to the entire lateral part of the dorsal aspect of the toe, surrounding the two mentioned locations.

Moxibustion
Use moxibustion to arrest bleeding in combination with Sp-1.

Magnets
Magnets can also be effectively applied to this location.

Use north pole on Liv-1 bilaterally, and south pole on GB-20, GB-21, Du-16 or Du-20 to draw down excessive yang and subdue internal wind, with symptoms affecting the head and neck.

Actions and indications
Liv-1 is an important point used to *subdue interior wind*, *restore consciousness* and *calm the mind*.

Other traditional functions include regulating Liver qi and harmonising the lower jiao and urogenital system.

Similarly to Sp-1, Liv-1 also helps *arrest bleeding*, and moxibustion can be used to decrease excessive or abnormal menstruation, particularly if it is due to Blood stasis.

Main Areas: Head. Nervous system. Uterus.

Main Functions: Subdues interior wind.
Calms the mind. Arrests bleeding.

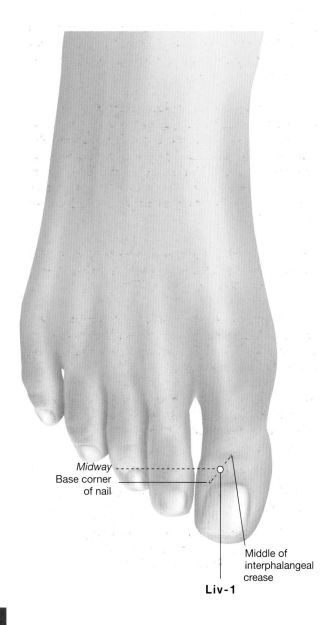

Midway
Base corner of nail

Middle of interphalangeal crease

Liv-1

Liv-2　Xingjian
Passing Between

行間

Spring-*Ying*, Fire (Tonification) point

On the dorsal aspect of the foot, on the web between the first and second toes, distal to the metatarsophalangeal joint. To aid location, Liv-2 is approximately 0.5 cun proximal to the margin of the web. When the toes are closed together it is at the end of the crease formed between the two toes. Furthermore, Liv-2 is also one of the M-LE-8 Bafeng points.

Best treatment positions
This location is best treated with the patient supine. However, side-lying or sitting can also be employed.

Needling
• 0.3 to 1 cun oblique insertion, directed toward the heel, between the first and second metatarsal bones.
• 0.3 to 0.5 cun perpendicular insertion.

! Do not puncture the dorsal digital artery, vein or nerve.

Manual techniques and shiatsu
Stationary perpendicular pressure is applied quite strongly into the space between the metatarsophalangeal joints of the first and second toe with the tip of the finger or thumb. Additionally, friction can be effective.

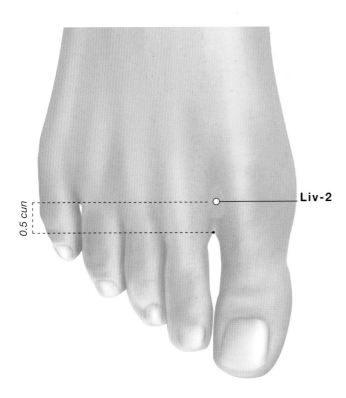

0.5 cun

Liv-2

Stretching the first and second toe downwards (flexion), opens this location. Additionally, mobilising the first and second toes helps release tension from this area.

Moxibustion
Cones: 3–5. Pole: 5–15 minutes. Rice-grain moxibustion is also applicable.

Magnets
Magnets are effective for problems of the metatarsophalangeal joints. Apply north and south poles alternately on the M-LE-8 Bafeng points.

Stimulation sensation
A deep numb ache usually spreads around the location and into the first or second metatarsophalangeal joint. An electric or tingling sensation extending toward the tip of the first or second toe is also common.

Actions and indications
Liv-2 is a powerful point to soothe the liver and is primarily employed to *clear heat and drain fire from the Liver*. It effectively *cools Blood, descends rising yang* and *subdues internal wind*.

Clinical manifestations include migraine, headache, red, painful and inflamed eyes, dizziness, hypertension, transient ischaemic attack, numbness of the face and limbs, convulsions, epilepsy, facial paralysis, fever, sore throat, soreness of the genital area, dysmenorrhoea, irregular menstruation, excessive or incessant menstruation, abnormal uterine bleeding, mental agitation, insomnia and irritability.

Liv-2 is also traditionally employed for urinary disorders including dysuria, hot or turbid urine, urethritis, cystitis, urinary retention and incontinence.

Other traditional indications include hypochondrial pain caused by liver disease, soft stool diarrhoea, abdominal distension and pain, indigestion, hernia, retching, spitting blood, chest and lumbar pain.

Additionally, Liv-2 is effective as a local point for disorders of the first and second metatarsophalangeal joint and is particularly indicated for inflammation and swelling.

Main Areas: Head Eyes. Nervous system. Abdomen.

Main Functions: Clears heat. Descends excessive yang and circulates Liver qi.

Liv-3 Taichong

Great Surge

太冲

Source-*Yuan* point
Stream-*Shu*, Earth point
Heavenly Star point

In the depression distal to the junction of the first and second metatarsal bones, approximately level with Sp-3. In the dorsal interosseous muscle, lateral to the tendon of extensor hallucis brevis. To aid location, palpate for the most reactive site.

Best treatment positions
With the patient in a supine position. However, side-lying or sitting up in a chair can also be employed.

Needling
• 0.3 to 1 cun perpendicular insertion in a slightly proximal-lateral direction, or 1.5 cun to join with Kd-1.

! Do not puncture veins of the dorsal cutaneous network, the terminal branch of the deep peroneal nerve, or the dorsal metatarsal artery.

Manual techniques and shiatsu
Perpendicular pressure and friction techniques are applicable with the fingertip or thumb. Additionally, mobilising the metatarsal bones can help relax this area. An effective shiatsu technique is to apply pressure to Liv-3 and Kd-1 simultaneously.

! Liv-3 can be extremely tight and painful. Ensure pressure is applied gently and carefully. Do not apply friction if there are visible cutaneous veins.

Moxibustion
Cones: 3–5. Pole: 5–10 minutes. Rice-grain moxibustion is also applicable.

! Do not overheat this location.

Magnets
Magnets are effectively employed at this location.

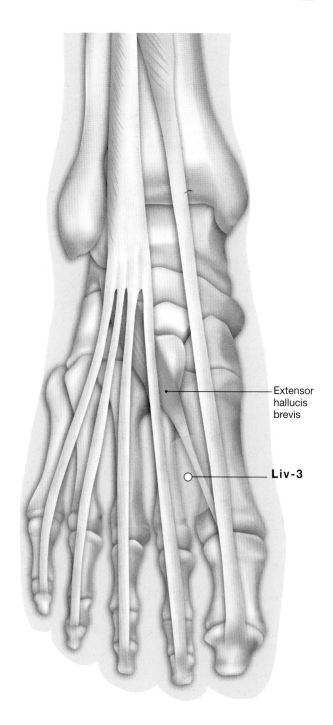

Extensor hallucis brevis

Liv-3

Stimulation sensation

Liv-3 is a powerful point and engenders strong reactions including aching, pain, numbness or electricity surrounding the location and spreading out across the dorsum of the foot and toward the toe. The sensation often extends proximally along the channel and may reach the abdomen and chest. Additionally, tingling or numbness may be perceived extending across the sole of the foot, around Kd-1.

For best results, a strong sensation should be achieved. Pain and other acute symptoms should be reduced after treatment.

Deqi at Liv-3 can make the person sigh, breathe deeper, cough or clear their throat. Also, when deqi arrives, there should be a noticeable change in the pulse, which should feel calmer, softer and usually slows down.

In many cases there may be emotional releases and the person may start talking about various issues that may or may not be directly relevant. In some cases the person may start crying.

! If there seems to be a strong reaction in response to treatment, discontinue manual stimulation or remove needles immediately.

! Liv-3 is a very strong point and can have powerful effects on the mind and body. It can engender strong physical or mental reactions and release emotions such as sadness or anger. In certain, albeit rare cases, treatment can bring to the surface excessive emotional states, indicating that the treatment was possibly inappropriate.

Additionally, excessive stimulation of Liv-3 can have an effect on the nervous system and cause a sudden drop in systemic blood pressure, leading to dizziness or fainting in sensitive patients.

Care should be taken not to overstimulate Liv-3, particularly in deficient patients and during pregnancy.

Actions and indications

Liv-3 is one of the most commonly used points with a wide area of applications in both excess and deficiency disorders.

It is a *primary point to smooth the Liver, dispel stasis and improve circulation of qi and Blood* throughout the Three Jiao. At the same time, Liv-3 is extremely important to *nourish Yin and Blood and cool the Liver.* It effectively *clears interior heat, sedates excessive Yang and subdues interior wind.*

Liv-3 has extremely *powerful qi moving qualities,* and alongside LI-4 is possibly the most *important point to alleviate pain* of any cause or location. These points are collectively known as the Four Gates, and combined are extensively used for pain relief and anaesthesia (see also LI-4).

Thus, it also has a powerful *calming and soothing effect on the mind* and is important to *release blocked emotional states* causing mental restlessness, psychological instability, mood swings, depression, fear or irritability. It has been extensively employed to treat a variety of *psychosomatic symptoms* including insomnia, dream disturbed sleep, frequent sighing, constriction of the chest, plum stone throat, addiction disorders and pain or other symptoms with no apparent medical cause.

Liv-3 also has a particularly powerful effect on the *head, eyes and nervous system* because it *clears heat and descends excess yang at the same time as nourishing and cooling the Liver yin and Blood.* Indications include headache, migraine, dizziness, pain and inflammation of the eyes, dry eyes, tired eyes, blurred vision, failing vision, glaucoma, Meniére's disease and tinnitus.

It is also commonly used to treat a variety of *neurological disorders* including symptoms following cerebro-vascular accident, paralysis, atrophy, spasticity, neuritis, disorders of the cranial nerves, facial paralysis, transient ischaemic attack, tremor, tick, spasm, epilepsy, seizures and vertigo.

In relation to the *cardiovascular system,* Liv-3 has been used to treat a variety of conditions including hypertension, coronary heart disease, angina pectoris, tightness, heaviness or pain of the chest, palpitations, swelling of the legs, circulation and vascular disorders, varicose veins, cold feet, bleeding disorders and anaemia.

Liv-3 has also been successfully employed in the treatment of disorders of the *respiratory system* and throat. Indications include cough, asthma, dyspnoea, tightness and constriction of the chest and throat, inflammation of the throat, pharyngitis, laryngitis, goitre, hyperthyroidism and swelling of the glands.

In relation to the *liver, gallbladder and digestive system,* Liv-3 has been extensively used to treat a variety of cases including liver and gallbladder disease, hepatitis, jaundice, gallstones, pancreatitis, hypochondrial distension and pain, epigastric pain, heartburn, indigestion, gastritis, oesophagitis, gastric ulceration, nausea, vomiting, abdominal distension and pain, abdominal rumbling, irritable bowel syndrome, diarrhoea, dysentery, blood in the stool and constipation.

Liv-3 is very extensively used to help *regulate menstruation* and is extremely important in the treatment of many gynaecological disorders, including dysmenorrhoea, premenstrual syndrome, breast swelling and pain, irregular menstruation, delayed menstruation, amenorrhoea, abnormal uterine bleeding, excessive or incessant menstruation, infertility and vaginal discharge. Treatment applied to Liv-3 before and during labour helps the cervix dilate (combine with Liv-5 and Sp-6 for this purpose), but also offers pain relief and relaxation for the mind and body during labour (combine with LI-4 and ear Shenmen for the latter functions).

Liv-3 has also been traditionally used to treat mastitis, insufficient lactation, uterine prolapse and to arrest severe sweating after childbirth.

It is also a significant point to *clear damp heat, harmonise the lower jiao and benefit the urogenital system.* Indications include dysuria, cystitis, urethritis, urinary incontinence or retention, itching, inflammation or pain of the external genitals, impotence and testicular pain, swelling or retraction.

Additionally, Liv-3 is important in the treatment of *musculo-skeletal disorders* including arthritis, muscle cramping, spasm tightness or contraction of the muscles, tics and tremors, tendinitis, pain, atrophy or weakness of the lower limbs and lumbar pain. As a local point, it effectively treats pain and swelling of the dorsum of the foot and area anterior to the medial malleolus.

Also, because Liv-3 increases qi and Blood circulation, it can be used to help support the musculo-skeletal system in persons who physically overexert themselves, including athletes and labourers. Treatment can help relax tight "sinews" and muscles throughout the entire body and is also of benefit during intensive sports and/or flexibility training. For the latter purpose, combine Liv-3 with GB-34, St-36 and LI-4.

Additionally, Liv-3 has been traditionally employed to treat a variety of other symptoms and disorders including swelling and pain of the axilla, inflammation of the sweat glands, excessive sweating, cold feet, and umbilical pain.

Combine Liv-3 with GB-34 for qi and Blood stagnation in the Liver, with LI-4 to treat stress, tension and pains anywhere in the body and addiction related problems and with Sp-4 and Ren-4 for Blood stasis in the uterus.

> **Main Areas:** Entire body. Abdomen. Digestive and reproductive systems. Chest. Head. Eyes. Nervous system. Mind.
>
> **Main Functions:** Circulates Liver qi and dispels stasis. Nourishes Yin and Blood. Cools the Liver. Regulates menstruation.

Liv-4 Zhongfeng

Mound Centre

中封

River-*Jing*, Metal point

In the depression anterior to the prominence of the medial malleolus, medial to the tibialis anterior tendon, when the foot is at a right angle to the tibia.

It is situated anterior to the great saphenous vein and posterior to the tendon of tibialis anterior. In its deep position and laterally, lies the extensor hallucis longus.

Needling
Note: palpate the saphenous vein and, if necessary, move it slightly posteriorly with the fingertip, so as to insert the needle anterior to it.

- 0.3 to 1 cun perpendicular insertion under the tibialis anterior tendon, toward St-41.
- 0 .5 to 1 cun oblique distal insertion in a slightly lateral direction under the tendon.

! Do not needle deeply in a posterior direction. Do not puncture the great saphenous vein or cutaneous branches of the crural nerve and deeper, the medial malleolar network of arteries and veins. Deeper still, in a lateral and slightly posterior direction, the anterior tibial artery and vein, and the deep peroneal nerve.

Manual techniques and shiatsu
Perpendicular pressure can be applied under the tibialis anterior tendon with the fingertip or thumb. Friction across the tibialis anterior and extensor hallucis longus tendon is also very effective.

Also, grasping and pressing these two tendons, with the thumb on Liv-4 and the fingers at St-41, is effective. Additionally, apply stationary pressure to Liv-4 and St-41 simultaneously.

! Do not apply friction across the great saphenous vein.

Moxibustion
Pole: 5–10 minutes with light-medium stimulation only. Direct moxibustion is not recommended at this location.

Stimulation sensation
Local numbness, aching or tingling is commonly experienced.

Actions and indications
Liv-4 is not as commonly used as other Liver points for its interior functions that include *spreading Liver qi* and *harmonising the lower jiao*. It does, however, effectively treat pain, swelling and stiffness of the ankle and medial aspect of the foot.

Other traditional indications include gynaecological complaints, dysmenorrhoea, abdominal pain, genital pain, hernia, retraction of the testicles, dysuria, retention of urine, jaundice and hepatitis.

> **Main Areas:** Ankle. Abdomen.
>
> **Main Functions:** Spreads Liver qi. Harmonises the lower jiao.

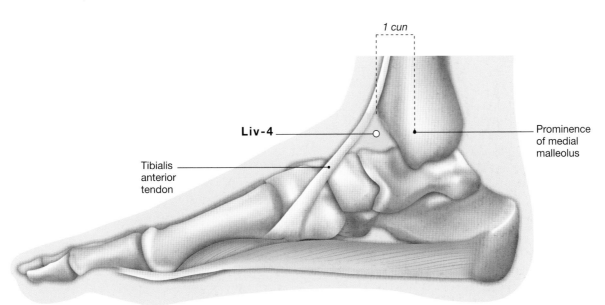

Liv-5 Ligou

Woodworm Channel

蠡溝

Connecting *Luo* point

5 cun above the medial malleolus, in a small depression just posterior to the medial tibial border.

To aid location, Liv-5 is one-third of the distance between the prominence of the medial malleolus and the popliteal (knee) crease. A visible depression normally appears at Liv-5 when the foot is dorsiflexed.

Best treatment positions

Treatment is best applied in a supine position with the knee flexed and the thigh laterally rotated. Use ample cushion support under the thigh, knee and leg.

Needling

- 0.5 to 1 cun perpendicular insertion along the posterior border of the tibia.
- 0.5 to 1.5 cun oblique proximal insertion, following the posterior border of the tibia.

! Do not puncture the cutaneous branches of the medial crural or saphenous nerve. More deeply and anteriorly, the tibial nerve, artery and vein.

Manual techniques and shiatsu

Pressure should be applied directly behind the medial tibial border with the fingertips or palms. Stretching the calf muscles is also effective.

Moxibustion

Cones: 3–5. Pole: 5–15 minutes with light-medium stimulation. Rice-grain moxa is also effective.

Magnets

Magnets may also be used effectively.

Stimulation sensation

Local aching, tingling or numbness, possibly extending proximally along the channel toward the abdomen.

Actions and indications

Liv-5 is an important point to *spread Liver qi* and clear dampness and heat. It is particularly indicated for *lower jiao disorders* affecting the *gynaecological and urogenital systems.*

Indications include pain, itching and inflammation of the external genitals or urethra, lower abdominal pain, dysuria, vaginal discharge, irregular menstruation, dysmenorrhoea, insufficient dilation of the cervix during labour, prolapse of the uterus, inguinal or scrotal hernia, testicular pain, prostatitis, testicular retraction, excessive libido, priapism and impotence.

It also effectively treats other symptoms of *Liver qi stagnation* such as hypochondrial pain, tightness of the chest, plum stone throat, poor vision, depression, mood swings and irritability. Liv-5 has a significant effect on the person's psycho-emotional state and can help release stuck emotions, particularly anger, depression and sadness. Liv-5 is also effective as a local point, and can be used to treat pain, swelling or restricted motility of the leg.

Main Areas: Genitourinary system. Mind. Liver.

Main Functions: Spreads Liver qi. Benefits the genitals and uterus. Clears damp heat.

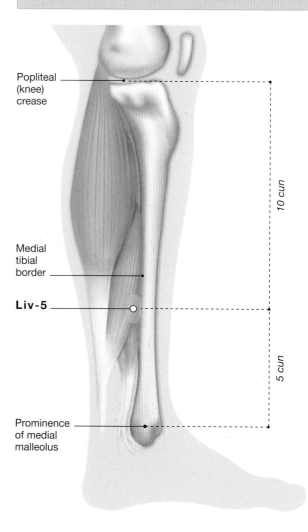

Popliteal (knee) crease

10 cun

Medial tibial border

Liv-5

5 cun

Prominence of medial malleolus

Liv-6 Zhongdu

中都

Central Pool

Accumulation Cleft-*Xi* point

7 cun above the medial malleolus, just posterior to the medial tibial border.

Best treatment positions
Similar to Liv-5.

Actions and indications
Liv-6 is the accumulation point of the Liver channel and therefore treats *acute pain* of the channel pathway as well as interior *Blood stasis* and heat. However, it is not as commonly used as other Liver points. Symptoms include abdominal pain, excessive menstruation, dysmenorrhoea and pain or swelling of the leg.

> **Main Areas:** Leg. Liver.
>
> **Main Function:** Dispels Blood stasis.

Liv-7 Xiguan

膝關

Knee Joint

With the knee flexed, locate Liv-7 posterior and inferior to the medial tibial condyle, in the upper portion of the medial head of the gastrocnemius muscle, 1 cun posterior to Sp-9.

Best treatment positions
Similar to Sp-9.

Needling
• 0.5 to 1 cun perpendicular insertion.

Actions and indications
Liv-7 is primarily used as a *local point* to dispel wind and damp, reduce swelling and relax the sinews. It helps treat pain, swelling and restricted motility of the knee.

> **Main Area:** Knees.
>
> **Main Function:** Dispels dampness.

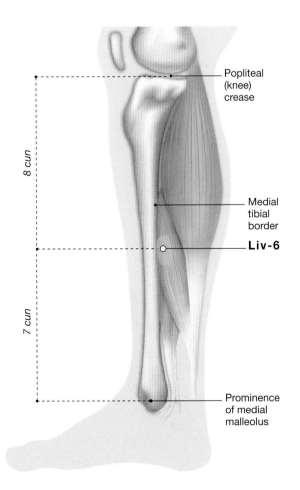

Popliteal (knee) crease

8 cun

Medial tibial border

Liv-6

7 cun

Prominence of medial malleolus

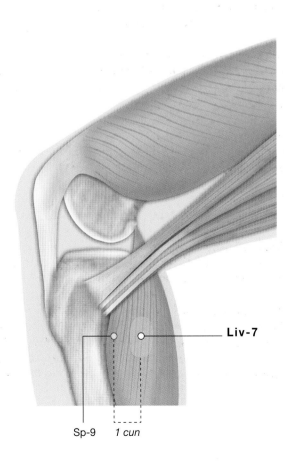

Liv-7

Sp-9   *1 cun*

Liv-8 Ququan

曲泉

Spring at the Bend

Uniting Sea-*He*, Water (Tonification) point

Anterior to the tendons attaching to the medial side of the knee, posterior to the medial femoral condyle when the knee is flexed. In a small depression, between the tendon of the gracilis and the posterior border of the sartorius muscle on, or slightly proximal to the medial end of the popliteal (knee) crease.

To aid location, grasp the flesh at the medial aspect of the knee, with the index finger placed on Kd-10. The thumb should automatically locate Liv-8.

Alternative locations
In cases where there is a lot of subcutaneous fat or the underlying muscles are flaccid, the small depression at the main Liv-8 location is not easily palpable. In these cases, locate it slightly anteriorly on the sartorius muscle, or just anterior to its border. Visually observe the large depression formed by the flesh at the medial aspect of the knee, and locate Liv-8 at its centre. If the depression is not visible due to swelling or excess fat, palpate gently with the palms to ascertain its centre.

Note: Other texts locate Liv-8 slightly more posteriorly between the semitendinosus and gracilis tendons.

Best treatment positions
Treatment is best applied in a supine position with the knee flexed and the thigh laterally rotated so that the medial aspect of the knee faces upwards. Use ample cushion support at the thigh, knee and leg.

Needling
• 0.5 to 1.5 cun perpendicular insertion.

! Do not puncture the great saphenous vein, the anterior branch of the femoral cutaneous nerve, the saphenous nerve, and more deeply, the genicular artery and vein.

Manual techniques and shiatsu
Stationary pressure is applicable with the fingertips or thumbs. However, palm pressure is often the most appropriate as the area may be sensitive or painful. Additionally, stretching the muscles posteriorly is also effective. Cross fibre friction can be applied across the gracilis, semimembranosus and semitendinosus tendons.

! This area can be extremely sensitive or painful, particularly if there is a lot of subcutaneous fat, swelling or varicosities in the area.

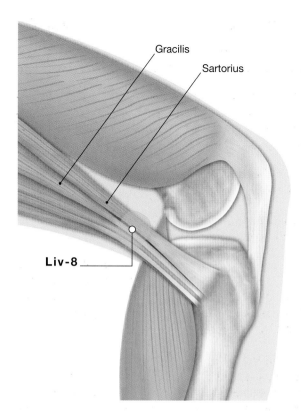

Gracilis
Sartorius
Liv-8

Moxibustion
Cones: 3–7. Pole: 5–15 minutes with light-medium stimulation. Rice-grain moxa can also be effective.

! Direct moxibustion is not recommended at this location in patients with varicosities.

Stimulation sensation
Distension, aching or numbness spreading out around the medial aspect of the knee, possibly extending proximally up the thigh, toward the genitals and abdomen.

Actions and indications
Liv-8 is a major point to *nourish Liver Blood and Yin* and *cool the Liver*. Moreover, it *dispels dampness, heat and blood stasis* from the lower jiao and benefits the Kidneys, uterus and urogenital system.

Indications include itching and inflammation of the genitals, dysuria, turbid urine, cystitis, urethritis, vaginal discharge, dysmenorrhoea, endometriosis, ovarian cysts, oligomenorrhoea, amenorrhoea, abdominal distension and pain, impotence, diarrhoea, headache and pain, swelling or restricted motility of the knee and leg.

Main Areas: Lower jiao. Genitals. Uterus.

Main Functions: Nourishes Blood and yin. Cools the Liver. Clears dampness and heat.

Liv-9　Yinbao 陰包

Yin Wrapping

On the medial aspect of the thigh, 4 cun proximal to the medial end of the popliteal (knee) crease, in the depression between the vastus medialis and sartorius muscles.

To aid location, if the knee joint is extended and the foot dorsiflexed, a groove appears between the muscles.

Needling
• 0.5 to 1.5 cun perpendicular insertion.

! Do not puncture the muscular branch of the femoral artery, or posteriorly, the muscular branch of the femoral nerve and the saphenous nerve. Further posteriorly lies the femoral artery and vein, and inferiorly the ascending genicular artery and vein.

Manual techniques and shiatsu
Perpendicular pressure and friction techniques are applicable with the fingers or thumbs. However, palm pressure is usually most effective here. Also, stretching the sartorius and adductor muscles in a posterior direction effectively relaxes the surrounding area.

! Do not apply friction to the great saphenous vein or the other deeper vasculature (see note above in the needling cautions section).

Moxibustion
Cones: 2–5. Pole: 5–10 minutes. Light-medium stimulation only. Rice-grain moxa is also applicable.

! Do not overheat this area. Direct moxibustion is not often recommended at this location and is contraindicated in patients with varicosities.

Actions and indications
Liv-9 is not a very commonly used point for its internal functions. However, it does help *regulate the lower jiao* and benefit menstruation. Symptoms include irregular menstruation, abdominal pain, lumbar pain, frequent urination, enuresis, incontinence and urinary retention.

Liv-9 can be useful in the treatment of channel disorders, in such cases as pain or swelling of the medial aspect of the knee, sciatica and thigh pain.

> **Main Areas:** Genitals. Uterus.
>
> **Main Functions:** Regulates qi. Benefits the lower jiao. Alleviates pain.

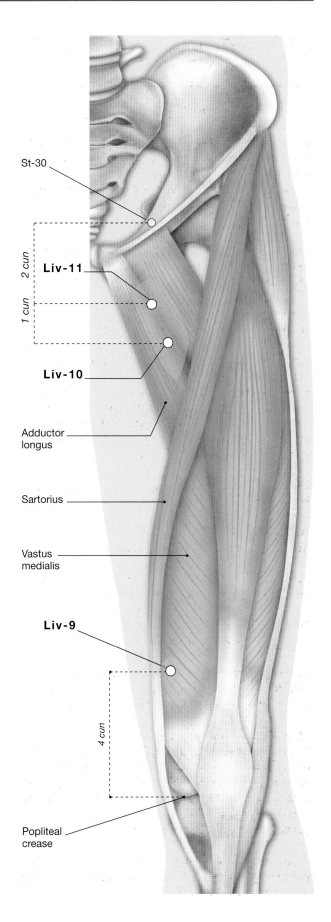

St-30

2 cun

1 cun

Liv-11

Liv-10

Adductor longus

Sartorius

Vastus medialis

Liv-9

4 cun

Popliteal crease

Liv-10 Zuwuli

Leg Five Miles

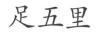

3 cun (one hand-width) distal to St-30, on the anterior border of the adductor longus muscle. Between the adductor longus and the pectineus muscles. In its deep position the adductor brevis and, deeper, the adductor minimus.

To aid location, the adductor longus tendon is the most prominent tendon in the groin.

!! Do not apply any form of treatment to this area if thrombosis has not been excluded.

Best treatment positions

This location is best treated with the patient lying in a supine position. The thigh and knee should be slightly flexed and laterally rotated so that the area is exposed. Use ample cushion support.

Needling

• 0.5 to 1.5 cun perpendicular insertion.

! Do not puncture the great saphenous vein or the anterior cutaneous branches of the femoral nerve. Deeper, branches of the medial femoral circumflex artery and vein and perforating branches of the deep femoral artery and vein. Medially, the obturator nerve, artery and vein. Do not puncture lymph nodes.

Manual techniques and shiatsu

Perpendicular pressure and friction techniques are applicable with the fingers or thumbs. However, palm pressure is usually most effective. Also, stretching the muscles posteriorly effectively relaxes the area.

! Do not apply friction to the great saphenous vein or the other deeper vasculature. Also, do not apply pressure to enlarged lymph nodes.

Moxibustion

Moxibustion is not often used at this location due to the underlying vasculature. However, indirect moxibustion can be effective to dispel cold and treat such cases as hernia, testicular pain, impotence and infertility.

Actions and indications

Choose between Liv-10 and Liv-11 depending on which is more reactive on pressure palpation (these points are used for similar purposes). Although neither point is very commonly used, they can be effective in such cases as *groin pain, hernia*, testicular pain or swelling, impotence, dysmenorrhoea, infertility, dysuria and prostatitis.

As *local points*, Liv-10 and Liv-11 can be used to treat injury, spasm or inflammation of the adductors.

> **Main Areas:** Thigh. Groin. Genitals.
>
> **Main Functions:** Regulates qi.
> Dispels stasis and pain.

Liv-11 Yinlian

Yin Corner

1 cun proximal to Liv-10, on the anterior border of the adductor longus muscle.

Best treatment positions

Similar to Liv-10.

Actions and indications

Liv-11 is used for similar purposes to Liv-10, although its traditional indications emphasise *gynaecological and fertility disorders*.

> **Main Areas:** Thigh. Genitals. Uterus.
>
> **Main Functions:** Dispels cold and pain.

Liv-12 Jimai

Urgent Pulse

On the inguinal groove, in the depression medial to the femoral artery and vein. Approximately 2.5 cun lateral to the anterior midline, distal and slightly lateral to St-30. Below the inguinal ligament in the depression of the saphenous hiatus. In its deep position lies the pectineus muscle.

To aid location, Liv-12 is about one finger-width medial to the palpable femoral artery and approximately 1 cun medial to Sp-12 (on the lateral side of the femoral artery).

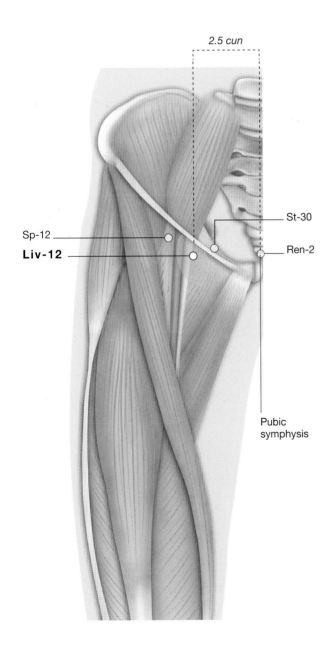

Best treatment positions
This location should be treated with the patient lying in a supine position. The thigh should be slightly flexed and laterally rotated so that this area is exposed. Use ample cushion support.

Important note
Traditionally, Liv-12 was treated by moxibustion rather than needling, because the latter was considered dangerous. However, moxibustion is not recommended at Liv-12, except in very rare cases, and direct moxibustion is contraindicated. Pressure techniques are easier to employ, and are thus more readily recommended.

! This is a sensitive location and any treatment applied should be carefully considered.

!! Do not apply any form of treatment to this area if there is any suspicion of thrombosis.

Needling
• 0.5 to 1 cun insertion medial to the femoral vein, in a perpendicular or slightly oblique and medial direction.

!! Do not puncture the cutaneous branches of the ilioinguinal nerve, the external pudendal artery and vein or the great saphenous vein; more deeply, the femoral artery and vein, and deeper still, branches of the medial femoral circumflex artery and vein. Medially, the obturator nerve, artery and vein. Furthermore, do not puncture lymph nodes.

Manual techniques and shiatsu
Perpendicular pressure with the fingertip or thumb, or palm is applicable. Also, stretching the adductor muscles in a medial and posterior direction, with the palm or heel of the hand is very effective. Additionally, friction to the pectineus insertion is beneficial in cases of injury.

! Do not apply friction to the saphenous hiatus area. Also, do not apply any form of pressure to enlarged lymph nodes.

Opening this point can be effectively achieved by stretching the thigh gently in a posterior direction. This helps improve circulation in the lower limbs and is an effective stretch for tight adductor muscles.

! Do not apply sudden or strong pressure to stretch the thigh because this can injure the hip joint.

A widely employed ancient Eastern technique is to apply pressure directly to the femoral artery for 30 to 60 seconds to occlude the blood flow, until the entire lower limb goes numb from the ischaemia.

Then, when the pressure is released, the blood rushes back through the arteries producing a sensation of heat throughout the entire limb. This technique can help *improve circulation* in the lower limbs and benefits athletes because the increase in pressure has a 'flushing' effect and helps detoxify the muscles following exercise. It is also very helpful for those who have poor circulation in the lower limbs, cold feet, cramps, and vascular disorders.

A more advanced technique is the simultaneous application of pressure to the axillary arteries at He-1 and the femoral arteries at Liv-12 to occlude blood flow to the four limbs. Although this technique can be dangerous and should not be applied in cases of advanced vascular disease or hypertension it can be of great benefit to those suffering from *circulation disorders* due to qi and Blood stagnation or qi and Blood deficiency.

!! Do not apply these occlusion techniques if there is any suspicion of thrombosis.

Stimulation sensation

Deqi at this location is often experienced as a strong tingling, or electric sensation, spreading distally along the medial aspect of the thigh and leg. Additionally the sensation may travel medially toward the genitals or upwards into the pelvis, sometimes reaching the lumbar area.

Moxibustion

Moxibustion is not often recommended because of the danger of overheating the underlying vasculature or burning the pubic hair. However, lightly applied indirect moxibustion can be cautiously employed to dispel cold from the liver channel and treat symptoms such as hernia or testicular pain and impotence.

Actions and indications

Treatment at Liv-12 can be useful to treat *disorders of the groin* area including hernia, testicular pain or swelling, impotence, dysmenorrhoea and uterine prolapse. It is also important in cases of poor circulation, vascular disorders and cold in the lower limbs.

Additionally, Liv-12 can be used to treat *injury* and inflammation of the adductors and sciatica.

> **Main Areas:** Groin. Genitals. Blood vessels. Entire lower limb.
>
> **Main Functions:** Improves qi and blood circulation. Dispels cold and pain from the channels.

Liv-13　Zhangmen　章門
Bright Gate

Alarm *Mu* point for the Spleen
Gathering *Hui* point for the five Yin Organs
Intersection of the Gallbladder and Liver

On the lateral side of the abdomen, below the free end of the eleventh rib. In the oblique abdominal muscles.

To aid location, if the arm is bent at the elbow and held down by the side, the tip of the elbow approximately touches the free end of the eleventh rib (near the mid-axillary line, just superior to the level of the umbilicus).

Alternative locations
Locate Liv-13 at the free end of the eleventh rib. This location may be better for manual techniques. Alternatively, palpate the entire area around the tip of and under the free end of the rib and treat where it is most reactive during pressure palpation.

Best treatment positions
Bilateral treatment is best applied in a supine position with the hips slightly flexed and the legs supported with cushions so that the abdomen and lower back can be as relaxed as possible. However, unilateral treatment can also be applied in a side-lying position.

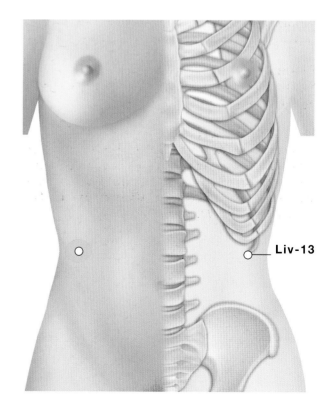

Liv-13

! Liv-3 is a sensitive location and can be tender or ticklish to the slightest touch.

Needling
• 0.3 to 1 cun perpendicular or slightly oblique insertion. However, in many cases there is a lot of subcutaneous fat requiring deeper needling to obtain deqi.
• 1 to 1.5 cun transverse insertion laterally, following the lower border of the rib, or direct the needle inferiorly.
• 0.5 to 1.5 cun oblique inferior insertion.

!! Needling deeply at this location holds a substantial risk of puncturing the liver, Spleen or colon, particularly if there is enlargement.

Manual techniques and shiatsu
Carefully applied gentle pressure or friction is applicable with the fingertips or thumbs.

Self-acupressure can also be applied with the thumbs or fingertips in a standing or sitting position while bending the trunk forward.

! Liv-13 can be very tender and should always be approached carefully. Avoid pressure on Liv-13 (and other abdominal points) if the abdomen is very painful and hard in cases of severe constipation or inflammation of the abdomen.

!! Do not apply strong pressure to the free ribs as they can fracture easily.

Moxibustion
Cones: 3–10. Pole: 5–20 minutes.

Cupping
Small or medium sized cups can be used with light or light-medium suction.

Stimulation sensation
A warm, spreading or tingling sensation can be felt radiating around the location or upwards under the ribs into the chest and/or across the epigastrium, intestines and down across the abdomen. However, deqi is often difficult to achieve at this location.

Actions and indications
Liv-13 is an important point to harmonise the middle jiao and Spleen.

It is effective to *boost Spleen qi* and *smooth the Liver*, particularly in relation to the *digestive system* and has been extensively employed in a variety of such disorders. These include indigestion, abdominal or epigastric distension, swelling and pain, abdominal rumbling, diminished appetite, belching, nausea and vomiting, hypochondrial distension and pain, jaundice, hepatitis, enlargement of the liver or spleen, gastroenteritis, flatulence, diarrhoea, loose or rough stools, undigested food in the stool and constipation.

Liv-13 also treats other manifestations of *Spleen and Liver disharmony*, including distension, fullness and pain of the chest, dyspnoea and coughing due to qi stagnation or phlegm-damp accumulation in the chest and abdomen.

Additionally, Liv-13 has been used to treat a variety of other symptoms, including chronic tiredness, weakness of the limbs and body, emaciation, mental agitation, fever, difficulty raising the arms due to contraction of the abdominal muscles, pain of the lumbar or thoracic spine and difficulty rotating or side-flexing the trunk.

Main Areas: Abdomen. Hypochondrium. Chest. Digestive system.

Main Functions: Harmonises the Liver and Spleen. Boosts Spleen qi.

Liv-14   Qimen

Qi Cycle Gate

期門

Alarm *Mu* point for the Liver
Intersection of the Spleen, Yin Wei Mai and Liver

Directly below the root of the breast on the mid-mamillary line in the sixth intercostal space, approximately 4 cun lateral to the anterior midline. In the oblique abdominal muscles and deeper, the intercostal muscles.

Alternative location
'Lower Qimen' is located directly below the main Liv-14 location, under the lower border of the costal cartilage, 4 cun lateral to the anterior midline.

Needling
· 0.3 to 0.8 cun oblique insertion, directed laterally along the intercostal space.
· Needling can also be applied in a medial direction along the intercostal space.

!! Do not needle deeply. This poses a considerable risk of puncturing the lung and inducing a pneumothorax.

Manual techniques and shiatsu
Perpendicular pressure is applicable with the fingertips. Also, deep friction of the intercostal space can be very useful to help release qi stagnation. Massage any nodules or spasms in the intercostal muscles until they soften.

!! Do not apply strong pressure to the rib cage.

Moxibustion
Although moxibustion is not commonly indicated at Liv-14, it can be employed lightly in certain cases.

Cupping
Use a small or medium cup size.

Magnets
Stick-on magnets can be effective.

Stimulation sensation
A distending sensation is felt extending out across the chest and epigastrium and into the thoracic cavity toward the liver, spleen, stomach, diaphragm and lungs.

Actions and indications
Liv-14 is a very important and widely used point as it *effectively spreads qi* and *dispels stasis from the Liver* and *cools Blood* and *nourishes the Liver*. It is particularly indicated for *diseases of the chest, hypochondrium and abdomen* caused by *qi and Blood stasis*.

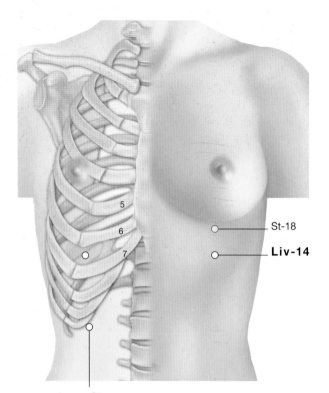

Lower Qimen

It has been extensively employed in disorders of the lungs, heart, breast and gynaecological system. Indications include breast pain, mastitis, fibrocystic breast disease, premenstrual syndrome, excessive uterine bleeding, failure to discharge the placenta, tightness and pain of the chest, intercostal neuralgia, dyspnoea, coughing, angina pectoris, palpitations, depression, irritability, mood swings and frequent sighing.

Liv-14 is also especially indicated to *harmonise the Liver and Stomach* and can be used in many digestive disorders, including hypochondrial pain and distension, jaundice, hepatitis, gallstones, palpable abdominal masses, enlargement of the liver or spleen, stomach ache, heartburn, hiccup, indigestion, nausea, vomiting, gastritis, gastric ulceration and distension, tightness or hardness of the epigastrium or abdomen.

Other traditional indications include tiredness, chills and fever, tidal fever, feeling of heat in the body, malaria, masses, swellings and nodules, stiffness and pain of the neck and skin diseases with redness and heat.

Main Areas: Hypochondrium. Chest. Breast. Abdomen.

Main Functions: Spreads Liver qi. Dispels stasis. Cools Blood.

Chapter 22

Points of the

Ren Mai
(Conception Vessel) Channel

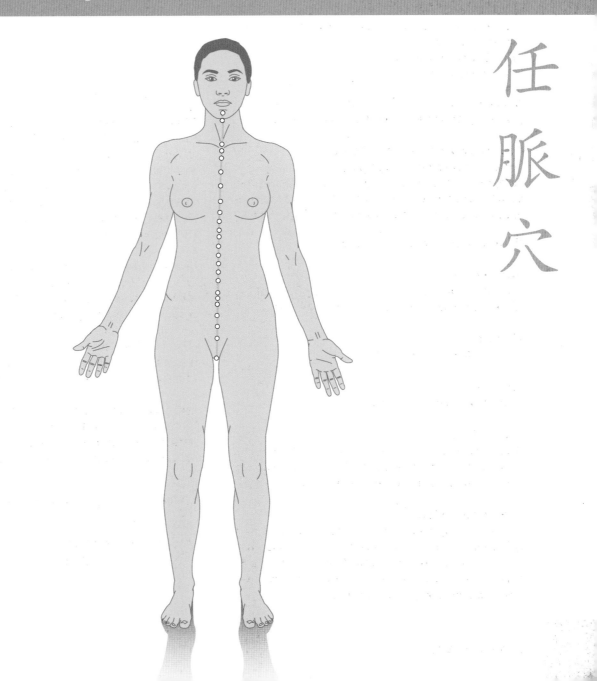

任
脈
穴

Ren-1   Huiyin

會陰

Meeting of Yin

Intersection of the Chong Mai and
Du Mai on the Ren Mai
Eleventh Ghost point

At the centre of the perineum, midway between the posterior border of the genitals and the anus.

Applications and treatment

Although Ren-1 is not commonly used in clinic due to its intimate location, it is considered very important for many reasons. It joins the Ren and Du channels, thus *balancing the flow of yin and yang qi throughout the body*. It is interesting to note that many traditional healing systems place great importance on this area and consider it to be the foundation of the body's energies.

Ren-1 is used *in many exercises as a focus point to contain and gather the yin qi and lift the yang qi*. Typical Qigong or Neigong and pelvic floor exercises employ mental focus or muscular contraction at this location. These exercises are beneficial to the health on many levels, and if done regularly, can be extremely useful to help *build and lift sinking qi* in cases of prolapses, particularly of the uterus or rectum. It is recommended that contraction of the pelvic floor muscles should be repeated at least 100 times per day. Results should be visible within a few days, but lifting of prolapsed organs requires daily practice for weeks or even months in very severe cases. Additionally, electro-stimulation devices can be employed at this location with impressive results.

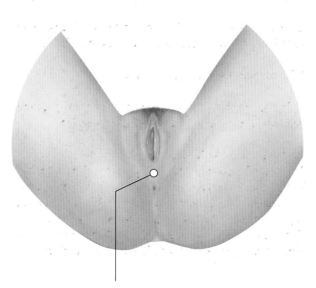

Ren-1

These exercises will also help any other symptoms caused by *deficiency of the lower jiao* including impotence, premature ejaculation, fertility disorders, vaginal dryness, diminished libido, frigidity, threatened miscarriage, postpartum haemorrhage, excessive uterine bleeding, blood in the stool or urine, chronic leucorrhoea, abdominal distension, chronic diarrhoea and haemorrhoids.

Additionally, these exercises greatly help many symptoms caused by *generalised deficiency*, including chronic tiredness, poor concentration, mental depression, dizziness, vertigo, poor circulation, low blood pressure and palpitations.

Another very effective method indicated for many of the above complaints is the application of magnets to this location on a regular basis. Apply north pole on Ren-1 and south pole on Ren-3, Ren-4 or Ren-6 and on Du-4 or bilaterally on Bl-35 Huiyang or other sacral points depending on which are more reactive on pressure palpation. Also apply opposite poles on Ren-1 and Du-1.

Moxibustion is also traditionally indicated for the above complaints and has also been employed to treat haemorrhage anywhere in the body. However, moxibustion is not recommended at this location.

Traditional functions of Ren-1 include *nourishing the Yin and benefitting the jing, resolving dampness and heat from the lower jiao*. Additionally, it is considered as the *Well-Jing point of the Ren Mai* and has been used to *calm the mind, clear the sense organs, treat epilepsy, restore consciousness* and is *traditionally indicated to resuscitate from drowning*.

In the clinic however, needling Ren-1 is only used in severe cases such as *paralysis of the perineum or lower limbs*, uterine prolapse, incontinence, testicular disorders including retraction, inflammation of the skin surrounding the genitalia caused by severe herpes or other infections.

Furthermore, Ren-1, is considered as opposite to Du-20 both in location and function.

Needling
• 0.5 to 1 cun perpendicular insertion.

Main Areas: Genitals. Mind.

Main Functions: Boosts the lower jiao.
Lifts sinking qi. Increases libido.

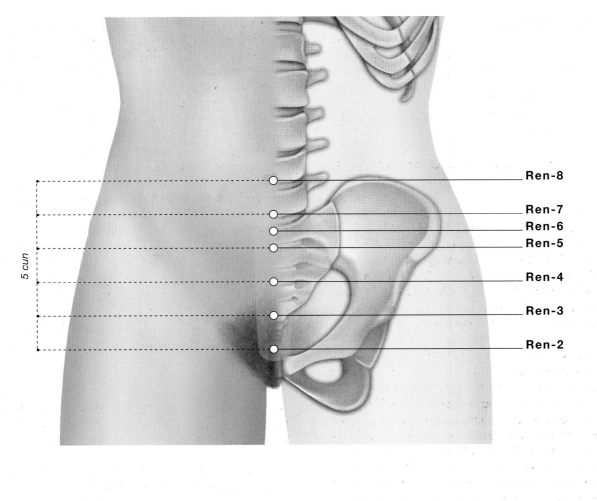

Ren-2 Qugu

曲骨

Curved Bone
(Pubic Symphysis)

Intersection of the Liver on the Ren Mai

Just above the superior border of the pubic symphysis on the anterior midline, 5 cun below the umbilicus.

! Contraindicated during pregnancy.

Best treatment positions
See Ren-3.

Actions and indications
Similar to Ren-3. Use Ren-2 instead of Ren-3 if it is more reactive on pressure palpation.

> **Main Areas:** Bladder. Genitals. Uterus.
>
> **Main Function:** Benefits the genitourinary system and lower jiao.

Ren-3 Zhongji

中極

Central Pivot

Alarm *Mu* point for the Bladder
Intersection of the Three Leg Yin and Ren Mai

On the anterior midline, 4 cun below the umbilicus, 1 cun superior to the upper border of the pubic symphysis.

! Contraindicated during pregnancy.

This site is often tender spontaneously or on pressure palpation if there is inflammation of the bladder.

Best treatment positions
Treatment is applied in a supine position. Generally, it is best to place the patient with the hips slightly flexed so that the abdomen can be as relaxed as possible (use cushion support under the thighs and legs). If the abdomen is very tight, or if there is lordosis of the lumbar spine, flex the hips more by placing extra cushions under the thighs.

Moreover, the qi comes closer to the surface if the person is lying down with the legs stretched out straight with minimal or no cushion support. Use the latter position if the abdomen is very flaccid or if deqi cannot be obtained.

! The bladder should be emptied before treating the lower abdominal points.

Needling
• 0.5 to 1.5 cun perpendicular insertion.

! Do not needle deeply. Do not puncture the peritoneum or a full bladder.

Manual techniques and shiatsu
Stationary pressure and circular friction techniques are applicable with the fingertips or thumbs. Deep stationary pressure is an effective tonifying technique and should be applied for at least 1 to 3 minutes with the patient's hips flexed, so that the lower back is pressing against the floor. Ensure that the abdomen is relaxed before applying this technique.

A useful technique is to gently stretch the linea alba toward the left and right, with the palms or fingertips, so that the abdominal wall of the opposite side is stretched. Hold the stretch for 10–30 seconds at least.

!! Avoid pressure on Ren-3 (and other abdominal points) if the abdomen is very painful or hard in cases of severe constipation, menorrhagia, or inflammatory conditions.

Moxibustion
Pole: 5–15 minutes. Burning moxa cones directly on the skin is not often recommended at this location. However, burning cones on ginger slices has been traditionally employed to warm the Bladder and lower jiao.

! Do not burn pubic hair.

Magnets
Stick-on magnets can also be beneficial (see also Ren-1). Use opposite poles on Ren-3 and St-29 or other adjacent Kidney or Stomach channel points.

Cupping
Medium-sized cups with light-medium cupping or empty cupping can be used effectively.

Stimulation sensation
Distension, warmth or numbness extending across the hypogastrium. Also, a tingling or electric sensation can extend inferiorly along the channel, sometimes reaching the tip of the urethra or clitoris.

Actions and indications
Ren-3 is an *important point for disorders of the urogenital and gynaecological systems*. Its main functions include *regulating the transformation of qi and fluids in the lower jiao*, *clearing dampness and heat*, *fortifying the Kidneys* and *benefitting the genitourinary system and uterus*. Common indications include dysuria, frequent urination, urinary retention, incontinence, cystitis, urethritis, prostatitis, impotence, premature ejaculation, lower abdominal pain and distension, leucorrhoea, genital itching and pain, uterine prolapse, infertility, dysmenorrhoea and irregular menstruation.

Moxa effectively *dispels cold and warms the lower jiao*. If deqi cannot be achieved at Ren-3, use Ren-2 or Ren-4 instead.

Main Areas: Bladder. Uterus. Lower jiao.

Main Functions: Dispels dampness. Heat and cold. Strengthens the genitourinary system.

Ren-4   Guanyuan   關原
Original Qi Gate

Alarm *Mu* point for the Small Intestine
Intersection of the Three Leg Yin and Ren Mai

On the anterior midline, 3 cun below the umbilicus.

! Contraindicated during pregnancy.

Best treatment positions
Similar to Ren-3 and Ren-6.

Needling
• 0.5 to 1.5 cun perpendicular insertion.
• 0.5 to 2 cun oblique inferior insertion.

! Do not needle deeper than 0.7 cun in thin recipients. Do not puncture the peritoneum.

Manual techniques and shiatsu
Similar to Ren-3. However, it is often possible to apply sustained pressure slightly deeper to Ren-4.

Moxibustion

Cones: 5–15. Pole: 10–30 minutes. Rice-grain moxibustion can also be useful. Using a small moxa box over the lower abdomen is effective to alleviate pain.

!! Do not apply moxibustion if there is inflammation in the abdomen or during heavy menstruation, because it can increase blood flow.

Magnets

Magnets can also be effectively employed at this location. Use opposite poles on Ren-4 and St-28 or other adjacent Kidney or Stomach channel points. Also, combine Ren-4 with Bl-26, the Back Transporting Shu point for the Gate of Original Qi.

Stimulation sensation

Regional distension and warmth, sometimes extending across the entire lower abdomen. Also, a tingling or electric sensation can travel inferiorly along the channel, sometimes reaching the tip of the urethra or clitoris.

Actions and indications

Ren-4 is the *intersection of the Liver, Spleen Kidney and Ren Mai*. It is an important point to *strengthen and regulate these organs*. Ren-4 is called *the Gate of Original Qi* because it has a direct effect on the Kidney qi and *strengthens the entire lower jiao*. It *nourishes yin, Blood and jing, and has a calming and grounding action on the mind* (it is often combined with Sp-6 for this purpose). Furthermore, it is effective to *dispel dampness, cold and heat from the lower jiao.*

Common indications include irregular menstruation, amenorrhoea, infertility, uterine fibroids, polycystic ovarian disease, endometriosis, dysmenorrhoea, excessive menstruation, postpartum haemorrhage, leucorrhoea, genital itching, dysuria, frequent urination, urinary tract infections, incontinence, impotence, prostatitis, abdominal distension and pain, irritable bowel syndrome, constipation, anxiety, restlessness, insomnia, palpitations, sore throat, tinnitus, diminishing vision and hearing, heat due to yin deficiency, emaciation, lumbar pain, chronic tiredness, weakness and exhaustion.

Main Areas: Entire body. Abdomen. Small Intestine. Bladder. Uterus.

Main Functions: Augments Yuan qi. Nourishes yin and Blood. Calms the mind. Reinforces the Kidneys. Regulates qi and Blood. Strengthens the lower jiao. Benefits the Small Intestine.

Ren-5 Shimen

石門

Stone Gate

Alarm Mu point for the Sanjiao

On the anterior midline, 2 cun below the umbilicus, 3 cun superior to the pubic symphysis.

! Contraindicated during pregnancy.

Best treatment positions

Similar to Ren-3, Ren-4 and Ren-6.

! Traditionally it was considered that needling this location could cause infertility in women, making the uterus 'cold like a stone'. This seems contradictory to its function of warming and mobilising the kidney energy and increasing fertility. One can rather consider this as a caution, implying that any form of excessively strong treatment can in fact dissipate rather than build up the energy. It is therefore recommended to use caution when applying any form of treatment to the lower abdomen.

Needling

• 0.5 to 1 cun perpendicular insertion.

Stimulation sensation

Local distension or warmth sometimes extending across the entire lower abdomen. Also, a tingling or electric sensation can extend inferiorly along the channel.

Main Areas: Abdomen. Uterus.

Main Functions: Mobilises Yuan qi. Warms and strengthens the lower jiao.

Ren-6   (Xia) Qihai   (下)氣海

(Lower) Sea of Qi

On the anterior midline, 1.5 cun below the umbilicus. In a small depression, at the lower border of the fleshy bulge formed by the subcutaneous fat deposit under the umbilicus (visible on most people, but more prominent on women).

To aid location, place the middle finger in the umbilicus and grasp the bulge in the flesh under the umbilicus with the thumb. The tip of the thumb should locate Ren-6. This fleshy bulge is formed by the subcutaneous fat cells deposited in a slightly thicker layer around the umbilicus in a 'U' shape. According to certain Japanese Hara diagnosis (abdominal diagnosis) models, this is the Kidney diagnostic area. Ren-6 lies close to the lower border of the Kidney diagnostic area.

! Contraindicated during pregnancy.

Best treatment positions
Treatment is applied in a supine position. Generally, it is best to place the patient with the hips slightly flexed (with cushion support under the thighs and legs) so that the abdomen can be as relaxed as possible. See also note for Ren-3.

! Ren-6 is often painful and hard.

Needling
• 0.5 to 1.5 cun perpendicular insertion.
• 0.5 to 2 cun oblique or transverse inferior insertion.

Palpate for the small gap at the bottom of the fatty bulge to insert the needle. If it feels tight and painful on insertion, do not manipulate the needle or insert deeper. If the pain continues during needle retention, or if deqi cannot be achieved, remove the needle and reinsert it in the nearest palpable gap further down the channel (palpate in an inferior direction toward Ren-5).

Manual techniques and shiatsu
Similar to Ren-3. However, because Ren-6 is usually palpable more superficially than the previous points, it is not easy to apply stationary pressure as deeply.

! This location can be quite painful and hard.

Moxibustion
Cones: 5–15. Pole: 10–30 minutes. Burning moxa cones on ginger slices effectively tonifies the yang qi. Rice-grain moxibustion is also effectively employed.

! Overstimulation of this location can overtonify the yang, causing symptoms of heat, dryness and psychological unrest, including insomnia, sweating and thirst.

!! Do not apply moxibustion to the lower abdomen in inflammatory conditions (such as appendicitis) or during heavy menstruation, because it increases blood flow.

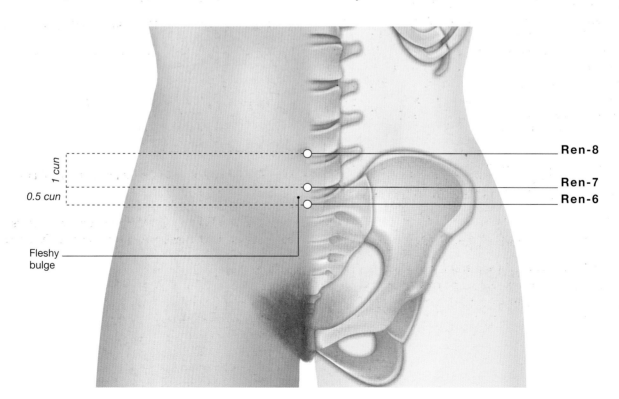

1 cun

0.5 cun

Fleshy bulge

Ren-8

Ren-7

Ren-6

Magnets

Magnet therapy can also be effective at Ren-6. Use opposite poles on Ren-6 and Bl-24, the Back Transporting-Shu point for the Sea of Qi. Also alternate poles with adjacent Ren, Kidney or Stomach channel points.

Stimulation sensation

Local distension, warmth or tingling. The sensation often extends inferiorly along the channel or laterally across the abdomen. In some cases deqi is achieved in an upward direction. However, it is not always possible to achieve strong deqi at Ren-6.

! Sharp pain is often perceived both during pressure palpation and needling. In such cases it is recommended to treat it with other methods such as moxibustion, cupping or magnets or choose another point further down the Ren channel (sometimes deqi is easier to achieve at Ren-5 or Ren-4).

Actions and indications

Ren-6 is the point of the Sea of Qi and is a *very important point to tonify and lift qi, warm and restore Yang* (with moxibustion) and *fortify the Kidneys*. It is a major point to *boost energy and is considered vital in the treatment of deficiency conditions* such as chronic tiredness, weakness, debility, exhaustion, old age or weakened immunity. It can be employed in *many chronic or serious diseases to help the general health and enliven the patient.*

It also effectively *regulates the abdominal qi and dispels dampness, particularly from the lower jiao*. It is an important point to *treat disorders of the abdomen and pelvis, including digestive, gynaecological and urogenital conditions*. Indications include abdominal distension and pain, bloating, IBS, diarrhoea, constipation, dysmenorrhoea, amenorrhoea, irregular menstruation, leucorrhoea, prolapse of abdominal or pelvic organs, frequent urination, male and female fertility disorders, impotence and frigidity.

It is commonly combined with St-36 for general weakness, with Sp-3 and Ren-12 for weakness of the Stomach and Spleen, and with St-36 and Du-20 for sinking qi.

> **Main Areas:** Entire body. Lower jiao.
>
> **Main Functions:** Tonifies and warms yang. Lifts sinking qi. Warms the abdomen. Regulates qi in the lower jiao.

Ren-7 Yinjiao
Yin Intersection

Intersection of the Kidney, Chong and Ren Mai

On the anterior midline, 1 cun below the umbilicus.

Best treatment positions
Similar to Ren-6.

Needling
• 0.5 to 1 cun perpendicular insertion.
• 0.5 to 1.5 cun oblique inferior insertion.

! Do not needle deeper than 1 cun in thin recipients. Do not puncture the peritoneum.

Actions and indications
Although Ren-7 is not as commonly employed as the previous points, it can be employed for similar purposes, including *regulating menstruation and qi in the abdomen*. Symptoms include abdominal distension and pain, leucorrhoea, infertility, excessive or irregular menstruation, and testicular retraction.

As a *local point*, Ren-7 is useful in cases of periumbilical pain and hernia.

> **Main Areas:** Abdomen. Umbilicus. Uterus.
>
> **Main Functions:** Regulates qi in the lower jiao. Alleviates pain.

Ren-8 Shenque
Spirit Palace Gate

On the anterior midline, at the centre of the umbilicus.

Contraindications
Needling is contraindicated. Although acupressure is also conventionally contraindicated, in certain cases it can be effectively employed.

Moxibustion

Burn 5–20 cones on salt. Also, use ginger over the salt to burn the cones. A moxa pole can be used for 10–30 minutes. Alternatively, a small moxa box can be placed over the navel.

Moxibustion should be applied until the entire body warms up, consciousness is revived and vital energy is increased.

! Overstimulation at this location can overtonify the yang, causing symptoms of heat, dryness and psychological unrest, including insomnia, sweating and thirst.

!! Do not apply moxibustion over an umbilical hernia.

Manual techniques and shiatsu

Stationary pressure can be applied carefully around the umbilical ring and inferiorly or superiorly along the linea alba.

! Ren-8 is usually sensitive and painful. Therefore, special care should be taken to ensure the correct angle and depth of pressure.

A useful technique to relax the entire abdomen is to gently mobilise the umbilicus toward the left and right with the palms or fingertips, so that the linea alba and abdominal wall of the opposite side is slightly stretched. Hold the stretch for at least 10 to 30 seconds.

Cupping

Light or medium suction and empty cupping can be effectively employed.

A very useful technique, also helpful in cases of acute abdominal pain due to qi stagnation, is to place a medium or large cup over the umbilicus with light or medium suction and rotate it clockwise or anticlockwise, depending on which of the two feels easiest, for at least one minute.

Also, place a small or medium cup over the umbilicus, *without suction*, and apply gentle stationary pressure so that the rim of the cup presses into the tissues around the umbilicus as far as is comfortable. Then, the cup is rotated clockwise or anticlockwise as described above. This technique has been used to treat umbilical hernia, strangulated hernia and inflammation of the intestine.

!! Do not apply suction over a hernia.

Stimulation sensation

Heat should be felt radiating around the navel, extending across the entire abdomen and warming the whole body. The colour should return to the person's face, the eyes should look brighter and the pulse should feel stronger.

Actions and indications

The application of moxibustion to Ren-8 is considered *very important to restore collapsed Yang* and *raise sinking qi*. It also effectively regulates *the flow of qi in the abdomen*. Indications include chronic or severe diarrhoea, abdominal swelling and oedema, abdominal pain, periumbilical pain, various prolapses, generalised weakness, loss of consciousness, wind stroke, arrhythmia, cardiac failure, cyanosis, profuse sweating and hypothermia.

Lightly applied indirect moxibustion over and around the navel is also useful for *infantile diarrhoea and colic*.

Traditionally, *burning large moxa cones on the umbilicus was used after all other treatment failed, in cases where imminent death was apparent*. The navel was considered the site where the spirit enters and leaves the body.

> **Main Areas:** Navel. Abdomen. Whole Body.
>
> **Main Functions:** Tonifies, warms, lifts and revives yang. Regulates qi in the abdomen.

Ren-9　Shuifen　水分
Water Separation

On the anterior midline, 1 cun above the umbilicus.

Best treatment positions

Similar to Ren-6 and Ren-12.

! According to certain classical texts, needling this point is contraindicated in cases of abdominal swelling. Moxibustion is recommended instead.

Needling

• 0.5 to 1 cun perpendicular insertion.

Actions and indications

Ren-9 is primarily used to promote *fluid transformation*. Indications include oedema, swelling and pain of the abdomen, diarrhoea, profuse urination and leucorrhoea.

> **Main Areas:** Abdomen. Whole Body.
>
> **Main Function:** Reduces oedema.

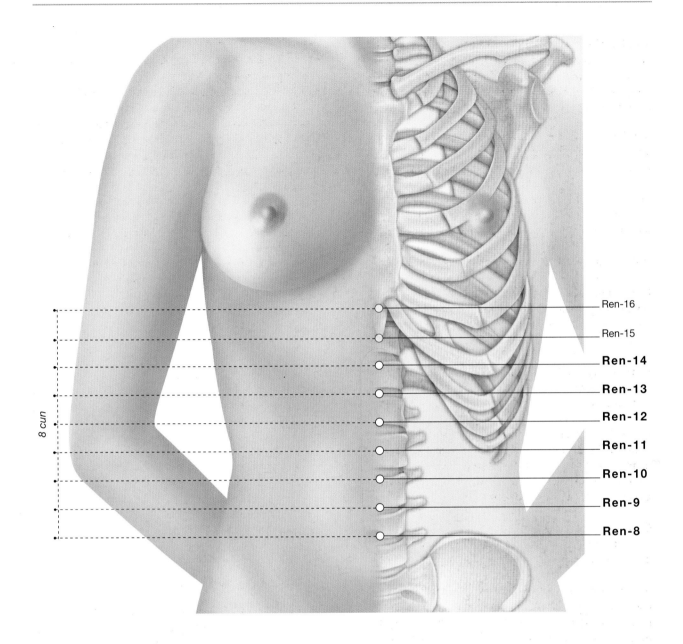

Ren-16
Ren-15
Ren-14
Ren-13
Ren-12
Ren-11
Ren-10
Ren-9
Ren-8

8 cun

Ren-10 Xiawan

下脘

Lower Stomach

Intersection of the Spleen on the Ren Mai

On the anterior midline, 2 cun above the umbilicus.

Best treatment positions
Similar to Ren-12 and adjacent Ren points.

Needling
• 0.5 to 1.5 cun perpendicular insertion.

Actions and indications
Ren-10 is an important point to *descend rebellious Stomach qi*. It is specifically indicated for disorders of *the lower part of the stomach*, therefore *relieving food retention*. Ren-10 also *tonifies the Spleen qi*.

Indications include, indigestion, nausea, heartburn, hiccup, fullness of the epigastrium and abdomen, abdominal rumbling, foul breath and belching.

Main Areas: Stomach. Abdomen.

Main Functions: Descends rebellious qi.
Relieves food stagnation.

Ren-11   Jianli

建里

Strengthen the Interior

On the anterior midline, 3 cun above the umbilicus.

Best treatment positions
Similar to Ren-12.

Needling
• 0.5 to 1 cun perpendicular insertion.

Actions and indications
Ren-11 *harmonises the middle jiao* and *regulates qi* in a similar way to Ren-10 and Ren-12. It should be chosen instead of the latter points if it is found to be more reactive on gentle pressure palpation.

Main Areas: Stomach. Middle jiao.

Main Function: Harmonises the middle jiao.

Ren-12   Zhongwan

中脘

Stomach Centre

Alarm *Mu* point for the Stomach
Gathering *Hui* point for the Yang organs
Intersection of the Small Intestine, Sanjiao
and Stomach channels on the Ren Mai
One of the nine points for Returning Yang

On the anterior midline, 4 cun above the umbilicus. To aid location, Ren-12 is midway between the umbilicus and the xiphisternal junction (the junction of the xiphoid process with the body of the sternum). It is usually found along one of the horizontal creases on the epigastrium, defined when the patient bends the trunk forward.

Best treatment positions
This location is treated with the person lying down supine. However, acupressure may also be employed with the person sitting in a chair.

! In many cases this area feels tight and hard, indicating that both perpendicular pressure and needling should be applied lightly and superficially. This is especially common in persons with a lot of stress or inflammation of the stomach. In these cases, superficial rubbing, light cupping or moxibustion may be more effective.

Needling
• 0.5 to 1.5 cun perpendicular insertion.

If it feels tight and painful on insertion, do not manipulate the needle and do not insert it deeper. If the pain continues during needle retention, or if deqi cannot be achieved, remove the needle and reinsert it in the nearest palpable gap further down or up the channel (palpate toward Ren-11 and Ren-13).

! Do not needle deeply, particularly in thin recipients. Do not puncture the peritoneum.

Moxibustion
Cones: 5–15. Pole: 10–30 minutes. Also, burn the cones on ginger or garlic slices. Additionally, a small moxa box can be placed over the epigastrium.

! Excessive moxibustion can dry out the body fluids and overheat the stomach causing symptoms of heat, including thirst, excessive hunger and insomnia.

Manual techniques and shiatsu
Stationary pressure is applicable with the fingertips or thumbs and the palm. Circular friction can also be applied. Always start by applying the pressure very lightly.

Stationary pressure should be released slightly during the inhalation and increased slightly during the exhalation.

A useful technique to tonify and warm the area is to apply superficial circular rubbing with the palm until the heat from the friction is felt extending across the epigastrium and abdomen. Traditionally, clockwise is considered more tonifying.

Also, in cases where the epigastrium is painful, open this area by gently stretching the abdominal muscles laterally with the palms. Furthermore, the linea alba can be 'opened' by applying gentle friction with the fingertips, laterally away from the point.

! Avoid excessive pressure on the epigastrium. In many cases this area feels tight and hard and pressure can only be applied lightly. This is especially common in persons with a lot of stress.

Actions and indications
Ren-12 is a *very important point to tonify the middle jiao*. It is used in many conditions caused by *deficiency of the Stomach and Spleen* and also helps *transform dampness and phlegm*. It is specifically indicated for disorders of the *middle part of the stomach* and also *descends rebellious qi*. Indications include poor appetite and digestion, nausea, morning sickness during pregnancy, loss of taste, fullness and heaviness of the epigastrium, stomach ache,

gastritis, gastric ulceration, heartburn, hiatus hernia, abdominal pain, abdominal rumbling, loose stools, dry stools, difficulty defecating, jaundice, productive cough, poor concentration and tiredness.

Ren-12 is also very important to *nourish Yin and body fluids*. Symptoms include thirst, dry mouth, dark and scanty urine, dry skin and mental restlessness.

Additionally, Ren-12 helps to *calm the heart and ease stress and tension*. Indications include mental restlessness, anxiety, heart pain and palpitations. It is important for digestive conditions caused by stress.

> **Main Areas:** Middle jiao. Stomach. Abdomen. Entire Body.
>
> **Main Functions:** Tonifies the Stomach and Spleen. Transforms dampness. Dispels cold. Harmonises the middle jiao and descends rebellious qi. Nourishes fluids and yin. Soothes the heart and calms the mind.

Ren-13   Shangwan   上脘
Upper Stomach

Intersection of the Small Intestine and Stomach on the Ren Mai

On the anterior midline, 5 cun above the umbilicus.

Best treatment positions
Similar to Ren-12 and Ren-14.

Actions and indications
Similar to Ren-12, but *more for acute cases*, particularly nausea and vomiting. Ren-13 is specifically indicated for disorders of the *upper part of the stomach*.

> **Main Area:** Stomach.
>
> **Main Function:** Harmonises the Stomach.

Ren-14   Juque   巨闕
Great Palace Gate

Alarm *Mu* point for the Heart

On the anterior midline, 6 cun above the umbilicus.

Best treatment positions
Treatment is applied in a supine position. Generally, it is best to place the patient with the hips slightly flexed (with cushion support under the thighs and legs) so that the abdomen can be as relaxed as possible. See also note for Ren-3.

! Ren-14 is a very sensitive point and all forms of treatment should be applied cautiously. Also, in certain cases, treatment can stir up the emotions and lead to an outburst.

Needling
• 0.5 to 1.5 cun perpendicular insertion.

If it feels tight and painful on insertion, do not manipulate the needle and do not insert it deeper. If the pain continues during needle retention, or if deqi cannot be achieved, remove the needle and reinsert it in the nearest palpable gap further down or up the channel (palpate toward Ren-13 and Ren-15).

! Do not needle deeply, particularly in thin recipients. Do not puncture the peritoneum. Do not needle in an upward direction.

Manual techniques and shiatsu
Similar to Ren-12.

! Never apply strong pressure directly to the xiphoid process, as it can fracture easily.

Stimulation sensation
Distension, dull aching, soreness or electricity may be perceived extending inferiorly along the channel toward the abdomen, and/or upward into the thoracic cavity toward the diaphragm and heart. Sometimes the sensation extends downwards and laterally. Additionally, the person may sigh or start talking.

! Ren-14 can engender an uncomfortable sensation of soreness and tightness, indicating that the stimulation applied is too strong.

Actions and indications

Ren-14 is the *Mu point for the Heart* and is used to treat *symptoms of heat and stagnation in the Heart and chest* including palpitations, dyspnoea, coughing, pain and constriction of the chest and epigastrium, insomnia, anxiety and emotional upsets in general.

Ren-14 also *descends rebellious Stomach qi* in cases of heartburn, nausea and vomiting.

> **Main Areas:** Heart. Chest. Epigastrium.
>
> **Main Functions:** Soothes the heart and calms the mind. Harmonises the Heart and Stomach.

Ren-15 Jiuwei

Turtledove Tail
(Xiphoid Process)

Connecting *Luo* point

On the anterior midline, 7 cun above the umbilicus, at the tip of the xiphoid process.

To aid location, if the xiphoid process is very long, find Ren-15 further inferiorly. It is always at the tip of the xiphoid process.

Needling
• 0.5 cun oblique inferior insertion just below the tip of the xiphoid process.

!! Do not needle deeper or upward. This poses considerable risk of puncturing the liver or an enlarged heart.

Manual techniques and shiatsu
Apply very gentle pressure or friction onto the entire xiphoid process and its tip.

! Never apply strong pressure directly to the xiphoid process, as it can fracture easily.

Moxibustion
Cones: 3–5. Pole: 5–10 minutes. Rice-grain moxibustion is also applicable.

Actions and indications
Ren-15 is the *Connecting Luo point of the Ren Mai* and is effective to *free up the entire abdomen when there is qi blockage*. It is *particularly indicated for psychosomatic disorders and diseases of the Heart, Lungs and chest.*

Indications include abdominal swelling or pain, itching or pain of the skin of the abdomen, difficulty swallowing, indigestion, heartburn, palpitations, heart pain, fullness of the chest, dyspnoea, coughing, haemoptysis, mental agitation, fright, abnormal behaviour, psychological disorders and epilepsy.

Furthermore, it *augments the functions of the Yin organs and boosts original (yuan) qi.*

> **Main Areas:** Chest. Abdomen.
>
> **Main Functions:** Regulates qi and dispels stasis. Calms and balances the mind.

Ren-16 Zhongting

Central Court

On the midline of the sternum, at the xiphisternal junction.

To aid location, the xiphisternal junction is a distinct depression, visible on thin patients.

Needling
• 0.5 cun oblique inferior insertion.

Manual techniques and shiatsu
Very gentle stationary pressure or friction is applicable.

! Do not apply strong pressure to the sternum.

Moxibustion
Cones: 3–5. Pole: 5–10 minutes. Rice-grain moxibustion is also applicable.

Actions and indications
Ren-16 is not as commonly used as other adjacent points. It can, however, help *relax the chest, harmonise the Stomach and descend rebellious qi.* Indications include fullness and heaviness of the chest, heartburn, difficulty swallowing, nausea, vomiting and epigastric pain.

> **Main Areas:** Chest. Abdomen.
>
> **Main Functions:** Regulates qi and dispels stasis. Calms and balances the mind.

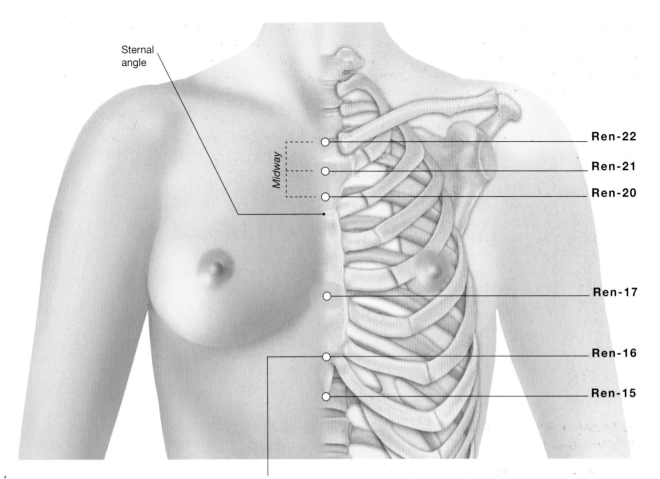

Sternal angle

Midway

Ren-22
Ren-21
Ren-20

Ren-17

Ren-16

Ren-15

Xiphisternal junction

Ren-17 Shanzhong (Shangqihai) 膻中

Chest Centre (Upper Sea of Qi)

Alarm *Mu* point for the Pericardium
Gathering *Hui* point for the Qi
Intersection of the Spleen, Kidney,
Small Intestine and Sanjiao on the Ren Mai
Point of the Sea of Qi

At the centre of the chest, on the anterior midline, level with the fourth intercostal space, between the nipples.

Best treatment positions
Treatment is applied with the patient supine or sitting. Use ample cushion support under the back and head.

! This is a very sensitive location and all forms of treatment should be applied cautiously. Also, treatment at this location can engender release or stir up the emotions, sometimes leading to an outburst.

Needling
• 0.3 to 1 cun transverse inferior or superior insertion.
• 0.5 to 1.5 cun transverse horizontal insertion, toward the breast.

! This location can be tight and painful. In such cases, manual techniques or moxibustion are preferred.

! According to certain classical sources, Ren-17 is contraindicated to needling. This may infer that it was accidentally needled deeply at a perpendicular angle through a gap in the sternum directly into the heart.

Manual techniques and shiatsu
Very gentle stationary perpendicular pressure or circular friction is applicable with the fingertips. Also, superficial rubbing of the sternum can help dissipate stagnant qi and warm the upper jiao.

! Do not apply strong pressure to the sternum.

Moxibustion
Cones: 2–5. Pole: 5–10 minutes. Rice-grain moxibustion is also applicable.

Magnets

Magnets can be successfully employed at this location.

Stimulation sensation

Deqi is generally not very strong or easy to achieve at Ren-17. Best results are obtained if a tingling sensation extends outward and upward across the chest.

Actions and indications

Ren-17 is a *major point to tonify and regulate chest qi* and is widely used for disorders of this area. Common indications include constriction, tightness, pain or heaviness of the chest, heart pain, palpitations, frequent sighing, plum stone throat, shortness of breath, dyspnoea, wheeze, cough, insufficient lactation and breast pain.

Ren-17 may also be thought of as the Mu point for the shen (mind) because it is used to treat many *psycho-emotional disorders* including depression, propensity for crying, sadness, hysteria and insomnia.

Additionally, Ren-17 is useful in chronic or serious diseases to enliven the qi throughout the body.

> **Main Areas:** Heart. Lungs. Chest. Breast. Entire body.
>
> **Main Functions:** Regulates qi and dispels stasis. Tonifies qi. Calms and balances the mind. Benefits the chest.

Ren-20   Huagai

Florid Canopy

華蓋

On the midline of the manubrium, just superior to the sternal angle, level with the first intercostal space.

To aid location, the sternal angle is palpable as the small bump of the manubrosternal articulation. Ren-20 is in the first palpable depression superior to the sternal angle.

Best treatment positions

Similar to Ren-17.

Needling

• 0.3 to 0.5 cun transverse inferior or superior insertion.

! This location can be tight and painful.

Actions and indications

Similar to other adjacent points, Ren-20 *regulates qi, descends rebellious qi and helps relax the chest*. It is used in such cases as cough, asthma, dyspnoea, pain and fullness of the chest, and angina pectoris.

> **Main Areas:** Heart. Lungs. Chest.
>
> **Main Function:** Regulates qi.

Ren-21   Xuanji

Jade Pivot

璇璣

In the shallow depression, slightly superior to the centre of the manubrium, about 1 cun inferior Ren-22.

To aid location, it is midway between Ren-20 and Ren-22.

Best treatment positions

Similar to Ren-20.

Actions and indications

Although Ren-21 is not very commonly used, it can *descend rebellious qi, relax the chest* and *benefit the throat*. Indications include sore throat, cough, dyspnoea, asthma, chest pain, epigastric fullness, nausea and vomiting.

> **Main Areas:** Chest. Throat.
>
> **Main Functions:** Relaxes the chest. Descends rebellious qi.

Ren-22   Tiantu

Celestial Prominence

天突

Intersection of the Yin Wei Mai on the Ren Mai

On the anterior midline, just superior to the suprasternal (jugular) notch.

To aid location, it is approximately 1 cun superior to Ren-21.

Best treatment positions

Needling is applied with the person lying supine and the head extended. However, acupressure can be more effective with the patient sitting up.

! Ren-22 is very sensitive and treatment here can occasionally make the person cough or feel nauseous.

Needling

• 0.3 cun perpendicular insertion.
• 0.5 to 1 cun inferior retrosternal insertion. Insert the needle perpendicularly about 0.3 cun and then direct it downward along the posterior border of the manubrium 0.5 to 1 cun.

!! Do not needle deeper perpendicularly, as this holds substantial risk of injuring the jugular venous arch, the inferior thyroid vein, and more deeply, the trachea. Also, the brachiocephalic vein and the arch of the aorta are situated slightly inferiorly.

Manual techniques and shiatsu

Pressure is applied downwards onto the superior aspect of the sternum.

! Do not press perpendicularly onto the throat.

Moxibustion

Pole: 3–5 minutes.

!! Do not use direct moxibustion.

Stimulation sensation

A gentle local sensation or slight pain is common. However, the deqi should extend downward retrosternally if the treatment is applied for diseases of the chest. Also the person may clear their throat or cough in response to deqi.

! Occasionally, the vomiting reflex can be activated, causing the person to feel nauseous.

Actions and indications

Ren-22 is primarily used to *descend rebellious qi, alleviate cough* and *benefit the throat and voice*. Indications include acute coughing, wheeze or asthma, acute dyspnoea, hoarseness, loss of voice, tightness, pain and swelling of the throat and goitre. Furthermore, it has been used to treat heartburn, nausea and vomiting.

Main Area: Throat.

Main Functions: Descends rebellious qi. Alleviates cough.

Ren-23 Lianquan

Corner Fountain
(Tongue Root)

Intersection of the Yin Wei Mai on the Ren Mai

On the anterior midline, just superior to the hyoid bone.

To aid location, it is where the chin joins with the throat. Palpate gently superior to the hyoid bone to find the small depression.

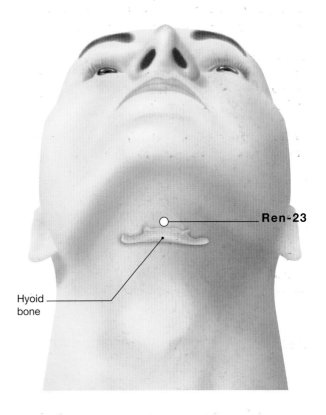

Ren-23

Hyoid bone

Best treatment positions

Ren-23 is best treated with the patient lying supine and the head slightly extended, without cushion support, or with a small roll under the neck.

! This location is very sensitive and should be approached carefully.

Needling

• 0.5 to 1.2 cun oblique insertion toward the base of the tongue.

! Do not puncture cutaneous branches of the transverse cervical nerve; more deeply, the branches of the hypoglossal nerve and the sublingual artery and vein. Slightly superiorly the arch of the anterior jugular vein.

Manual techniques and shiatsu
Gentle pressure and friction is applicable with the fingertips.

Moxibustion
Moxibustion is not recommended at this location.

Magnets
Magnet therapy can be used effectively.

Stimulation sensation
Regional tingling or electricity, giving way to numbness extending out across the submandibular area, toward the root of the tongue and down the throat.

Actions and indications
Ren-23 is a *useful point to treat in disorders of the tongue, throat and submandibular glands*. Indications include swelling and inflammation of the submandibular glands, paralysis of the tongue, speech disorders, loss of voice, soreness or swelling of the throat, and goitre.

> **Main Areas:** Tongue. Throat.
>
> **Main Functions:** Resolves phlegm and clears heat. Descends rebellious qi.

Manual techniques and shiatsu
Stationary perpendicular pressure or very small circular friction is applicable with the fingertips.

Magnets
Magnets can also be effectively employed.

Actions and indications
Ren-24 is an effective point to treat *various disorders of the region* including *facial paralysis* and pain, deviation of the mouth, swelling of the face and *disorders of the gums, salivary glands and teeth*. Furthermore, it *clears and brightens the eyes*.

Additionally, Ren-24 is an *important beauty point to improve appearance*. Needling horizontally into, or pressing across, the wrinkle of the mentolabial groove is effective. Furthermore it helps *release tension* from the entire chin area and cheeks.

Furthermore, it *clears heat from the face* and treats acne, distended capillaries and red blotchy skin.

> **Main Areas:** Chin. Face.
>
> **Main Functions:** Dispels wind and clears heat. Treats paralysis.

Ren-24   Chengjiang
Saliva Receptacle

承漿

Intersection of the Stomach, Large Intestine and Du Mai on the Ren Mai
Eighth Ghost point

On the anterior midline, in the depression at the centre of the mentolabial groove, approximately midway between the lower lip and the chin.

To aid location, palpate the mentolabial groove for the small, but distinct, depression between the orbicularis oris and mentalis muscles.

Needling
· 0.2 to 0.3 cun upward oblique insertion.
· Transverse horizontal insertion along the mentolabial groove, toward jiachengjiang M-HN-18 (see page 325).

! Do not puncture branches of the mental nerve, the inferior labial artery and vein.

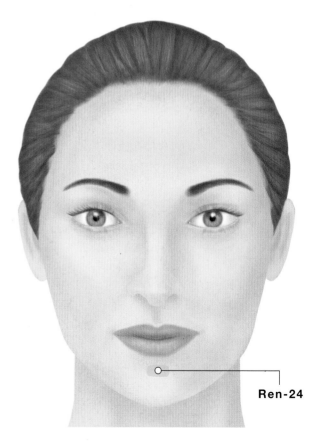

Ren-24

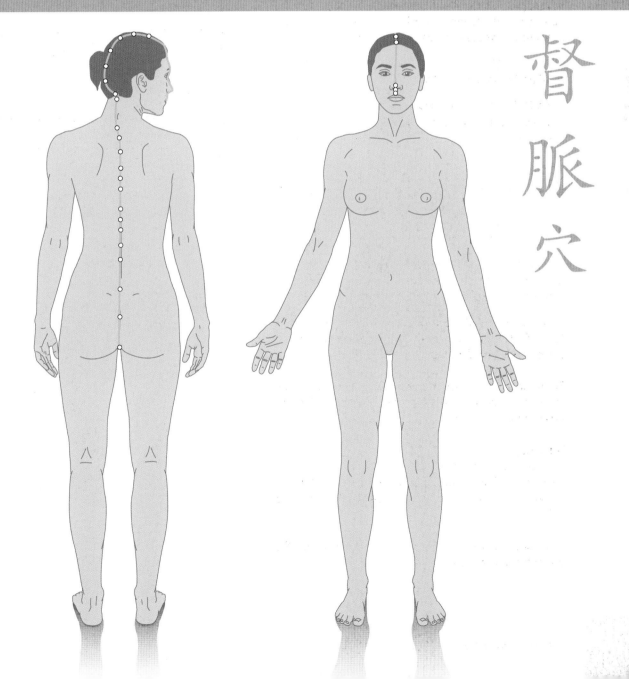

Chapter 23

Points of the
Du Mai
(Governing Vessel) Channel

督脈穴

Du-1   Changqiang   長強
Long Strength

Connecting Luo point
Meeting point of the Ren Mai Gallbladder and
Kidney on the Du Mai

Midway between the tip of the coccyx and the anus.

Best treatment positions
Du-1 is often treated with the patient lying prone.
However, needling and moxibustion may be better applied
with the person lying sideways and the knees bent and
drawn up toward the chest. Furthermore, a 'child's pose'
can be employed. Ask the patient to kneel down and then
lean the trunk forward (use cushion support for the upper
body and arms).

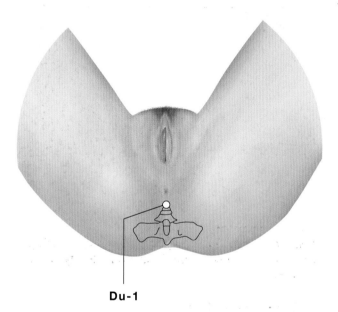

Du-1

Needling
• 0.5 to 1 cun perpendicular or upward oblique insertion,
  between the coccyx and anus.

! Do not needle deeper or at different angle. Do not
puncture the middle rectal artery and vein or branches of
the coccygeal or anal nerves.

Manual techniques and shiatsu
Although carefully applied finger pressure and friction
can be applied to the tip of the coccyx, in a shiatsu
context, pressure is best applied with the palm or sole of
the foot.

A useful technique to tonify and lift the yang qi is to
apply a gentle pulsating movement by pushing the tip of
the coccyx in a superior direction, until the movement is
perceived moving up the spine. Use the palm of the hand
or sole of the foot.

!! Do not apply strong pressure to the coccyx.

Moxibustion
Pole: 5–10 minutes. Direct moxibustion is not
recommended at this location.

Magnets
Apply opposite poles to Du-1 and Bl-35 or Ren-1.

Stimulation sensation
Regional distension, tingling or ache, extending across
the anal region, into the rectum or superiorly along the
channel pathway.

Actions and indications
Du-1 is primarily used for *disorders of the anus and
rectum* including haemorrhoids, diarrhoea, blood in the
stool, constipation, rectal pain and prolapse.

It also *regulates the spine and tonifies the Yang of the
whole body* and can be used to treat pain or swelling of
the coccyx, lumbar pain, spermatorrhoea and painful or
turbid urination.

Du-1 has also been *traditionally used to calm and clear
the mind* and treat spasm and epilepsy.

Furthermore, it is an important *focus point for energy
circulation* in Qigong practices.

> **Main Areas:** Anus. Coccyx. Spine.
>
> **Main Functions:** Benefits the anus and rectum.
> Regulates qi. Benefits the spine.

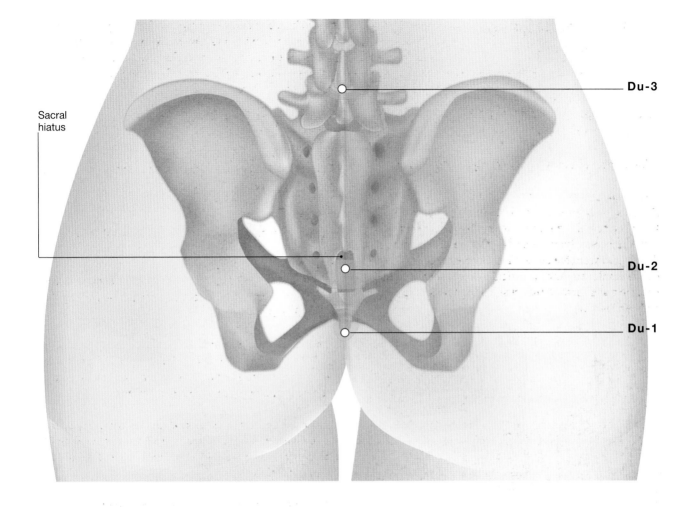

Sacral
hiatus

Du-3

Du-2

Du-1

Du-2　Yaoshu　腰俞

Lumbar Point

On the posterior midline, at the sacrococcygeal hiatus.

To aid location, it is in the depression inferior to the fourth sacral spinous process, if it can be palpated.

Needling
• 0.3 to 1 cun perpendicular or transverse oblique superior insertion.

Manual techniques and shiatsu
Sustained pressure and friction of the hiatus area is applicable.

Moxibustion
Cones: 3–10. Pole: 10–20 minutes.

Magnets
Magnets can also be effectively used here.

Stimulation sensation
Regional distension, tingling or ache, possibly extending inferiorly toward the anus or laterally across the sacrum.

Actions and indications
Du-2 helps to *move qi and Blood, dispel wind and dampness and alleviate pain from the channel pathway.* It is of particular benefit to the *sacrum, lumbar area and legs*.

It is also useful in the treatment of rectal pain, diarrhoea, dysuria and rectal prolapse, in common with Du-1.

It is also mentioned as one of the *Seven Points to Clear Heat from the Extremities* alongside Lu-2, LI-15 and Bl-40.

Main Areas: Sacrum. Coccyx. Lumbar spine.

Main Functions: Regulates qi and Blood. Alleviates pain. Benefits the spine.

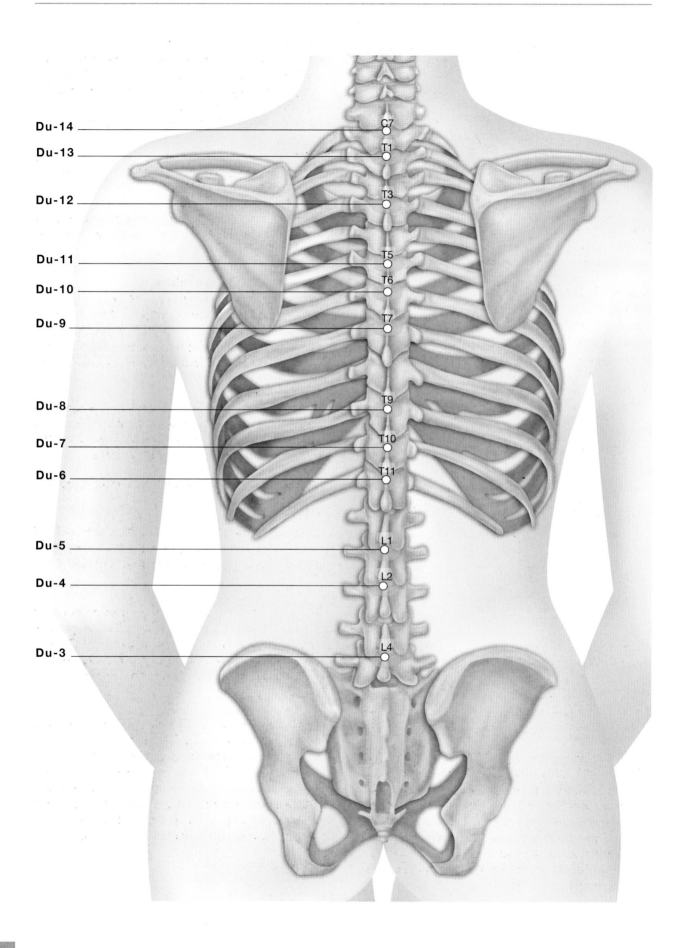

Du-14 ———————————————— C7
Du-13 ———————————————— T1
Du-12 ———————————————— T3
Du-11 ———————————————— T5
Du-10 ———————————————— T6
Du-9 ———————————————— T7
Du-8 ———————————————— T9
Du-7 ———————————————— T10
Du-6 ———————————————— T11
Du-5 ———————————————— L1
Du-4 ———————————————— L2
Du-3 ———————————————— L4

Du-3 Yaoyangguan 腰陽關

Yang Lumbar Gate

On the posterior midline, below the spinous process of L4.

Note: To aid in understanding its location and function, Du-3 is level with the Large Intestine Back Transporting-Shu point (Bl-25).

Best treatment positions

Similar to Du-4. However, traditionally, burning fewer moxa cones is recommended at this location.

Actions and indications

Du-3 can be used to *dispel cold and regulate the lower jiao, benefit the lumbar area and legs* and treat *disorders of the urogenital and gynaecological systems.* Indications include pain, weakness or paralysis of the lower limbs, lumbar pain, dysuria, urinary tract infections, diarrhoea, irregular menstruation, leucorrhoea, infertility, premature ejaculation and impotence.

> **Main Areas:** Lumbar area. Spine. Lower limbs. Urogenital system. Uterus.
>
> **Main Functions:** Dispels dampness, heat and cold. Benefits the genitourinary system.

Du-4 Mingmen 命門

Life Gate

On the posterior midline, below the spinous process of L2.

Note: To aid in understanding its location and function, Du-4 is level with the Kidney Back Transporting-Shu point (Bl-23).

Best treatment positions

This location is best treated with the patient in a prone position. If there is lumbar lordosis, place a cushion under the abdomen so that the lumbar spine is lifted up slightly and the space between the spinous processes opens. Also, the child's pose can be very effective for the application of manual techniques, because the space between the spinous processes widens in this posture (ask the patient to kneel and bend the trunk forward).

Needling

· 0.4 to 1.2 cun perpendicular insertion between the spinous processes of L2 and L3. The needle follows the angle defined by the shape of the spinous processes in a slightly superior direction.
· 0.4 to 1 cun laterally directed oblique insertion.

Alternatively, needle from a location approximately 3–6 mm laterally, in an oblique medial direction until deqi is perceived.

!! Do not needle deeper because the spinal canal lies at a depth that can be as little as 1.5 cm in persons of a small build.

Manual techniques and shiatsu

Sustained perpendicular pressure can be applied to the space between the spinous processes with the thumbs or fingertips. Also, gentle cross-fibre friction can be applied to the supraspinal ligament, and in some cases slightly deeper into the interspinal ligament and small interspinal muscle.

Alternatively, pressure can be applied bilaterally in a medial direction from two points slightly lateral to Du-4. This is useful in cases where the point is too tight due to malformation or injury to the vertebrae.

! Do not apply strong pressure to the spinous processes.

Moxibustion

Cones: 3–15. Pole: 10–30 minutes. A moxa box placed on the lumbar area covering Du-4 and Bl-23 is one of the most effective treatments to warm and tonify the Kidney Yang.

! According to a number of classical texts, moxibustion is contraindicated in patients younger than 20 years of age. This may be because it powerfully tonifies the yang qi, which in such cases, can overheat the Mingmen and injure the jing, as well as cause mental disorders.

Cupping

Empty cupping can be very effective. Apply the cup with strong suction so that Du-4 is at the centre. Often a dimple appears between the spinous processes when the suction is applied, indicating there is a lot of tension. In such cases, turn the cup gently in a clockwise and anticlockwise direction. Continue rotating the cup toward the easier of the two directions for 1 to 2 minutes. Ensure adequate lubricant has been applied to the skin.

Magnets

Magnet therapy can be effectively applied. Place north pole on Du-4 and two south poles at 0.5 to 3 cm laterally on either side, or vice-versa. Also, use opposite poles on Du-4 and Du-2 or Du-1 and/or Du-14 or Du-16, depending on the treatment principle. Furthermore, for disorders of the lower limbs, use opposite poles on Du-4 and distal points such as Bl-40.

Similar techniques can be applied at any location along the lumbar and thoracic spine.

Stimulation sensation

Regional ache and distension. However, deep needling induces numbness, tingling or electricity extending to the lower limbs. Furthermore, deqi can extend laterally, reaching the abdomen.

Actions and indications

Du-4 is one of the *most powerful points to tonify the Kidney jing and Kidney yang*, because of its location at the Gate of Life (also known as the *Gate of Vitality*). For these purposes, moxibustion is the treatment of choice.

Common indications for treatment at Du-4 include chronic lumbar pain, stiffness of the spine, tinnitus, poor memory, chronic tiredness, irregular menstruation, amenorrhoea, leucorrhoea, abnormal uterine bleeding, infertility, impotence, spermatorrhoea, dysuria, incontinence, abdominal pain, haemorrhoids, diarrhoea and prolapse of the rectum.

Du-4 is also important to *clear heat of interior, exterior, excess or deficient nature.* It treats such disorders as steaming bone syndrome, fevers, headaches, epilepsy and spasm.

Furthermore, it is an *important focus point for energy circulation* in the Du Mai in Qigong practices.

> **Main Areas:** Lumbar area. Spine. Lower limbs. Urogenital system. Uterus. Whole body.
>
> **Main Functions:** Tonifies Kidney jing and Kidney yang. Dispels cold and dampness. Alleviates pain. Clears heat. Benefits the lower jiao and genitourinary system. Increases fertility and vitality. Treats chronic diseases.

Du-5 Xuanshu
Suspended Pivot

On the posterior midline, below the spinous process of L1.

Note: To aid in understanding its location and function, Du-5 is level with the Sanjiao Back Transporting-Shu point (Bl-22).

Best treatment positions

Similar to Du-4. However, needling should not be applied as deeply as at Du-4.

Actions and indications

Du-5 is used to *strengthen the spleen* and *benefit the lumbar spine and the lower jiao.* Symptoms include abdominal distension, diarrhoea, undigested food in the stool, rectal prolapse and pain or stiffness of the lumbar spine.

> **Main Areas:** Lumbar area. Spine.
>
> **Main Functions:** Strengthens the lumbar area. Alleviates pain. Boosts Spleen qi and harmonises the Stomach.

Du-6 Jizhong 脊中
Spine Centre

On the posterior midline, below the spinous process of T11.

Note: To aid in understanding its location and function, Du-6 is level with the Spleen Back Transporting-Shu point (Bl-20).

Best treatment positions

Similar to Du-4. However, needling should not be applied as deeply as at Du-4.

! Moxibustion is contraindicated at this location according to some classical sources.

Actions and indications

Du-6 can be used to *strengthen the Spleen, drain dampness and benefit the spine*. Symptoms include diarrhoea, jaundice, abdominal distension or pain, anorexia, epilepsy and disorders of the spine, including pain and stiffness.

Main Areas: Spine. Middle jiao.

Main Functions: Strengthens the spine and alleviates pain. Boosts Spleen qi.

Du-7 Zhongshu
Central Pivot
筮樞

On the posterior midline, below the spinous process of T10.

Note: To aid in understanding its location and function, Du-7 is level with the Gallbladder Back Transporting-Shu point (Bl-19).

Best treatment positions
Similar to Du-6 and Du-4.

! Moxibustion is contraindicated at this location according to several classical texts.

Actions and indications
Similar to Du-6 and Bl-19.

Main Areas: Spine. Stomach.

Main Functions: Strengthens the Spine. Alleviates pain.

Du-8 Jinsuo
Sinew Contraction
筋縮

On the posterior midline, below the spinous process of T9.

Note: To aid in understanding its location and function, Du-8 is level with the Liver Back Transporting-Shu point (Bl-18).

Best treatment positions
Similar to Du-6 and Du-4.

Actions and indications
The main actions of Du-8 are to *promote circulation of Liver qi, calm the spirit, subdue wind and relieve spasm*. Indications include psychological disturbances, dizziness, epilepsy, fever, spasm and stiffness or pain of the spine.

Main Areas: Spine. Liver.

Main Functions: Relaxes the Spine and alleviates pain. Smoothes the Liver.

Du-9 Zhiyang
Reaching Yang
至陽

On the posterior midline, below the spinous process of T7.

Note: To aid in understanding its location and function, Du-9 is level with the Diaphragm Back Transporting-Shu point (Bl-17).

Best treatment positions
Similar to Du-4.

Needling
- 0.4 to 1 cun perpendicular insertion between the spinous processes of T7 and T8. The needle follows the angle defined by the shape of the spinous processes in a slightly superior direction.
- 0.4 to 0.8 cun laterally directed oblique insertion.

Alternatively, needle from a location approximately 3–6 mm laterally, in an oblique medial direction until deqi is induced.

!! Do not needle deeper because the spinal canal lies at a depth of 1.5–3 cm to the skin surface.

Actions and indications

Du-9 is an *important point to clear dampness and heat, particularly from the middle jiao*. It has been traditionally employed to treat *disorders of the Liver and Gallbladder* with such symptoms as tightness and heaviness of the chest, hypochondrium and abdomen, pain and swelling of the breasts, jaundice, nausea, dyspnoea and cough.

Du-9 also *fortifies the Spleen* and treats generalised weakness and emaciation.

As *a local point,* it helps treat pain and stiffness of the spine.

> **Main Areas:** Spine. Diaphragm. Liver. Middle jiao.
>
> **Main Functions:** Clears dampness and heat. Smoothes the Liver. Harmonises the middle jiao.

Du-10   Lingtai
Spirit Tower
靈台

On the posterior midline, below the spinous process of T6.

Note: To aid in understanding its location and function, Du-10 is level with the Back Transporting-Shu point for the Du Mai (Bl-16).

Best treatment positions
Similar to Du-9 and Du-4.

! According to many classical texts, this point should not be needled.

Stimulation sensation
Ache, distension or tingling locally, or extending outward across the chest, or downward to the lumbar area.

Actions and indications
Although Du-10 is not very commonly employed, it can *benefit the breathing* and *alleviate cough*. It has also been employed to *clear heat* and *detoxify poison* in the treatment of purulent boils (furuncles).

As *a local point,* it helps treat pain and stiffness of the spine.

> **Main Areas:** Chest. Lungs. Spine.
>
> **Main Functions:** Treats cough. Clears heat.

Du-11   Shendao
Spirit Path
神道

On the posterior midline, below the spinous process of T5.

Note: To aid in understanding its location and function, Du-11 is level with the Heart Back Transporting-Shu point (Bl-15).

Best treatment positions
Similar to Du-9 and Du-4.

! According to many classical texts, this point should not be needled.

Actions and indications
The actions of Du-11 are primarily associated with *functions of the upper jiao organs*. Indications include dyspnoea, cough, asthma, depression, sadness, poor memory, fright palpitations, heart pain, epilepsy and spasm.

As *a local point,* it helps treat pain and stiffness of the upper back and spine.

> **Main Areas:** Chest. Heart. Spine.
>
> **Main Functions:** Regulates upper jiao qi. Calms the mind.

Du-12   Shenzhu   身柱
Body Pillar

On the posterior midline, below the spinous process of T3.

Note: To aid in understanding its location and function, Du-11 is level with the Lung Back Transporting-Shu point (Bl-13).

Best treatment positions
Similar to Du-9 and Du-4.

Actions and indications
Similar to Bl-13 and Du-11.

> **Main Areas:** Chest. Lungs. Spine.
>
> **Main Function:** Regulates upper jiao qi.

Du-13   Taodao   陶道
Way of Happiness

Intersection of the Bladder on the Du Mai

On the posterior midline, below the spinous process of T1.

Best treatment positions
Similar to Du-14.

Actions and indications
In common with adjacent Du Mai and Bladder channel points, Du-13 *releases the exterior*, *clears heat* and *alleviates cough*.

Furthermore, it may be used as a *local point* to treat pain and stiffness of the upper back and neck.

> **Main Areas:** Chest. Lungs. Spine.
>
> **Main Function:** Regulates upper jiao qi.

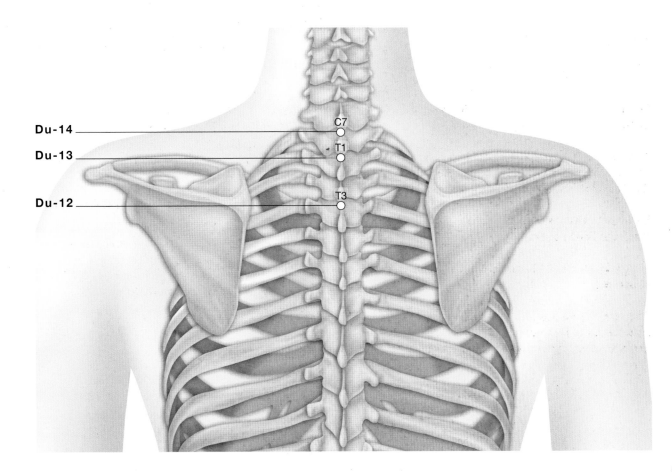

Du-14   Dazhui

大椎

Great Vertebra

Intersection of the six yang channels on the Du Mai

On the posterior midline, below the spinous process of C7.

Best treatment positions
In general, sitting up is the posture of choice for many techniques. Prone and side-lying can also be used. However, never leave a patient unattended with needles in a sitting position.

Needling
• 0.5 to 1.2 cun perpendicular insertion between the spinous processes of C7 and T1. The needle follows the angle defined by the shape of the spinous processes, i.e. in a slightly superior direction.
• 0.4 to 1 cun laterally directed oblique insertion.

Alternatively, needle from a location approximately 3–6 mm lateral to Du-14, in an oblique medial direction.

!! Do not needle deeper because the spinal canal lies at a depth of 1.5–3 cm to the skin surface. If an electric or numb sensation is felt in the limbs, remove the needle immediately.

Manual techniques and shiatsu
Sustained pressure and friction can be successfully employed, and are best applied in a sitting position. Open Du-14 by stretching the neck forward and bending the head (flexion). See also Du-4.

Moxibustion
Cones: 3–10. Pole: 5–20 minutes. Rice-grain moxa is also effectively employed.

Cupping
Place a medium- or large-sized cup over the spinous processes of C7 and T1 with medium or strong suction. Empty cupping is also useful. Also, needle cupping or moxa cupping is commonly employed.

Guasha
Guasha is effectively applied across the spinous processes and interspinal ligaments. Also, it may be applied downward or upward along the channel pathway, or outward across the trapezius fibres.

Magnets
Magnets can also be very effectively employed. Place south pole on Du-14 and north poles on Dingchuan M-BW-1b to treat dyspnoea and cough. Place south pole on Du-14 and north poles on GB-21, or vice-versa to treat pain and stiffness of the neck.

Stimulation sensation
Regional numbness, aching and distension, possibly extending laterally toward the shoulders, upward toward the back of the head, or down the spine. Furthermore, deqi can induce a sensation of coolness or heat.

Actions and indications
Du-14 is one of the *most important and commonly used points*. It is the intersection of all the Yang channels and is *important to regulate the movement of Yang qi throughout the whole body*. It can *tonify or sedate the Yang qi* and *regulates the ascending and descending of Yang qi*. It is *widely used to sedate excessive or rising yang, subdue internal wind and clear heat*. Indications include acute headache, migraine, high fever, convulsions, epilepsy, spasms, dizziness, hemiplegia, hypertension, tinnitus, pain and redness of the eyes and redness of the face.

Furthermore, it can *help to lift the yang qi*, particularly when treated with moxibustion. Indications include tiredness, poor concentration and memory, depression, dull headache, tinnitus and diminished hearing or sight.

Du-14 also effectively *calms the Heart and the mind*. Indications include palpitations, tachycardia, heart pain, tightness and pain of the chest, insomnia, mental restlessness, depression and emotional disturbances.

Du-14 is *equally important to release the exterior* in cases of *wind-heat and wind-cold*. Symptoms include chills and fever, runny nose, cough and sore throat. It also *clears and tonifies the Lungs* and is useful to treat asthma, wheeze, dyspnoea, shortness of breath, haemoptysis and other symptoms of interior or chronic lung disease.

It is a very important *local point* for *acute or chronic disorders of the cervical spine and upper back*. Symptoms include pain and stiffness of the neck, upper back and shoulders, kyphosis, excessive protrusion of C7, stooped posture, and difficulty flexing the head and neck.

Main Areas: Tai Yang area. Lungs. Chest. Heart. Mind. Cervical spine. Head.

Main Functions: Regulates ascending and descending of Yang qi. Clears heat. Subdues internal wind. Releases the exterior. Regulates qi and Blood. Benefits the spine.

Du-15   Yamen   啞門

Gate of Muteness

Intersection of the Yang Wei Mai on the Du Mai
One of the nine points for Returning Yang
Point of the Sea of Qi

On the posterior midline, 0.5 cun inferior to Du-16, in the depression 0.5 cun within the posterior hairline. Superior to the spinous process of C2.

Best treatment positions
See Du-16.

Actions and indications
Du-15 *dissipates wind of both exterior and interior origin* and is an important point to *open the sense organs* and *treat the back of the head, neck and brain*. It is particularly indicated for *disorders of the tongue* including paralysis, numbness, aphasia and other speech disorders.

Other indications include windstroke, loss of consciousness, epilepsy, poor concentration and memory, heaviness of the head, deafness, headache, epistaxis, stiffness and pain of the neck and degenerative disorders of the cervical spine.

> **Main Areas:** Tongue. Head. Spine.
>
> **Main Functions:** Subdues wind. Benefits the tongue. Opens the sense organs and benefits the brain.

Du-16   Fengfu   風府

Wind Mansion

Intersection of the Yang Qiao Mai on the Du Mai
sixth Ghost point
Point of the Sea of Marrow
Window of Heaven point

Directly below the external occipital protuberance, in the depression between the attachments of the trapezius muscle.

To aid location, it is approximately 1 cun within the posterior hairline.

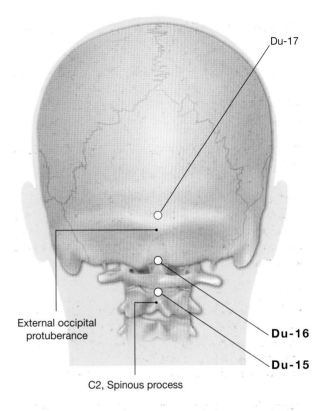

External occipital protuberance

Du-17

Du-16

Du-15

C2, Spinous process

Best treatment positions
Manual pressure techniques are generally best applied with the patient lying supine, without cushion support. However, sideways, sitting and prone postures can also be employed (in the latter case the head must be suitably supported in an anatomically shaped cushion or couch). Needling can be applied with the patient lying supine, prone or sideways. Sitting is not recommended, except for very superficial needling.

Important note: If there is a lot of tension in the neck, the head will be in a slightly extended position, requiring needling and pressure to be applied slightly more superficially. In all cases, the head should be comfortably supported so that the neck muscles can be relaxed.

Needling
• 0.5 to 1 cun perpendicular insertion, directed slightly inferiorly. Do not apply strong manipulation.

! Do not puncture the third occipital nerve and branches of the occipital artery and vein.

!! Do not needle deeply or in a superior direction because this poses considerable risk of injuring the spinal cord, which lies at a depth that may be as little as 2 cm in patients with a small build. If there is a strong electric sensation spreading to the limbs, remove the needle immediately (this means the tip is touching the spinal cord).

!!! Needling deeply in a superior direction may puncture the medulla oblongata and cause death.

Manual techniques and shiatsu
Sustained perpendicular pressure should be applied reasonably deeply into the large depressions of Du-16 and Du-15. Also, friction is effective across the nuchal ligament.

A favourite for Du-15 and Du-16 is to apply the pressure under the occipital protuberance with the patient lying supine (without cushion support). The chin should lift up slightly as the pressure is applied. Also try curling the fingers under the occipital bone.

To open and stretch Du-15 and Du-16, flex the head in an anterior direction.

! Do not apply stretching in cases of degenerative disorders of the cervical spine.

Moxibustion
Lightly applied indirect moxibustion can be beneficial in certain cases.

! According to a number of classical texts, moxibustion at Du-16 is contraindicated.

Guasha
Guasha can be applied to the nuchal fascia.

Magnets
The application of magnets at Du-15 and Du-16 can be beneficial in chronic disorders and pain. Also, use opposite poles on adjacent points such as GB-20 and Bl-10.

Stimulation sensation
Regional warmth, distension, tingling, ache or numbness. The sensation may extend upward or downward and in some cases, may lead to the whole body feeling numb.

! If a strong electric sensation is perceived during needling, remove the needle immediately.

Actions and indications
Du-16 is a very important point for many disorders of the head, brain and spine. Its main functions are to *dispel exterior wind, descend excessive yang, subdue interior wind and release cramp, nourish the Sea of Marrow* and *clear the sense organs*. Indications include sequela of wind stroke, transient ischaemic attack, hemiplegia, numbness of the head and body, flaccidity or deviation of the tongue, aphasia, hypertension, dizziness, epilepsy, spasticity, vertigo, blurred or diminishing vision, headaches, epistaxis, tinnitus, sore throat, chills and fever, vomiting and dyspnoea.

Du-16 is also very *important to calm the mind* and has been employed to treat such cases as mental confusion, restlessness, agitation, insomnia, depression, suicidal tendencies and even madness.

As *a local point*, it is helpful for stiffness and pain of the back of the neck, degenerative disorders of the cervical spine, difficulty rotating or bending the head forward or backward, and occipital headache.

Furthermore, it is an important focus point for energy circulation in the Du Mai in Qigong practices.

> **Main Areas:** Head. Brain. Sense organs. Spine.
>
> **Main Functions:** Dissipates wind. Regulates qi and Blood. Alleviates stiffness and pain. Clears the sense organs. Relaxes the body and calms the mind. Balances the NS.

Du-17　Naohu　　脑戶
Brain Door

Intersection of the Bladder on the Du Mai

In the depression directly superior to the external occipital protuberance, 1.5 cun superior to Du-16.

To aid location, Du-17 is one quarter of the distance from Du-16 to Du-20.

Needling
• 0.1 to 0.3 cun perpendicular insertion.
• 0.3 to 1 cun transverse insertion upward or downward along the course of the channel.

! According to a number of classical texts, needling is contraindicated at Du-17.

Manual techniques and shiatsu
Sustained perpendicular pressure and friction is applicable with the tips of the fingers. Also, mobilise the epicranial fascia upward, downward and laterally to loosen and relax this area.

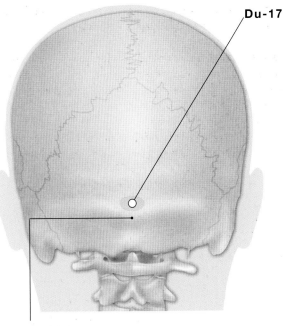

Du-17

External occipital
protuberance

Moxibustion
Lightly applied moxibustion can be beneficial in certain cases.

! According to a number of classical texts, moxibustion at Du-17 is contraindicated.

Guasha
Guasha can be applied gently downward across the external occipital protuberance.

Actions and indications
Although Du-17 is not as commonly used as adjacent points, it can be effectively employed to *dissipate wind, clear heat, clear the sense organs and benefit the eyes, regulate qi and Blood and alleviate pain*. Indications include headache, chills and fever, stiffness and pain of the neck, diminishing vision, redness and pain of the eyes and excessive lacrimation.

Furthermore, it helps *clear and calm the mind* in cases of dizziness, epilepsy, depression, anxiety and insomnia.

> **Main Areas:** Head. Sense organs.
>
> **Main Functions:** Dispels wind. Clears heat.

Du-20 Baihui 百會
One Hundred
Convergences

Intersection of the sixth Yang Channels and
Du Mai Point of the Sea of Marrow

At the vertex of the head, on the mid-saggital line, 7 cun superior to the posterior hairline, 5 cun posterior to the anterior hairline, at the midpoint of the line connecting the apex of the two ears (fold the ear forward carefully to find the apex precisely).

To aid location, Du-20 is usually at the centre of the visible spiral of the hair growth.

Best treatment positions
Du-20 can be treated with the patient sitting or lying (supine is best).

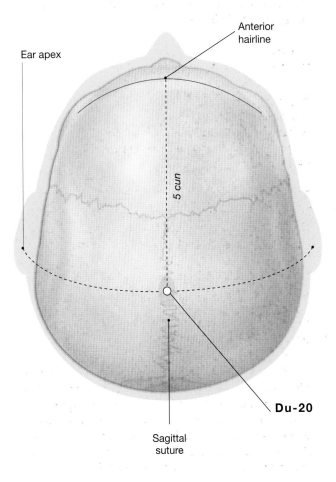

Ear apex

Anterior
hairline

5 cun

Du-20

Sagittal
suture

Needling
• 0.3 to 1 cun transverse insertion posteriorly or anteriorly along the course of the channel.

! Do not puncture the anastomotic branches of the superficial temporal and occipital artery and vein.

!! Do not needle Du-20 in cases where the fontanelle has not properly fused or in patients with hydrocephalus.

Manual techniques and shiatsu
Sustained perpendicular pressure and friction is applicable with the tips of the fingers. Also, mobilising the epicranial fascia posteriorly and anteriorly, to the left and right, or in a circular motion, is effective to loosen and relax the area.

A useful technique, particularly for sinking qi syndromes, is to apply stationary perpendicular pressure to the vertex with the palm of the hand (the patient should be sitting up). Simultaneously the patient pushes upwards against the resistance of the practitioner's palm whilst imagining the spine elongating upward and the qi lifting up.

! Do not apply strong pressure to the vertex, particularly in cases of degeneration of the spine or herniated discs.

Furthermore, self-acupressure or tapping the vertex of the head can be beneficial.

Moxibustion
Pole: 5–20 minutes. Direct moxibustion is not recommended.

Guasha
Guasha can be applied along the course of the channel and in a lateral direction.

Stimulation sensation
Regional ache or tingling, possibly extending across the vertex and possibly posteriorly or anteriorly along the course of the channel.

Actions and indications
Du-20 is a *very important and dynamic point*. It is considered the *most yang point of the body* (in this respect it is opposite to Ren-1 and Kd-1) and has the function of *descending excessive Yang* and *subduing interior wind*. It is *very important to clear the head and sense organs* and also to *calm the mind*.

Indications include headache, pain of the vertex, heavy sensation in the head, dizziness, vertigo, windstroke, loss of consciousness, numbness of the head and body, transient ischaemic attack, hemiplegia, spasticity, clenched jaw, hypertension, palpitations, feeling of heat,

redness of the face, deafness, tinnitus, epistaxis, loss of sense of smell or taste, eye pain, blurred or diminishing vision, blindness, epilepsy, sadness, fright, mental agitation, depression and even madness.

Additionally, Du-20 is *extensively employed to raise sinking qi*, *increase yang* and *benefit the Sea of Marrow*. Indications include prolapse of the uterus, rectum or other organs, haemorrhoids, chronic diarrhoea, hypotension, poor memory and concentration, and mental exhaustion.

Furthermore, Du-20 is extensively employed in beauty treatment protocols to aid the raising of qi and help 'lift' flaccid areas. Also, moxibustion at Du-20 helps bring the colour back to a pale face.

Du-20 is also an important point of focus for vertically aligning the posture during qigong practice.

> **Main Areas:** Head. Sense organs. Rectum. Uterus. Whole body.
>
> **Main Functions:** Descends excessive yang and subdues wind. Lifts sinking qi. Clears the head and sense organs. Calms the mind.

Du-23   Shangxing   上星
Upper Star

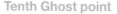

Tenth Ghost point

On the mid-saggital line, 1 cun posterior to the anterior hairline.

To aid location, the hairline is 3 cun superior to the glabella.

Best treatment positions
Du-23 can be treated with the patient sitting or lying (supine is best).

Needling
• 0.3 to 1 cun transverse insertion posteriorly or anteriorly along the course of the channel.

! Do not puncture the frontal branches of the superficial temporal artery and vein.

Manual techniques and shiatsu

Sustained perpendicular pressure and friction is applicable with the tips of the fingers. Also, mobilising the epicranial fascia forward, backward and to the left and right, or in a circular motion, is effective to loosen and relax this location.

Moxibustion

Lightly applied moxa pole therapy can be used for up to 5 minutes.

Guasha

Guasha can be applied in certain cases.

Stimulation sensation

Regional ache or tingling, possibly extending anteriorly toward the nose.

Actions and indications

Du-23 is an *important and widely used point for many disorders of the nose*. Its traditional functions include *dissipating wind, reducing swelling, clearing heat, arresting bleeding* and *clearing the head and face.*

Indications include blocked nose, nasal discharge, rhinitis, sinusitis, epistaxis, loss of sense of smell, headache, dizziness, diminishing vision, eye pain and swelling or redness of the face.

Furthermore, Du-23 has been traditionally employed to *calm the mind* and treat such cases as epilepsy, depression and even madness.

Main Areas: Nose. Eyes. Face. Head.

Main Functions: Dispels wind, clears heat and reduces swelling. Benefits the nose. Clears the face and eyes. Calms the mind.

Du-24　Shenting　神庭

Spirit Court

Intersection of the Bladder and Stomach on the Du Mai

On the mid-saggital line, 0.5 cun within the anterior hairline.

To aid location, the hairline is 3 cun superior to the eyebrows and the glabella.

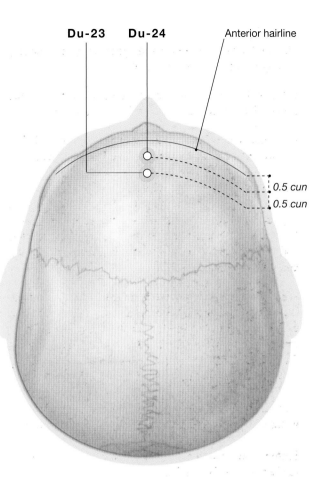

Du-23　Du-24　Anterior hairline

0.5 cun
0.5 cun

Best treatment positions

See Du-23.

Actions and indications

Du-24 is an important point to *descend rising yang, subdue internal wind, clear the head* and *calm the mind.*

Indications include blocked or runny nose, epistaxis, eye pain, excessive lacrimation, chills and fever, headaches, vomiting, dizziness, windstroke, hemiplegia, epilepsy, loss of consciousness, insomnia, depression, fright and even madness.

Main Areas: Head. Mind. Nose. Eyes.

Main Functions: Descend rising yang and subdues wind. Calms the mind. Benefits the nose. Clears the face and eyes.

Du-25   Suliao

素髎

White Crevice

At the tip of the nose, in the small depression between the two greater alar cartilages.

! Du-25 is a sensitive location.

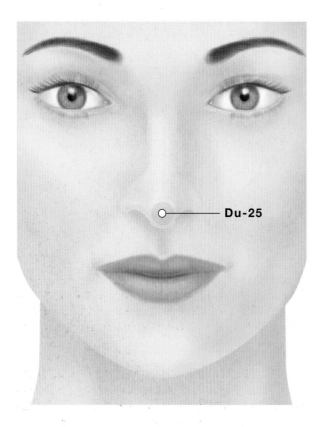

Du-25

Best treatment positions
Du-23 is usually treated with the patient lying supine.

Needling
• 0.1 to 0.4 cun perpendicular insertion between the greater alar cartilages.
• 0.5 to 1 cun upward transverse insertion.
• Prick to bleed.

Manual techniques and shiatsu
Du-25 is very rarely used in bodywork treatments, because it is difficult to treat manually. Although pressure and friction cannot be applied, pinching the tip of the nose with two or four fingers can effectively stimulate the nose and breathing, as well as help to revive consciousness.

Moxibustion
! Contraindicated.

Stimulation sensation
Deqi is often perceived as a strong tingling or electric sensation going into the nose, possibly extending upward toward the eyes. The sensation often leads to numbness. Deqi at Du-25 also gives rise to other reactions such as lacrimation, watery nasal discharge, tickly eyes, nose and throat, and sneezing.

Actions and indications
Du-25 is a *very dynamic and effective point to clear the sense organs, awaken the mind* and *restore consciousness.* However, because it is a sensitive location and treatment brings on intense reactions, it is rarely treated.

It *stimulates the lungs and breathing,* and effectively aids the body in the *detoxification process.* It is used extensively in *smoking cessation prescriptions* and is also indicated to *detoxify the blood, particularly following alcohol consumption.*

Du-25 is very effective to *dispel wind, clear heat and dissipate stasis from the face,* and is particularly indicated to *open the nose and brighten the eyes.* Indications include acute or chronic disorders of the nose (including epistaxis, blocked nose, polyps, loss of sense of smell, rhinitis, and redness or swelling of the nose), dyspnoea, excessive lacrimation, and dryness, inflammation or swelling of the eyes.

Du-25 *revives yang, restores qi* and *powerfully stimulates the mind.* Indications include hypotension, palpitations, loss of consciousness and other manifestations of shock.

Although Du-26 and not Du-25 is categorised as 'The Command Point for the Consciousness', Du-25 may be equally, if not more, effective.

> **Main Areas:** Nose. Lungs. Eyes. Mind.
>
> **Main Functions:** Benefits the nose. Clears the face and eyes. Revives yang, stimulates the mind and restores consciousness.

Du-26 Shuigou (Renzhong)

水溝
人中

Philtrum (Man Centre)

Intersection of the Large Intestine and
Stomach on the Du Mai
First Ghost point

On the anterior midline, below the nose, approximately
one third of the distance between the bottom of the nose
and the top of the lip, a little above the midpoint of the
philtrum. In the orbicularis oris muscle.

Needling

• 0.2 to 0.4 upward oblique insertion.

! Do not puncture the superior labial artery and vein.

Manual techniques and shiatsu

Sustained perpendicular pressure and friction is applicable
with the fingertip. The pressure is applied through the
orbicularis oris muscle so that it reaches the maxilla and
Du-28 (Du-28 is directly under Du-26, thus pressure at
this site affects both points).

Press quite strongly to resuscitate consciousness and to
'alert' the mind. If pressure doesn't work, rub strongly
across the philtrum.

Applying friction at Du-26, and lateral to it, reaching
the nasolabial line with an appropriate lubricant or anti-
wrinkle preparation, is very effective to diminish wrinkles
and tonify the orbicularis oris muscle.

Moxibustion

! Contraindicated.

Actions and indications

Du-26 is a *dynamic and important point to clear the
face and nose, dissipate wind, clear heat, open the sense
organs* and *restore consciousness.* Indications include
loss of consciousness, windstroke, coma, spasticity,
epilepsy, epistaxis, loss of sense of smell, runny nose,
facial paralysis, deviation of the mouth, swelling of
the face, thirst, halitosis, chills and fever, hypertension,
depression, psychological disorders, hysteria and even
madness.

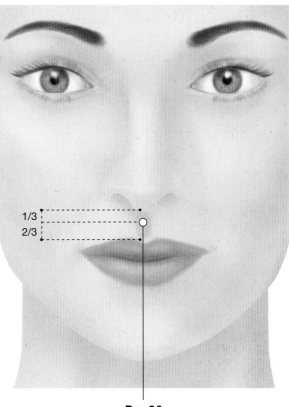

1/3
2/3

Du-26

Since Du-26 *strongly activates the Du Mai,* it is also
effective for *disorders of the spine,* and is especially
indicated for *acute lower backache and injury to
the spine.*

As a *local point,* GV-26 *is effective to improve the
appearance* and can help treat swelling or twitching
of the upper lip, flaccidity or excessive tightness or the
orbicularis oris muscle and wrinkles of the upper lip.

Main Areas: Mind. Nose. Face. Spine.

Main Functions: Benefits the nose. Clears the
face and eyes. Restores consciousness and
stimulates the mind. Regulates qi and Blood.
Alleviates lumbar pain.

Du-28   Yinjiao

Gum Intersection

齦交

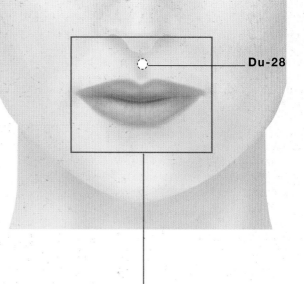

Du-28

Intersection of the Du Mai with the Ren Mai and Stomach channel

Inside the mouth on the frenulum, at the junction of the upper lip and gum.

To aid location, the frenulum is the thin vertical band of tissue connecting the upper lip and gum at the midline.

Best treatment positions
Although Du-28 is effective in a variety of mouth and gum disorders, it is not often treated with acupuncture. Other forms of treatment should not be used directly upon it (although it may be accessed with pressure from Du-26).

Needling
• 0.1 to 0.3 cun upward oblique insertion.
• Prick to bleed.

Actions and indications
Du-28 is primarily used to *clear heat* and treat *disorders of the gums and mouth*, although it also has a beneficial effect on the nose and eyes.

Indications include acute inflammation of the gums, mouth ulcers, periodonditis, stomatitis and disorders of the nose such as rhinitis and chronic blocked nose.

Main Areas: Gums. Mouth. Nose.

Main Functions: Benefits the gums. Clears heat.

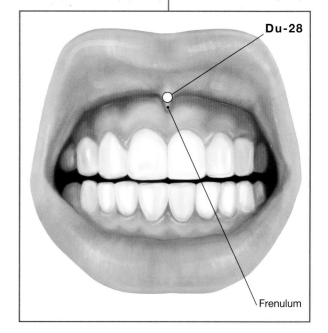

Du-28

Frenulum

Chapter 24

Extraordinary (Miscellaneous) Non-channel Points

Miscellaneous and New Points of the Head and Neck

M-HN-1 Sishencong 四神聰
Four Spirit Brightness

Four points either side of the vertex, 1 cun anterior, posterior and lateral to Du-20.

To aid location, Du-20 is 5 cun posterior to the anterior hairline.

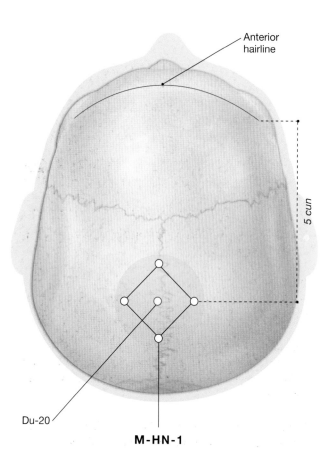

M-HN-1

Best treatment positions
Similar to Du-20.

Needling
• 0.2 to 1 cun transverse insertion toward Du-20 (needle all four points).

Alternatively, insert needle at Du-20 and direct it toward one of the four points.

! Do not puncture the branches of the superficial temporal artery and vein or the occipital artery and vein.

Actions and indications
In common with Du-20, these four points are effective to *subdue interior wind, descend yang, clear the ears, eyes and nose,* and *calm the mind.*

Indications include headache, dizziness, vertigo, numbness, hemiplegia, windstroke, aphasia, epilepsy, insomnia, depression, psychological disorders, poor memory, disorders of the ears, eyes and nose, epistaxis, tinnitus and deafness.

> **Main Areas:** Head. Mind.
>
> **Main Functions:** Clears the head and calms the mind. Subdues wind.

M-HN-3 Yintang 印堂
Seal Hall

Midway between the eyebrows, on the anterior midline, at the glabella. Situated in the procerus muscle.

Best treatment positions
M-HN-3 can be treated with the patient lying supine or sitting.

Needling
• 0.3 to 0.7 cun oblique inferior insertion into the corrugator muscle. Pick up the muscle to insert the needle.
• 0.4 to 1 cun oblique or transverse insertion medially toward Bl-2 or Bl-1.

! Apply pressure to the point after removing the needle.

Manual techniques and shiatsu
Perpendicular pressure and friction can be applied gently or quite strongly. Sometimes a very light touch can be more effective to calm the mind.

Also, picking up, pressing and squeezing the corrugator muscle is very effective to relax the area and brighten the eyes. Furthermore, friction applied superiorly, inferiorly and laterally, with an appropriate lubricant, effectively diminishes lines and furrows.

Magnets

Small magnets can be successfully used on Yintang (M-HN-3). Use opposite poles on Bl-2 and Yintang to treat frontal headache.

Stimulation sensation

Deqi is usually perceived as a pleasant, heavy or tingling sensation, often extending to the eyes, forehead and possibly across the entire face and head. Sometimes the sensation feels like coolness spreading across the forehead. The body and mind should relax, and the patient may feel sleepy.

! Sometimes needling can be sharp and painful and deqi difficult to achieve.

Actions and indications

Yintang is *an important and extensively used point to calm the mind* and *dispel wind, clear heat* and *alleviate pain from the face.* It effectively treats *disorders of the eyes, sinuses and nose.*

Indications include anxiety, insomnia, depression, psycho-emotional disorders, hypertension, dizziness, epilepsy, frontal headache, tiredness and heaviness of the eyes, inflammation of the eyes, sinusitis, disorders of the nose such as rhinitis and nasal congestion.

Yintang (M-HN-3) also helps *regulate the endocrine system* by stimulating the hypophysis and pineal gland, and can be used to treat hormonal imbalances.

Furthermore, it is a useful distal point for lumbar back ache. Additionally, Yintang (M-HN-3) is *an important beauty point* for the area between the eyebrows.

Main Areas: Mind. Forehead. Eyes. Nose. Whole body.

Main Functions: Calms the mind and relaxes the body. Clears wind and heat from the face. Benefits the eyes and nose. Subdues wind.

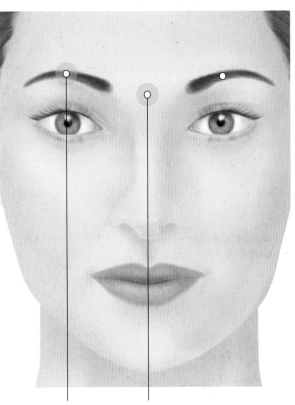

M-HN-6　　　**M-HN-3**

M-HN-6　Yuyao　　　魚腰

Fish Waist

In the depression at the centre of the eyebrow, directly above the pupil.

Best treatment positions

M-HN-3 can be treated with the patient lying supine or sitting.

Needling

• 0.3 to 1 cun transverse insertion medially or laterally along the eyebrow. Pick up the skin to insert the needle into the muscle.

! Apply pressure to the point after removing the needle. Do not puncture the supraorbital artery, vein or nerve.

Manual techniques and shiatsu

Sustained perpendicular pressure and friction can be applied gently or quite strongly. Sometimes a very light touch can be more effective to calm the mind.

Magnets

Small magnets can be successfully used on Yuyao. Use opposite poles on Bl-2 and Yintang to treat frontal headache.

Actions and indications

Yuyao (M-HN-6) is an excellent point to *regulate qi, alleviate pain* and *benefit the eyes*. Indications include spasm of the eye muscles, flaccidity of the upper eyelid, paralysis of the orbicularis oculi, inflammation and swelling of the eyes, frontal headache, migraine, facial pain and trigeminal neuralgia.

> **Main Areas:** Eyes. Forehead.
> **Main Functions:** Regulates qi and Blood. Alleviates pain and swelling. Benefits the eyes.

M-HN-8　Qiuhou

球后

Behind the Eye Ball

Between the eyeball and the infraorbital ridge, halfway between St-1 and the lateral edge of the orbit.

Best treatment positions

Similar to St-1.

Needling

!! Qiuhou is one of the most sensitive and dangerous points to needle and therefore requires special skill and experience. Great care should be taken as wrongly angled insertion can damage the eye. Use the thinnest needle possible.

- 0.5 to 1.2 cun perpendicular insertion angled between the eyeball and inferior orbital ridge.

Support the eyeball with the tip of the finger and insert the needle slowly and carefully, whilst the patient looks upward. Angle the needle slightly downward and then perpendicularly along the inferior orbital wall under the eyeball. Do not manipulate the needle.

! Qiuhou can bruise easily, see first aid for bruising for St-1.

Manual techniques and shiatsu

Light, sustained pressure may be applied carefully onto the infraorbital ridge with the tip of the finger.

Actions and indications

Benefits the eyes, similar to St-1.

> **Main Area:** Eyes and area below.
> **Main Function:** Benefits the eyes and improves vision.

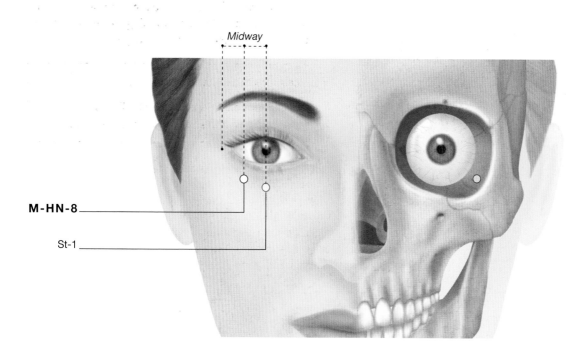

M-HN-9 Taiyang

太陽

The Sun
(Supreme Yang)

In the depression of the temporal fossa, approximately 1 cun posterior to the midpoint between the outer canthus of the eye and the tip of the eyebrow.

To aid location, Taiyang is at the site of most tenderness on pressure palpation.

M-HN-9

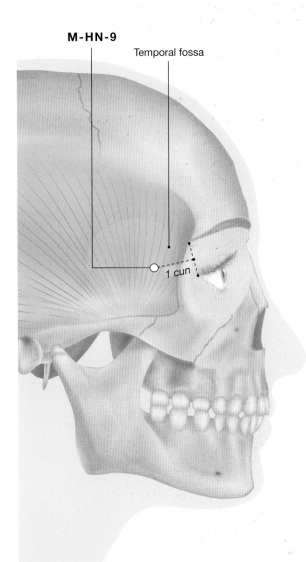

Temporal fossa

1 cun

Best treatment positions
Taiyang M-HN-9 can be treated with the patient lying supine or sideways, or sitting up.

Needling
- 0.3 to 0.8 cun perpendicular insertion.
- 0.5 to 1.5 cun transverse posterior insertion.
- 0.5 to 1 cun oblique insertion.
- Prick to bleed.

! Do not puncture the branches of the zygomaticoorbital and superficial temporal artery, or the branches of the facial nerve; more deeply, the middle temporal vein and the zygomaticotemporal nerve; in its deep position, the deep temporal artery and nerve.

Manual techniques and shiatsu
Whilst sustained pressure and friction are equally applicable in acute pain conditions, friction applied lightly is usually the best choice (with or without a lubricant). For best results, apply friction to the entire temple for at least 5 minutes and then use sustained perpendicular pressure on the site of most tenderness.

Magnets
Small magnets can be used to treat pain.

Actions and indications
Taiyang M-HN-9 is an *extremely useful and widely used point* for temporal headache and disorders of the eyes. Its traditional functions include *regulating qi and Blood, dissipating wind and clearing heat.*

Indications include temporal headache, migraine, acute or chronic eye pain, redness, itching or swelling of the eyes, tired eyes, redness or swelling of the face, facial pain, trigeminal neuralgia and facial paralysis.

Main Areas: Temples. Eyes. Head.

Main Functions: Regulates qi and Blood. Alleviates pain and swelling. Benefits the eyes.

M-HN-10   Erjian   耳尖

Ear Apex

At the apex of the ear. Fold the ear forward to locate the apex precisely.

M-HN-10

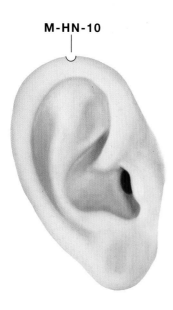

Needling
• 0.1 to 0.2 cun perpendicular insertion.
• Prick to bleed (let 2 to 5 drops).

Manual techniques and shiatsu
The ear apex can be pinched reasonably strongly.

Moxibustion
Pole: 3 to 5 minutes. Rice-grain moxibustion is also effective.

Actions and indications
The Ear tip point is a *dynamic point to clear heat* and *descend rising yang*. It also *soothes inflammation* and *dissipates swelling from the eyes and throat*. Furthermore it has a *calming and pain reducing effect*.

Indications include high fever, hypertension, painful, inflamed eyes, sore, swollen throat, loss of consciousness, migraine, various pain conditions and mental agitation.

> **Main Areas:** Eyes. Head. Liver. Whole body.
>
> **Main Functions:** Descends yang and clears heat. Alleviates pain.

M-HN-14   Bitong   鼻通

Nose Passage

In the depression below the nasal bone, at the superior end of the nasolabial sulcus.

Best treatment positions
Similar to LI-20.

Needling
• 0.3 to 0.5 cun transverse insertion toward the bridge of the nose.

In many cases, needling Bitong through from LI-20 is most effective.

Manual techniques and shiatsu
Self-acupressure is most effective applied regularly until symptoms subside.

Stimulation sensation
Regional ache and distension extending into the nose. The sensation often gives way to numbness.

Actions and indications
Bitong, also known as *Shangyingxiang*, *Upper LI-20*, is an *important and widely used point for disorders of the nose*.

It has *similar functions to LI-20*, and is especially indicated for nasal congestion, rhinitis, sinusitis, nasal polyps, nasal discharge and epistaxis.

Furthermore, Bitong soothes and clears the eyes.

> **Main Area:** Nose.
>
> **Main Functions:** Clears wind and heat. Opens the nose.

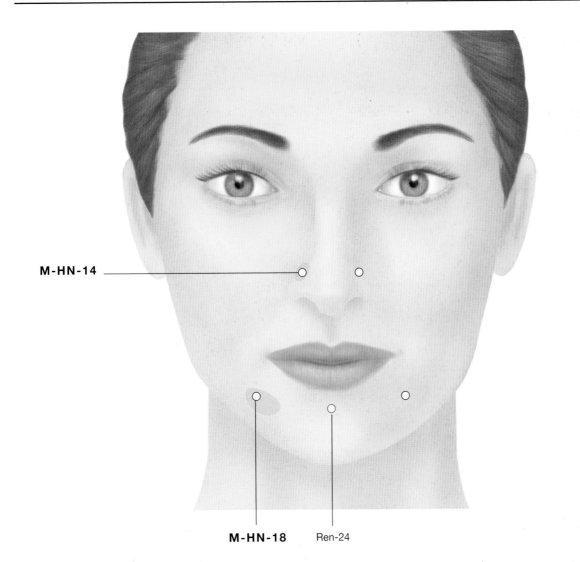

M-HN-14

M-HN-18   Ren-24

M-HN-18 Jiachengjiang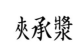

Adjacent to Ren-24

Approximately 1 cun lateral to Ren-24, in the depression of the mental foramen.

To aid location, it is approximately below St-4.

Best treatment positions
Similar to Ren-24.

Needling
• 0.3 to 0.5 cun perpendicular insertion.
• 0.5 to 1.5 cun transverse insertion.

Actions and indications
Jiachengjiang is an *effective point to dissipate wind* and *regulates qi and Blood* in the region. Its main indications include trigeminal neuralgia, facial pain, toothache, inflammation of the gums, deviation of the mouth and facial paralysis.

Main Areas: Mouth. Chin.
Main Functions: Regulates qi and Blood.
Dispels wind. Alleviates pain.

M-HN-30 Bailao 百勞

Hundred Labours

1 cun lateral to the posterior midline and 1 cun inferior to the posterior hairline (2 cun superior to the level of Du-14).

Best treatment positions
Similar to Bl-10.

Needling
• 0.5 to 1 cun perpendicular insertion.

Manual techniques and shiatsu
Stationary pressure and friction is applicable with the finger and thumb tips. For more techniques see Bl-10.

! Always apply pressure carefully to the neck area.

Moxibustion
Cones: 2–5. Pole: 5–15 minutes.

Magnets
Stick-on magnets can be very helpful.

Guasha
Guasha can be successfully employed across or down the trapezius fibres.

Stimulation sensation
Aching, distension and tingling, extending superiorly to the head or inferiorly down toward the upper back and shoulders.

Actions and indications
Bailao has been traditionally used to *tonify the energy* and *treat exhaustion,* especially in *chronic disorders and the elderly.* It is particularly indicated for *weakness of the neck muscles* leading to *difficulty in keeping the head upright, dizziness, poor concentration* as well as *pain and chronic stiffness of the neck.*

It also effectively treats *phlegm accumulation* and *Lung deficiency* with symptoms such as dyspnoea, cough, wheeze, spontaneous sweating, night sweating and lymphadenopathy. Traditionally, it was used to treat tuberculosis and other severe or chronic diseases.

> **Main Areas:** Chest. Lungs. Spine.
>
> **Main Function:** Regulates upper jiao qi.

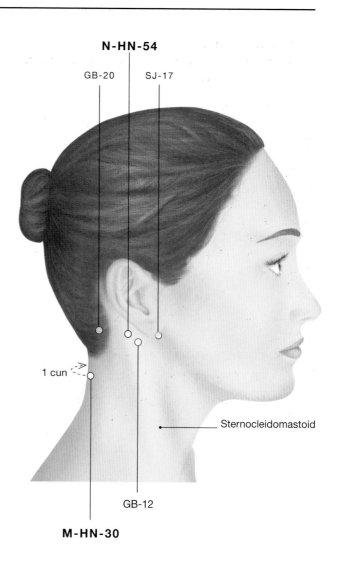

N-HN-54

GB-20   SJ-17

1 cun

Sternocleidomastoid

GB-12

M-HN-30

N-HN-54 Anmian 安眠

Peaceful Sleep

At the posterior border of the mastoid process, midway between GB-20 and SJ-17, slightly posterior and superior to GB-12. At the centre of the insertion of the sternocleidomastoid muscle. More deeply, it is situated in the splenius capitis, and deeper still, in the obliquus capitis superior muscle.

Best treatment positions
Similar to GB-12.

Needling
• 0.5 to 1 cun perpendicular insertion.
! Do not puncture the branches of the greater auricular nerve and the posterior auricular artery and vein, and more deeply, the occipital artery and vein.

Manual techniques and shiatsu

Stationary pressure and friction is applicable with the finger and thumb tips.

Stimulation sensation

Aching, distension and tingling, extending into the head or down the neck.

Actions and indications

In common with adjacent points such as GB-12 and GB-20, Anmian *promotes relaxation by soothing Liver qi* and is *extensively used to treat insomnia*. It also *clears heat and dispels wind from the head*. Indications include mental restlessness, pain conditions, depression, dizziness, vertigo, migraine, hypertension, epilepsy and tinnitus.

Furthermore, Anmian clears *the eyes and improves vision*.

> **Main Areas:** Mind. Head. Eyes.
>
> **Main Functions:** Promotes relaxation and sleep. Smoothes Liver qi. Benefits the eyes.

Miscellaneous and New Points of the Back and Waist

M-BW-1A Chuanxi
Gasping

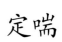

M-BW-1B Dingchuan
Relieve Dyspnoea

M-BW-1A *Chuanxi* is situated 1 cun lateral to Du-14. M-BW-1B *Dingchuan* is 0.5 cun lateral to Du-14.

To aid location, palpate superficially and then deeply to determine the most reactive site.

Best treatment positions
Similar to the upper Back-Shu points.

Needling
• 0.5 to 1 cun medial oblique insertion toward Du-14.

Manual techniques and shiatsu
Sustained pressure and friction should be applied quite strongly for 2 to 5 minutes to treat dyspnoea and wheezing.

Cupping
Cupping with medium or strong suction is effective. Also needle cupping can be very effective for asthma.

Guasha
Guasha can be effectively employed.

Magnets
For breathing disorders, alternate poles between adjacent and distal points, including Bl-12, Bl-13, Lu-7, Lu-9 and LI-4.

Actions and indications
Both Chuanxi (M-BW-1A) and Dingchuan (M-BW-1B) are widely employed to treat a variety of breathing complaints including acute wheezing, dyspnoea, cough and asthma.

> **Main Areas:** Chest. Lungs. Neck. Upper back.
>
> **Main Functions:** Benefits breathing and alleviates cough.

Paravertebral Points
and Other Miscellaneous Points of the Back and Waist

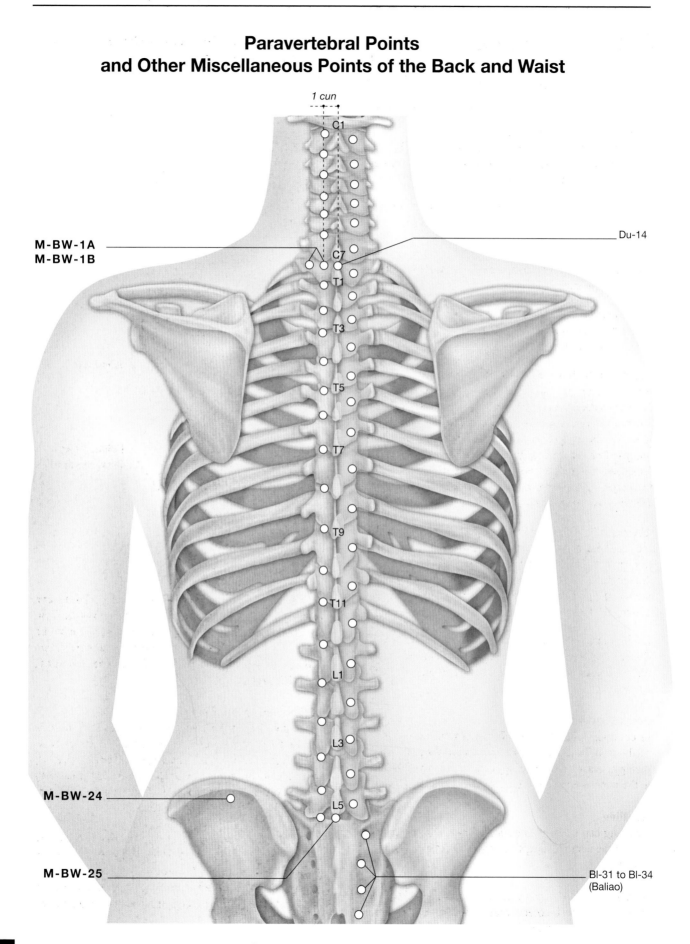

1 cun

C1

C7

Du-14

M-BW-1A
M-BW-1B

T1

T3

T5

T7

T9

T11

L1

L3

M-BW-24

L5

M-BW-25

Bl-31 to Bl-34
(Baliao)

EXTRAORDINARY (MISCELLANEOUS) POINTS

M-BW-35 Huatuojiaji

Hua Tuo's Para-
vertebral Points

In the paraspinal groove, approximately 0.5 cun lateral to the posterior midline. Lateral either to the lower borders, or the tips of the spinous processes of the cervical, thoracic and lumbar vertebrae.

The points shown on the left are level with the facet joints. Those on the right are approximately over the spinal nerves.

To aid location, apply pressure palpation to determine the most reactive sites.

Some sources place these points slightly more medially, others more laterally, at a distance of 0.8 or 1 cun from the posterior midline.

These points may be approximately *located over the facet joints* or over the *spinal nerves emerging from the intervertebral foramina.* Therefore, in general, the former are more effective for *disorders of the vertebrae,* and the latter are *more effective to regulate the nervous system and for interior disorders and neurological conditions.* However, the entire spine varies greatly from person to person, and furthermore, the spinous processes and vertebrae are all different from one another.

The term *Jiaji* or *Paravertebral points* was assigned to the 17 pairs of points situated along the thoracic and lumbar spine by the renowned doctor *Hua Tuo* during the 2nd century. This group of points has been expanded to include the points lateral to the 7 cervical vertebrae, thus making 24 sets of points.

Furthermore, the 8 sacral foramina points (called *Baliao 'Eight Bone-holes'*), can be considered part of the paravertebral point group (Bl-31, Bl-32, Bl-33 and Bl-34).

Best treatment positions
In common with the Back Transporting-Shu points, all methods of treatment, including moxibustion, magnet therapy, guasha and cupping, can be effectively applied to the paravertebral points.

Needling
Needling can be *applied obliquely in a medial direction* toward the spine to a depth of approximately 0.5 to 1 (or 1.5) cun.

Also, *perpendicular needling* can be applied 0.5 to 1 cun in the cervical and thoracic regions and up to 2 cun in the lumbar and sacral spine.

General functions of the paravertebral points in relation to the vertebrae:

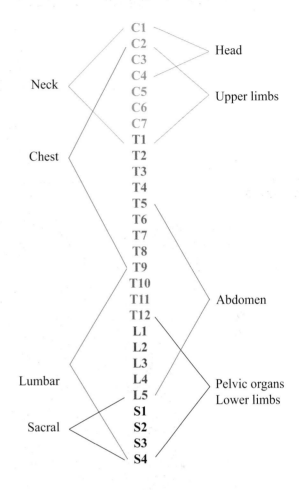

! These techniques apply to points located 0.3 to 0.8 cun lateral to the midline. Points at a 1 cun distance from the midline between T1 and L1 should not be punctured perpendicularly to a depth of more than 0.6 cun in thin patients, to avoid the possibility of puncturing the lungs and other organs.

Actions and indications
These points are *very important and extensively used in a wide range of disorders*. From a Chinese point of view, they are particularly *effective to dispel qi and Blood stasis, clear interior heat* and *regulate the internal organs.* They can be considered *alternative Back Transporting-Shu points*, whose functions they share.

They *effectively regulate the nervous system* and *are very useful in many disorders of the limbs and internal organs.* They are also *extensively employed to treat disorders of the spine* and *spinal nerves* and are very useful in the *treatment of pain* (they are used in acupuncture anaesthesia).

Furthermore, they *calm the mind* and *induce physical relaxation*. They have also been employed in a *variety of severe stubborn diseases* including aphasia, hemiplegia, lupus erythematosus, ankylosing spondylitis and multiple sclerosis.

Additionally, the paravertebral points are *useful diagnostically* both in terms of zangfu imbalance, and of spinal nerve or visceral referred pain.

> **Main Areas:** Entire body. Spine. Nervous system. Internal organs.
>
> **Main Functions:** Alleviates pain. Regulates the pertaining internal organs and the nervous system. Relaxes the body and mind.

M-BW-24   Yaoyan   腰眼
Lumbar Eyes

At the centre of the large depressions inferior to the iliac crests, 3 to 4 cun lateral to the posterior midline, level with the lower border of the spinous process of L4 (Du-3). In the gluteus medius muscle.

To aid location, in many people the 'eyes' are visible depressions, just over a hand's width from the midline. Apply pressure palpation to determine the most reactive location. These depressions are formed by the iliac crests (superiorly), the lateral margin of the gluteus maximus (medially) and the attachment of the gluteus minimus muscle (inferiorly, under the gluteus medius).

Some sources place this point superior to the iliac crests, lateral to the third lumbar vertebra.

Actions and indications
Yaoyan is an important point to strengthen the lumbar spine and reinforce the Kidneys. It is very effective to alleviate acute or chronic low back pain, irrespective of the cause.

Needling
• 1 to 1.5 cun perpendicular insertion.

! Do not puncture the superior cluneal nerve or the dorsal branch of the twelfth thoracic nerve, or more deeply, the branches of the superior gluteal artery, vein and nerve.

Moxibustion
Cones: 5–10. Pole: 10–20 minutes.

Cupping
Medium, strong or empty cupping is effective. Also, moving a medium-sized cup over and below the iliac crest in the upper gluteal region is very effective.

Actions and indications
M-BW-24 is a very effective point to *regulate qi in the lower jiao* and *alleviate pain*. Indications include chronic or acute lower back pain, sciatica, irregular menstruation and frequent urination.

> **Main Areas:** Lower back. Uterus. Urinary system.
>
> **Main Functions:** Alleviates pain. Regulates qi in the lower jiao.

M-BW-25   Shiqizhui   十七椎
Seventeenth Vertebra Point

On the posterior midline, between the spinous process of L5 and the sacrum.

Note: In some cases, L5 and S1 are fused making it seem that there are six sacral vertebrae. In these cases, use Du-3, between L4 and L5 instead. Also, in some cases there are six lumbar vertebrae, and in others, S1 is not fused with S2, making it appear there are six lumbar vertebrae. In these cases, palpate the points between L5–L6 and L6–S1 or L5–S1 and S1–S2 to determine which is more reactive on pressure palpation.

Manual techniques and shiatsu
Pressure is best applied in a prone position with cushions under the abdomen so that the pelvis is raised and the lumbosacral joint opens up.

Needling
• 0.5 to 1.2 cun perpendicular insertion into the space between L5 and S1.

!! Do not needle deeply because this poses considerable risk of injuring the spinal cord, which lies at a depth that may be as little as 1.5 cm.

Moxibustion
Cones: 5–10. Pole: 5–15 minutes.

Cupping

Medium, strong or empty cupping is effective.

Actions and indications

This point is very effective to treat *acute or chronic pain and weakness of the lumbosacral joint*. It is also *widely used to treat acute dysmenorrhoea and pelvic pain*.

It has also been traditionally employed to *fortify the Kidneys* and *benefit the genitourinary system*.

> **Main Areas:** Lower back. Uterus. Urinary system.
>
> **Main Functions:** Alleviates pain. Regulates qi in the lower jiao.

Miscellaneous and New Points of the Chest and Abdomen

M-CA-23　Sanjiaojiu　三角灸

Moxibustion Triangle

Three points on each corner of an equilateral triangle, with the apex point at the navel (Ren-8). The sides of the triangle are measured as equal to the width of the patient's smile.

Best treatment positions

These points are treated with moxibustion only. Use 5–10 cones, directly placed on the skin, or on ginger or garlic. Also use rice-grain moxibustion.

Actions and indications

These points *effectively regulate qi in the abdomen, alleviate abdominal pain and stop diarrhoea*. They are also indicated to treat *hernias* and other *symptoms of upsurging qi* such as nausea and thoracic oppression. See also Ren-8.

Furthermore, it is common to treat the point on the left side for disorders of the right, and vice-versa.

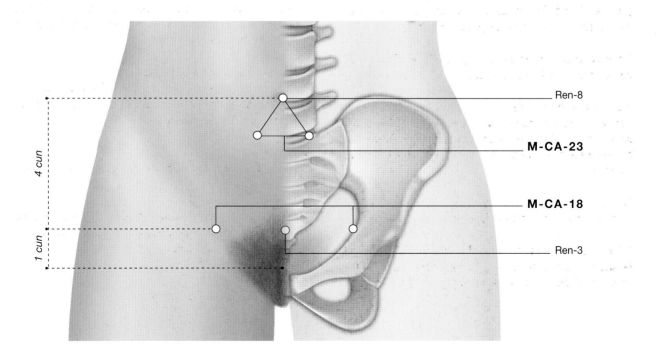

M-CA-18 Zigong

子宫

Child's Palace (Uterus)

3 cun (one hand-width) lateral to Ren-3, 4 cun below the umbilicus.

Best treatment positions
Similar to St-29.

Needling
• 0.5 to 1.5 cun perpendicular insertion.

! Do not puncture branches of the superficial epigastric artery and vein.

!! Needling deeply will puncture the peritoneum.

Manual techniques and shiatsu
Sustained pressure can be applied perpendicularly, or in a medial direction toward the uterus.

Moxibustion
Cones: 5–10. Pole: 5–15 minutes. Rice-grain moxa is also applicable.

Cupping
Medium- or small-sized cups with light or medium suction are applicable.

Magnets
Magnets can be successfully employed to treat chronic blood stasis in the uterus.

Stimulation sensation
Regional distension and warmth extending into the lower abdominal area.

Actions and indications
Zigong M-CA-18 is an *important point for disorders of the ovaries and uterus*, including infertility, irregular menstruation, abnormal uterine bleeding, leucorrhoea, endometriosis, uterine prolapse and abdominal pain.

> **Main Areas:** Uterus. Ovaries. Abdomen.
>
> **Main Functions:** Increases fertility. Regulates menstruation. Benefits the uterus.

Miscellaneous and New Points of the Upper Limb

M-UE-1 Shixuan

十宣

Ten Diffusions

Ten points, at the tip of each finger, 0.1 cun from the centre of the free margin of the nail.

Needling
Most texts recommend pricking these points with a three-edged needle to draw a little blood, and then applying moxibustion.

However, shallow perpendicular needling, sustained pressure or strong tapping of the fingertips can also be effectively employed. Furthermore, moxa-pole therapy and rice-grain moxibustion can be useful.

M-UE-1

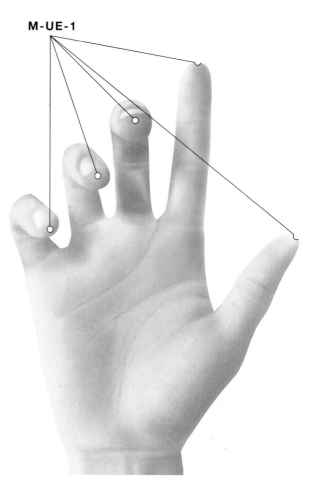

Actions and indications

These points are *very dynamic* and have similar functions to the Well-*Jing* points, including *clearing the sense organs, face, head and throat, dispelling exterior wind and heat, subduing interior wind, clearing interior heat and restoring consciousness*. Furthermore, they are also *employed to treat children*.

Indications include loss of consciousness, fainting, windstroke, hypertension, heat stroke, high fever, seizures, infantile convulsions, acute pain or swelling of the throat, vomiting and diarrhoea.

Additionally, these points can be useful to treat *numbness and pain of the fingers*.

> **Main Areas:** Brain. Senses. Abdomen.
>
> **Main Functions:** Restores consciousness. Subdues wind and stops seizures. Clears the brain and sense organs. Clears heat and dispels exterior wind.

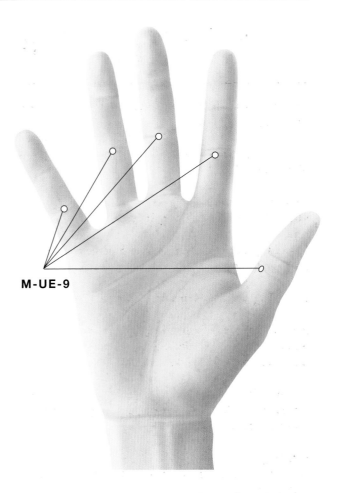

M-UE-9

M-UE-9   Sifeng   四縫

Four Seams

Four points at the midpoint of the transverse creases of the proximal interphalangeal joints of the second to fifth fingers, on the palmar aspect of the hands.

Usually there are two main creases; these points are located at the deeper of the two creases, which is usually the proximal one.

To aid location, define the creases by flexing the fingers.

Needling
Most texts recommend pricking these points to draw a little blood or thin yellow fluid. However, acupressure and moxibustion can also be employed.

Actions and indications
These points are extensively used to treat a *wide range of paediatric disorders*, particularly in relation to *nutrition and the digestive system*. They *boost the middle jiao and Spleen* helping *improve the transformation and transportation of food essences and body fluids*, thus *helping nourish the body* and *relieve accumulation and abdominal swelling*.

Indications include eating disorders in children, malnutrition, emaciation, swelling and pain of the abdomen, diarrhoea, vomiting, food retention, lack of appetite, infantile colic and indigestion, and respiratory disorders such as cough and asthma.

Furthermore, they effectively treat *pain and stiffness of the fingers*.

> **Main Areas:** Abdomen. Chest.
>
> **Main Functions:** Boosts the middle jiao and tonifies the Spleen. Relieves accumulation.

M-UE-22 Baxie

Eight Evils

八邪

Eight points on the webs between each of the fingers, distal to the metacarpophalangeal joints and approximately 0.5 cun proximal to the margin of the webs. They are usually located and treated with the hand in a loose fist.

To aid location, when the fingers are closed together (adducted), the points are at the end of the creases between each finger.

This group of points also includes SJ-2 and LI-4 (approximately).

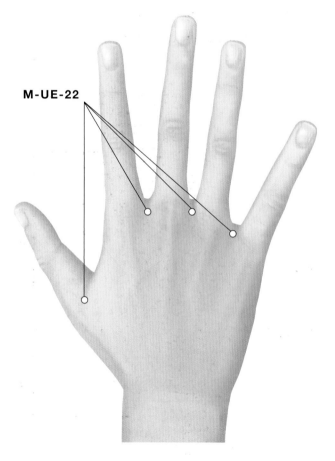

M-UE-22

Needling
• 0.5 to 1 cun perpendicular insertion between the shafts of the metacarpal bones. Needle with the fingers relaxed in a loose fist.
• Prick to bleed.

Manual techniques and shiatsu
Sustained perpendicular pressure and friction is applicable with the tips of the fingers.

Moxibustion
Pole: 2–5 minutes. Rice-grain moxa is also effectively employed.

Actions and indications
These are important points for *disorders of the fingers and metacarpophalangeal joints*, including arthritis and injury, swelling, stiffness and contraction of the fingers.

They are also used to *clear heat* and treat headache, earache, toothache, sore throat, pain of the eyes and fever.

> **Main Areas:** Fingers. Head.
>
> **Main Functions:** Regulates qi and Blood. Alleviates swelling, stiffness and pain. Clears heat.

M-UE-24 Luozhen (Wailaogong)

Stiff Neck (Outer P-8)

落枕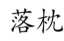

On the dorsum of the hand, between the second and third metacarpal bones about 0.5 cun proximal to the metacarpophalangeal joints.

To aid location, it is at the site of most tenderness (often, there is a small palpable 'nodule' at the epicentre that can be very painful on pressure).

Also, if the patient makes a loose fist, the skin is stretched and a visible depression appears. M-UE-24 is usually at the epicentre of this depression.

Best treatment positions
M-UE-24 can be treated easily in most positions. To release stiffness more quickly, mobilise the neck as you stimulate the point with acupressure or needling. The patient should be sitting in a chair.

Needling
• 0.3 to 1 cun perpendicular or oblique proximal insertion.

! Avoid the dorsal cutaneous veins, and more deeply, the dorsal metacarpal arteries.

Manual techniques and shiatsu
Friction and sustained pressure should produce a fairly strong sensation to be effective. Apply friction to the nodules until they soften or disappear entirely.

Moxibustion

Cones: 1–3. Pole: 5–10 minutes. Rice-grain moxibustion is also effective.

Guasha

Guasha can be applied gently.

Stimulation sensation

Both pressure and needling induce a strong sensation both regionally and extending toward the shoulder and chest.

Actions and indications

Luozhen is a very dynamic and effective point to *release pain and stiffness of the neck and arm*.

> **Main Areas:** Neck. Upper limbs.
>
> **Main Functions:** Regulates qi and Blood. Alleviates pain and stiffness.

M-UE-29   Erbai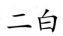

Two Whites

Two points, 4 cun proximal to the wrist crease, either side of the flexor carpi radialis tendon.

Best treatment positions

Similar to P-5 and P-4.

Needling

• 0.3 to 1 cun perpendicular insertion.

Actions and indications

M-UE-29 is an effective point for *disorders of the rectum and anus*, including rectal prolapse and haemorrhoids.

> **Main Areas:** Rectum and anus.
>
> **Main Function:** Benefits the rectum.

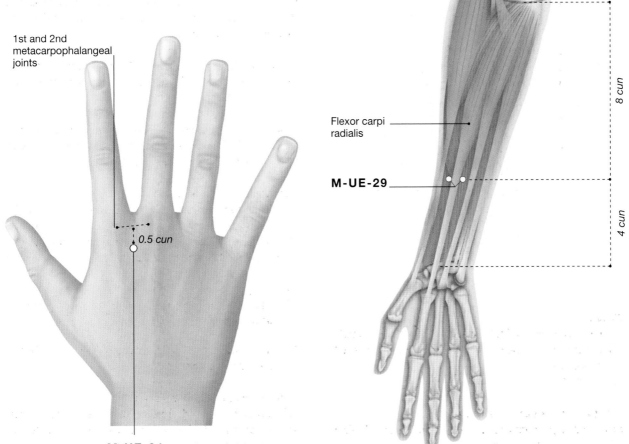

1st and 2nd metacarpophalangeal joints

0.5 cun

M-UE-24

Flexor carpi radialis

M-UE-29

8 cun

4 cun

M-UE-48 Jianqian (Jianneiling)

肩前

Front of the Shoulder

In the depression between the coracoid process and the head of the humerus, midway between the end of the anterior axillary fold and LI-15.

M-UE-48 is usually located with the arm hanging down freely at sides. However, if the arm is abducted, it is sometimes easier to find the tender point.

Needling

• 0.5 to 1 cun perpendicular insertion.
• 1 to 1.5 cun oblique inferior insertion.

! Do not puncture the supraclavicular nerve, and more deeply, the anterior humeral circumflex artery and vein.

Manual techniques and shiatsu

Sustained pressure and friction can be applied into the space between the coracoid process and the humeral head.

Moxibustion

Cones: 3–7. Pole: 5–15 minutes.

Cupping, guasha and magnets

These forms of treatment can be extremely effective to alleviate pain and stiffness of the shoulder. Combine M-UE-48 with adjacent points around the shoulder.

Actions and indications

This is a very useful point for chronic or acute stiffness and pain of the shoulder joint.

> **Main Areas:** Shoulder. Upper arm.
>
> **Main Functions:** Regulates qi and Blood. Alleviates stiffness and pain.

N-UL-19 Yaotongdian

腰痛點

Lumbar Pain Point

Three points on the dorsum of the hand, in the depressions between the second, third, fourth and fifth metacarpal bones. Approximately 1 cun distal to the transverse wrist crease, in the depressions just distal to the bases of the metacarpals.

To aid location, there are often one or more small palpable 'nodules' in the region between the metacarpals. The best treatment site is usually at the most painful 'nodule'.

Furthermore, points (a) and (c) are more effective for stiffness or injury to the paraspinal muscles in the lower back and pain next to the spine, whereas the middle point (b) is more effective for pain on the spine itself.

Best treatment positions

N-UE-24 can be treated easily in most positions.

For the best results, ask the patient to gently bend and turn the trunk. For this purpose, the patient must be standing up or sitting in a chair.

Needling

• 0.5 to 1 cun perpendicular insertion.

! Avoid the dorsal cutaneous veins, and more deeply, the dorsal metacarpal arteries.

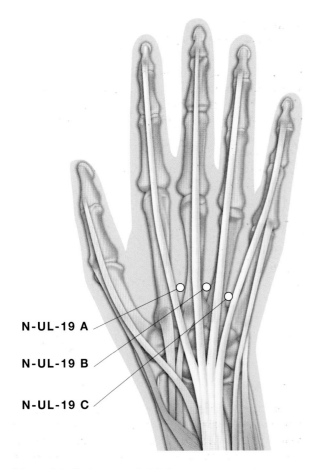

N-UL-19 A

N-UL-19 B

N-UL-19 C

Manual techniques and shiatsu
Friction and sustained pressure should produce quite a strong sensation to be effective. Apply friction to the nodules until they soften or disappear entirely.

Moxibustion
Cones: 1–3. Pole: 5–10 minutes. Rice-grain moxibustion is also effective.

Stimulation sensation
Both pressure and needling induce a strong sensation.

Actions and indications
These points are very *effective to treat acute lower backache.*

Main Area: Lower back.

Main Functions: Regulates qi and Blood. Alleviates stiffness and pain.

Miscellaneous and New Points of the Lower Limb

M-LE-8 Bafeng
Eight Winds

Eight points, on the dorsal surface of the foot, located in the webs between each of the toes, distal to the metatarsophalangeal joints. Approximately 0.5 cun proximal to the margin of the webs.

To aid location, when the toes are closed together (adducted), the points are at the end of the creases between the toes.

The Bafeng point group includes Liv-2, St-44 and GB-43.

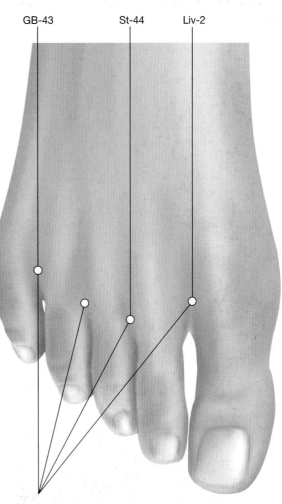

GB-43   St-44   Liv-2

M-LE-8

Needling
- 0.3 to 1 cun oblique insertion, directed between the metatarsal bones.
- 0.3 to 0.5 cun perpendicular insertion.

Manual techniques and shiatsu
Stationary perpendicular pressure is applied quite strongly into the space between the metatarsophalangeal joints with the tip of the finger or thumb. Additionally, friction can be effective.

Stretching the toes downwards (flexion) opens these points. Additionally, mobilising the toes also helps release tension from the surrounding area.

Moxibustion
Cones: 3–5. Pole: 5–15 minutes. Rice-grain moxa effective.

Magnets
Magnet therapy can be very effective for disorders of the metatarsophalangeal joints. Alternate poles on each of the Bafeng points to treat pain, stiffness or swelling of the metatarsophalangeal joints and toes.

Stimulation sensation
A deep numb ache extends into the metatarsophalangeal joints. Also, an electric or tingling sensation can spread toward the tips of the toes.

Actions and indications
These are all *very dynamic points*, and are *extensively employed to clear interior heat and descend excessive yang.* They have been used in a *large variety of disorders* including headache, tinnitus, inflammation of the eyes, toothache, hypertension, fever, hepatitis, gastritis, constipation, seizures and menstrual disorders (see also Liv-2, St-44 and GB-43).

However, they are of *primary importance as local points for pain, swelling and stiffness of the metatarsophalangeal joints and toes.* They also *improve qi and Blood circulation in the entire lower limbs* and may be useful in the treatment of atrophy and paralysis.

Main Area: Lower back.

Main Functions: Regulates qi and Blood. Alleviates stiffness and pain.

M-LE-13   Lanweixue   闌尾

Appendix Point

Approximately 2 cun below the right St-36, at the most tender site during pressure palpation.

However, this location can be treated bilaterally for channel disorders and pain.

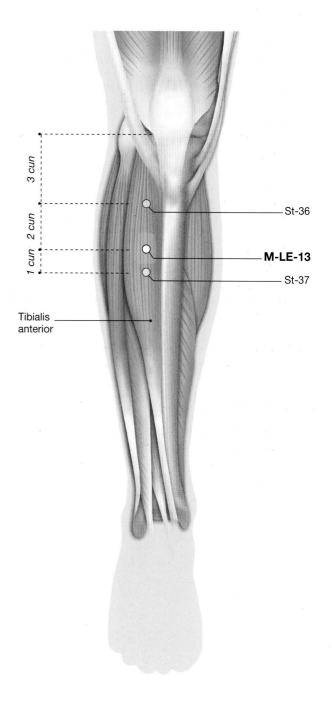

St-36

M-LE-13

St-37

Tibialis anterior

3 cun

2 cun

1 cun

Best treatment positions
Similar to St-36 and St-37.

Needling
• 0.5 to 1.5 cun perpendicular insertion.

Manual techniques and shiatsu
Perpendicular pressure and friction techniques can be applied quite strongly.

Moxibustion
Cones: 3–10. Pole: 5–15 minutes. Rice-grain moxa is also effectively applied.

Cupping and guasha
Both cupping and guasha can be effectively applied.

! Avoid areas with distended vessels.

Magnets
Use opposite poles on M-LE-13 and locally on the abdomen over the appendix.

Actions and indications
This is a *very important and extensively used point for the treatment of acute and chronic appendicitis.*

Furthermore, it may be used to treat other digestive symptoms such as bloating and indigestion.

It is also *useful diagnostically*, because it becomes tender if there is inflammation of the intestine.

As *a local point*, it can be treated (on both sides) for cases of pain, weakness or paralysis of the lower limbs.

> **Main Areas:** Appendix and large intestine.
>
> **Main Functions:** Clears heat, dampness and fire poisons from the Large Intestine.

M-LE-16 Xiyan 膝眼
Eyes of the Knee

A pair of points, just below the patella, one in the medial and one in the lateral depression formed by the patellar tendon when the knee is flexed.

To aid location, these points are approximately one finger's width from the border of the patellar tendon.

The medial point is known as *Nei Xiyan (Inner Eye of the Knee),* and the lateral one, *Wai Xiyan (Outer Eye of the Knee),* is also called *Dubi (Calf's Nose)* or *St-35.*

Best treatment positions
These points are best treated with the patient in a supine position, with the knee flexed and supported with cushions. However, treatment can also be applied in other positions.

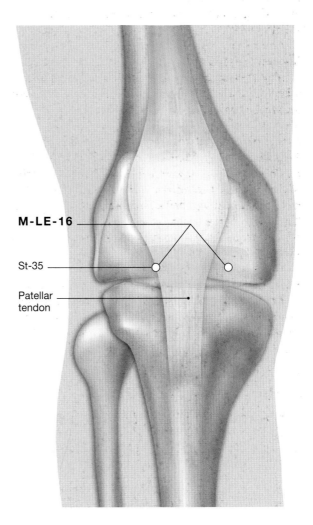

M-LE-16

St-35

Patellar tendon

Needling

- 1 to 2 cun perpendicular insertion toward the centre of the knee joint, or Bl-40.
- 1 to 1.5 cun horizontal insertion, through or under the patellar tendon to connect the two points.
- 1 to 2 cun oblique superior medial insertion under the patella.

! Do not puncture arteries and veins of the genicular network.

Manual techniques and shiatsu

Perpendicular pressure can be applied quite strongly to these points, and is most effective in a supine position with the knee flexed. Friction is effectively applied to the patellar tendon and other soft tissues and insertions surrounding the knee joint.

Furthermore, mobilising the leg and knee is very beneficial.

Moxibustion

Cones: 3–7. Pole: 5–15 minutes. Rice-grain moxa is also effectively applied.

Cupping

Medium or strong suction, with small cups, can be very effective.

Guasha

Guasha applied across the patellar tendon is very effective.

Magnets

Use opposite poles on the medial and lateral eyes of the knee.

Actions and indications

These points are *extremely helpful in many disorders of the knees*, including chronic or acute pain, stiffness and swelling. Treatment applied here is *beneficial to the cartilages and menisci* and helps in cases of degenerative conditions and inflammation.

> **Main Areas:** Knees. Lower limbs.
>
> **Main Functions:** Regulates qi and Blood. Alleviates stiffness, swelling and pain.

M-LE-23 Dannangxue 膽囊穴
Gallbladder Point

On the right leg, 1 to 2 cun distal to GB-34, at the most tender site on pressure palpation.

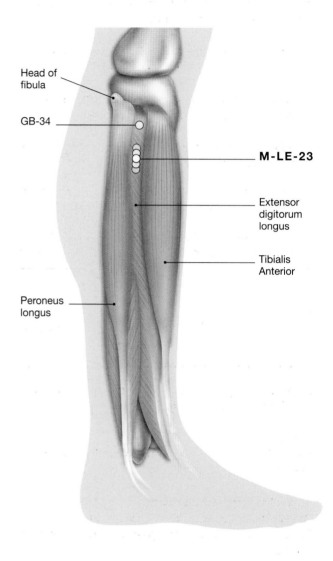

Head of fibula

GB-34

M-LE-23

Extensor digitorum longus

Tibialis Anterior

Peroneus longus

Best treatment positions
Similar to GB-34.

Needling
- 0.5 to 1.5 cun perpendicular insertion.

Manual techniques and shiatsu
Perpendicular pressure and friction techniques can be applied quite strongly.

Guasha
Guasha can be very effective.

Magnets

Use opposite poles on M-LE-23 and GB-24 (or other point in the region of the gallbladder).

Actions and indications

Dannangxue *is a very important and extensively used point for many disorders of the gallbladder and bile duct* and is especially indicated for both acute and chronic cholelythiasis and cholecystitis.

It also treats such symptoms as nausea, poor digestion of fats, obesity and pain of the hypochondrial area.

Furthermore, it is *useful diagnostically*, because it often becomes tender in cases of gallbladder disharmony.

As *a local point*, it can be treated bilaterally in cases of pain, weakness or paralysis of the lower limbs.

> **Main Areas:** Gallbladder. Digestive system.
>
> **Main Functions:** Regulates qi, dispels stasis and alleviates pain. Benefits the gallbladder.

M-LE-27 Heding 鶴頂

Crane's Summit

In the small depression just above the midpoint of the superior border of the patella.

Needling
• 0.5 to 1 cun perpendicular or transverse insertion under the patella.

Manual techniques and shiatsu
Perpendicular pressure and friction are applicable. Furthermore, mobilising the patella gently helps ease stiffness.

Actions and indications
This is an effective point for disorders of the knee and patella, including swelling, stiffness and pain.

> **Main Area:** Knees.
>
> **Main Function:** Alleviates stiffness and pain.

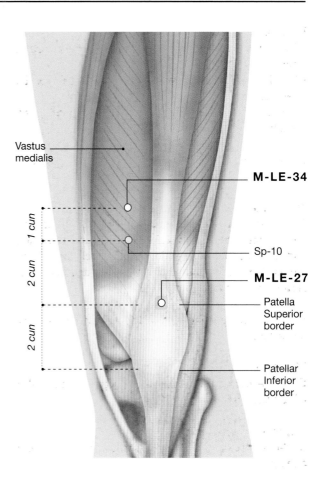

Vastus medialis — M-LE-34 — Sp-10 — M-LE-27 — Patella Superior border — Patellar Inferior border — 1 cun — 2 cun — 2 cun

M-LE-34 Baichongwo 百蟲窩

Hundred Insect Nest

3 cun proximal to the superior medial border of the patella, 1 cun proximal to Sp-10. Locate with the knee flexed.

To aid location, this point is at a tender spot on the bulge of the vastus medialis muscle.

Best treatment positions
Similar to Sp-10.

Actions and indications
M-LE-34, also known as *Sp-10 and a Half*, is *an important point to cool the Blood, dissipate wind and dampness from the skin and alleviate itching*. It is extensively employed to treat skin diseases with itching, redness and blistering such as urticaria and eczema, and insect bites.

> **Main Area:** Skin.
>
> **Main Function:** Alleviates itching and pain.

Resources

Cheng, Xinhong.: 1999. *Chinese Acupuncture and Moxibustion.* Foreign Languages Press, Beijing.

Clemente, C.: 1985. *Gray's Anatomy of the Human Body, thirtieth edition.* Lippincott, Williams & Wilkins, Baltimore.

Deadman, P., Baker, K., Al-Khafaji, Mazin.: 2007. *A Manual of Acupuncture, second edition.* Journal of Chinese Medicine Publications, Brighton.

Ding, Li, Professor.: 1991. *Acupuncture, Meridian Theory and Acupuncture Points.* English translation by You Benlin and Wang Zhaorong, Nanjing College of Traditional Chinese Medicine and Nanjing International Acupuncture Training Centre. Foreign Languages Press, Beijing.

Ellis, A., Wiseman, N., Boss, K..: 1989. *Grasping the Wind.* Paradigm Publications, Brookline, Massachusetts.

Ellis, A., Wiseman, N., Boss, K.: 1991. *Fundamentals of Chinese Acupuncture, revised edition.* Paradigm Publications, Brookline, Massachusetts.

Hecker, Hans-Ulrich, Steveling, Angelika, Peuker, Elmar, Kastner, Jorg, Liebchen, Kay.: 2001. *Color Atlas of Acupuncture: Body Points, Ear Points, Trigger Points.* Thieme Medical Publishers, Germany.

Hoppenfeld, S.: 1976. *Physical Examination of the Spine and Extremities.* Appleton-Century-Crofts, a Publishing Division of Prentice-Hall, USA.

Jarmey, C.: 1999. *Shiatsu: a Complete Guide.* Harper Collins, London.

Jarmey, C.: 2004. *The Atlas of Musculo-skeletal Anatomy.* Lotus Publishing/ North Atlantic Books, Chichester/ Berkeley.

Jarmey, C.: 2006. *The Foundations of Shiatsu.* Lotus Publishing/ North Atlantic Books, Chichester/ Berkeley.

Kendall, F. P., McCreary, E. K. & Provance, P. G.: 1993. *Muscles: Testing and Function, 4th edition.* Lippincott, Williams & Wilkins, Baltimore.

Lade, A.: 1989. *Acupuncture Points: Images and Functions.* Eastland Press, Seattle, Washington.

Lian, Yu-Lin, Chen, Chun-Yan, Hammes, M., Kolster, B. C. *The Pictorial Atlas of Acupuncture: an Illustrated Manual of Acupuncture Points.* Edited by Hans P. Ogal and Wolfram Stor. Translation from German by Colin Grant. Konemann Publishers.

Longmore, M., Wilkinson, I., Torok, E.: 2001. *Oxford Handbook of Clinical Medicine, fifth edition.* Oxford University Press.

Maciocia, Giovanni.: 1989. *The Foundations of Chinese Medicine: a Comprehensive Text for Acupuncturists and Herbalists, first edition.* Churchill Livingstone, Edinburgh.

McCracken, T.: 2005. *Black's Concise Atlas of Human Anatomy.* A & C Black, London.

Netter, F. H.: 1995. *Atlas of Human Anatomy.* Ciba-Geigy Corporation, Summit, New Jersey.

Platzer, W.: 2003. *Color Atlas and Textbook of Human Anatomy, Vol. 1: Locomotor System.* Thieme Medical Publishers, Germany.

Putz, R., Pabst, R., Weiglein, A. H.: 2001. *Sobotta Atlas of Human Anatomy, thirteenth edition.* Lippincott, Williams & Wilkins, Baltimore.

Rohen, Johannes W., Yokochi, Chihiro, Lutjen-Drecoll, Elke.: 2002. *Color Atlas of Anatomy: a Photographic Study of the Human Body, fifth edition.* Lippincott, Williams & Wilkins, Baltimore.

Schuenke, M., Schulte, E., & Shumacher, U.: 2005. *General Anatomy and Musculo-skeletal System.* Thieme Medical Publishers, Germany.

Shanghai College of Traditional Medicine.: 1981. *Acupuncture: a Comprehensive Text.* Translated and edited by John O'Connor and Dan Bensky. Eastland Press, Seattle, Washington.

Wang, Deshen.: 1993. *Manual of International Standardization of Acupuncture (Zhenjiu) Point Names.* The Higher Education Press of China.

Zhong, Yi Xue, Chu, Ji.: 1995. *Fundamentals of Chinese Medicine, revised edition.* Translated and amended by Nigel Wiseman and Andrew Ellis. Paradigm Publications, Brookline, Massachusetts.

Index of Points

Point Name-Number

Bladder channel

Bl-1 160
Bl-2 161
Bl-3 162
Bl-4 163
Bl-5 163
Bl-6 164
Bl-7 164
Bl-8 165
Bl-8 165
Bl-9 165
Bl-10 165
Bl-11 170
Bl-12 170
Bl-13 170
Bl-14 171
Bl-15 171
Bl-16 172
Bl-17 172
Bl-18 173
Bl-19 173
Bl-20 174
Bl-21 174
Bl-22 174
Bl-23 175
Bl-24 175
Bl-25 176
Bl-26 176
Bl-27 176
Bl-28 177
Bl-29 178
Bl-30 178
Bl-31 178
Bl-32 179
Bl-33 179
Bl-34 179
Bl-35 179
Bl-36 180
Bl-37 180
Bl-38 181
Bl-39 181
Bl-40 182
Bl-41 183
Bl-42 183
Bl-43 185
Bl-44 185

Bl-45 185
Bl-46 186
Bl-47 186
Bl-48 186
Bl-49 187
Bl-50 187
Bl-51 188
Bl-52 188
Bl-53 188
Bl-54 189
Bl-55 190
Bl-56 190
Bl-57 191
Bl-58 192
Bl-59 193
Bl-60 194
Bl-61 195
Bl-62 196
Bl-63 197
Bl-64 198
Bl-65 199
Bl-66 199
Bl-67 200

Du mai channel

Du-1 304
Du-2 305
Du-3 307
Du-4 307
Du-5 308
Du-6 308
Du-7 309
Du-8 309
Du-9 309
Du-10 310
Du-11 310
Du-12 311
Du-13 311
Du-14 312
Du-15 313
Du-16 313
Du-17 314
Du-20 315
Du-23 316
Du-24 317
Du-25 318
Du-26 319
Du-28 320

Extraordinary points

M-HN-1 322
M-HN-3 322
M-HN-6 323
M-HN-8 324
M-HN-9 325
M-HN-10 326
M-HN-14 326
M-HN-18 327
M-HN-30 328
M-HN-54 328
M-BW-1A 329
M-BW-1B 329
M-BW-35 331
M-BW-24 332
M-BW-25 332
M-CA-23 333
M-CA-18 334
M-UE-1 334
M-UE-9 335
M-UE-22 336
M-UE-24 336
M-UE-29 337
M-UE-48 338
N-UL-19 338
M-LE-8 339
M-LE-13 340
M-LE-16 341
M-LE-23 342
M-LE-27 343
M-LE-34 343

Gallbladder channel

GB-1 240
GB-2 241
GB-3 242
GB-4 243
GB-5 244
GB-6 244
GB-7 244
GB-8 245
GB-9 245
GB-12 245
GB-13 247
GB-14 247
GB-15 248
GB-20 249
GB-21 251
GB-22 254
GB-23 254
GB-24 255
GB-25 256
GB-26 257
GB-27 258

GB-28 258
GB-29 259
GB-30 260
GB-31 261
GB-32 262
GB-33 262
GB-34 263
GB-35 264
GB-36 264
GB-37 265
GB-38 266
GB-39 266
GB-40 267
GB-41 268
GB-42 269
GB-43 269
GB-44 270

Heart channel

He-1 136
He-3 137
He-4 138
He-5 139
He-6 140
He-7 140
He-8 142
He-9 143

Kidney channel

Kd-1 202
Kd-2 203
Kd-3 204
Kd-4 205
Kd-5 206
Kd-6 207
Kd-7 208
Kd-8 209
Kd-9 209
Kd-10 210
Kd-11 211
Kd-16 211
Kd-18 212
Kd-19 212
Kd-21 213
Kd-22 213
Kd-25 213
Kd-27 214

Large intestine channel

LI-1 60
LI-2 60
LI-4 61
LI-5 64

LI-6 65
LI-7 66
LI-10 66
LI-11 68
LI-12 70
LI-14 71
LI-15 72
LI-16 73
LI-18 74
LI-20 75

Liver channel

Liv-1 272
Liv-2 273
Liv-3 274
Liv-4 277
Liv-5 278
Liv-6 279
Liv-7 279
Liv-8 280
Liv-9 281
Liv-10 282
Liv-11 282
Liv-12 283
Liv-13 284
Liv-14 286

Lung channel

Lu-1 48
Lu-2 50
Lu-5 51
Lu-6 52
Lu-7 53
Lu-8 54
Lu-9 55
Lu-10 57
Lu-11 58

Pericardium channel

P-1 216
P-3 217
P-4 218
P-5 219
P-6 220
P-7 222
P-8 223
P-9 224

Ren mai channel

Ren-1 288
Ren-2 289
Ren-3 289

Ren-4 290
Ren-5 291
Ren-6 292
Ren-7 293
Ren-8 293
Ren-9 294
Ren-10 295
Ren-11 296
Ren-12 296
Ren-13 297
Ren-14 297
Ren-15 298
Ren-16 298
Ren-17 299
Ren-20 300
Ren-21 300
Ren-22 300
Ren-23 301
Ren-24 302

Sanjiao (triple burner) channel

SJ-1 226
SJ-2 226
SJ-3 227
SJ-4 228
SJ-5 229
SJ-6 230
SJ-7 231
SJ-10 232
SJ-14 232
SJ-15 234
SJ-16 235
SJ-17 236
SJ-20 237
SJ-21 237
SJ-23 238

Small intestine channel

SI-1 146
SI-3 146
SI-4 148
SI-5 148
SI-6 149
SI-8 150
SI-9 151
SI-10 152
SI-11 152
SI-12 153
SI-13 154
SI-14 154
SI-15 155
SI-17 156
SI-18 157
SI-19 158

Spleen channel

Sp-1 116
Sp-2 117
Sp-3 118
Sp-4 119
Sp-5 121
Sp-6 122
Sp-7 124
Sp-8 124
Sp-9 126
Sp-10 127
Sp-12 128
Sp-13 129
Sp-14 129
Sp-15 130
Sp-16 131
Sp-17 132
Sp-18 132
Sp-19 133
Sp-20 133
Sp-21 134

Stomach channel

St-1 78
St-2 79
St-3 80
St-4 81
St-5 82
St-6 83
St-7 84
St-8 85
St-9 86
St-10 88
St-11 89
St-12 89
St-13 90
St-14 91
St-15 92
St-16 92
St-17 92
St-18 93
St-19 94
St-20 94
St-21 96
St-22 96
St-23 96
St-24 97
St-25 97
St-26 98
St-27 98
St-28 99
St-29 99
St-30 99

St-31 100
St-32 101
St-33 102
St-34 102
St-35 103
St-36 104
St-37 106
St-38 107
St-39 108
St-40 108
St-41 109
St-42 110
St-43 111
St-44 112
St-45 113

Chinese Point Name (Pinyin)

Bladder channel

Baihuanshu 178
Baohuang 188
Chengfu.. 180
Chengguang . . .. .164
Chengjin.. 190
Chengshan.. 191
Ciliao 179
Dachangshu.. 176
Danshu . . .. .173
Dazhu 170
Dushu 172
Feishu.. 170
Feiyang 192
Fengmen. 170
Fufen 183
Fuxi.. 181
Fuyang. 193
Ganshu . . .. .173
Gaohuangshu 185
Geguan 186
Geshu.. 172
Guanyuanshu 176
Heyang 190
Huangmen 188
Huiyang.. 179
Hunmen.. 186
Jinggu.. 198
Jingming. 160
Jinmen.. 197
Jueyinshu 171
Kunlun.. 194
Luoque 165
Meichong 162
Pangguangshu 177
Pishu.. 174
Pohu . . .. .183
Pucan 195
Qihaishu . . .. .175
Quchai.. 163
Sanjiaoshu 174
Shangliao 178
Shenmai.. 196
Shenshu.. 175
Shentang. 185
Shugu 199
Tianzhu 165
Tongtian 164
Weicang.. 187
Weishu.. 174
Weiyang 181
Weizhong 182

Wuchu.. . .. .163
Xialiao.. . .. .179
Xiaochangshu.. 176
Xinshu. 171
Yanggang . . .. .186
Yinmen 180
Yishe 187
Yixi 185
Yuzhen.. 165
Zanzhu.. 161
Zhibian 189
Zhishi 188
Zhiyin.. . .. .200
Zhonflushu 178
Zhongliao 179
Zutonggu 199

Du mai channel

Baihui.. 315
Changqiang . . .. .304
Dazhui . . .. .312
Fengfu . . .. .313
Jinsuo . . .. .309
Jizhong . . .. .308
Lingtai . . .. .310
Mingmen . . .. .307
Naohu.. 314
Shangxing . . .. .316
Shendao.. 310
Shenting 317
Shenzhu.. 311
Shuigou (Renzhong) 319
Suliao 318
Taodao. 311
Xuanshu . . .. .308
Yamen 313
Yaoshu. 305
Yaoyangguan 307
Yinjiao. 320
Zhiyang.. 309
Zhongshu 309

Extraordinary points

Anmian 328
Bafeng. 339
Baichongwo 343
Bailao.. 328
Baxie 336
Bitong.. 326
Chuanxi.. 329
Dannangxue 342
Dingchuan 329
Erbai. 337
Erjian . .. .326

Heding. .343
Huatuojiaji. .331
Jiachengjiang .327
Jianqian (Jianneiling).. .338
Lanweixue. .340
Luozhen (Wailaogong) .336
Qiuhou. .324
Sanjiaojiu .333
Shiqizhui .332
Shixuan .334
Sifeng. .335
Sishencong .322
Taiyang .325
Xiyan .341
Yaotongdian .338
Yaoyan. .332
Yintang .322
Yuyao .323
Zigong. .334

Gallbladder channel

Benshen.. .247
Daimai. .257
Diquhui . .269
Fengchi . .249
Fengshi . .261
Guangming .265
Hanyan . .243
Huantiao. .260
Jianjing .251
Jingmen.. .256
Juliao . .259
Qiuxu . .267
Qubin . .244
Riyue . .255
Shangguan. .242
Shuaigu . .245
Tianchong.. .245
Tinghui . .241
Tongziliao . .240
Toulinqi . .248
Waiqiu . .264
Wangu . .245
Weidao . .258
Wushu . .258
Xiaxi. .269
Xiyangguan . .262
Xuanli.. .244
Xuanlu. .244
Xuanzhong (Juegu) . .266
Yangbai . .247
Yangfu . .266
Yangjiao . .264
Yanglingquan .. .263
Yuanye. .254

Zhejin .254
Zhongdu .262
Zulinqi. .268
Zuqiaoyin .270

Heart channel

Jiquan .136
Lingdao .138
Shaochong. .143
Shaofu . .142
Shaohai . .137
Shenmen. .140
Tongli .139
Yinxi. .140

Kidney channel

Bulang. .213
Dazhong. .205
Fuliu. .208
Henggu .211
Huangshu .211
Jiaoxin .209
Rangu .203
Shencang .213
Shiguan . .212
Shufu . .214
Shuiquan .206
Taixi . .204
Yindu .212
Yingu .210
Yongquan .202
Youmen . .213
Zhaohai .207
Zhubin. .209

Large intestine channel

Binao .71
Futu. .74
Hegu. .61
Jianyu . .72
Jugu.. .73
Pianli .65
Quchi .68
Sanjian. .60
Shangyang. .60
Shousanli .66
Wenliu. .66
Yangxi. .64
Yingxiang.. .75
Zhouliao .70

Liver channel

Dadun.. .. .. .272
Jimai.. .. .. .283
Ligou 278
Qimen.. .. .. .286
Ququan 280
Taichong. ... ... .274
Xiguan.. .. .. .279
Xingjian.. .. .. .273
Yinbao. .. .. .281
Yinlian. .. .. .282
Zhangmen . ... .284
Zhongdu . ... .279
Zhongfeng . ... .277
Zuwuli.. .. .. .282

Lung channel

Chize 51
Jingqu.. 54
Kongzui.. 52
Lieque 53
Shaoshang 58
Taiyuan 55
Yuji 57
Yunmen 50
Zhongfu.. 48

Pericardium channel

Daling.. .. .. .222
Jianshi . ... .219
Laogong . ... .223
Quze . ... .217
Neiguan.. .. .. .220
Tianchi . ... .216
Ximen.. .. .. .218
Zhongchong . ... .224

Ren mai channel

Chengjiang . ... .302
Guanyuan.. .. .. .290
Huagai . ... .300
Huiyin . ... .288
Jianli . ... .296
Jiuwei . ... .298
Juque . ... .297
Lianquan . ... .301
Qugu. ... ... .289
Shangwan.. .. .. .297
Shanzhong (Shangqihai) . ... .299
Shenque.. .. .. .293
Shimen . ... .291
Shuifen . ... .294

Tiantu .. .. .300
(Xia) Qihai .. .. .292
Xiawan . ... .295
Xuanji.. . ... .300
Yinjiao. ... ... .293
Zhongji . ... .289
Zhongting.. .. .. .298
Zhongwan . ... .296

Sanjiao (triple burner) channel

Ermen.. .. .. .237
Guanchong . ... .226
Huizong.. .. .. .231
Jianliao . ... .232
Jiaosun. ... ... .237
Sizhukong . ... .238
Tianjing . ... .232
Tianliao . ... .234
Tianyou . ... .235
Waiguan . ... .229
Yangchi . ... .228
Yemen . ... .226
Yifeng . ... .236
Zhigou . ... .230
Zhongzhu . ... .227

Small intestine channel

Bingfeng. ... ... .153
Houxi . ... .146
Jianwaishu. ... ... .154
Jianzhen.. . ... .151
Jianzhongshu . ... .155
Naoshu . ... .152
Quanliao. ... ... .157
Quyuan . ... .154
Shaoze . ... .146
Tianrong . ... .156
Tianzong. ... ... .152
Tinggong . ... .158
Wangu . ... .148
Xiaohai . ... .150
Yanggu . ... .148
Yanglao . ... .149

Spleen channel

Chongmen. ... ... .128
Dabao .. .. .134
Dadu . ... .117
Daheng . ... .130
Diji . ... .124
Fuai . ... .131
Fujie . ... .129
Fushe . ... .129

Gongsun 119
Lougu 124
Sanyinjiao 122
Shangqiu 121
Shidou 132
Taibai 118
Tianxi 132
Xiongxiang 133
Xuehai 127
Yinbai 116
Yinlingquan 126
Zhourong 133

Xiangu 111
Yingchuang 92
Yinshi 102
Zusanli 104

Stomach channel

Biguan 100
Burong 94
Chengman 94
Chengqi 78
Chongyang 110
Daju 98
Daying 82
Dicang 81
Dubi (Waixiyan) 103
Fenglong 108
Futu 101
Guanmen 96
Guilai 99
Huaroumen 97
Jiache 83
Jiexi 109
Juliao 80
Kufang 91
Liangmen 96
Lianqiu 102
Lidui 113
Neiting 112
Qichong 99
Qihu 90
Qishe 89
Quepen 89
Renying 86
Rugen 93
Ruzhong 92
Shangjuxu 106
Shuidao 99
Shuitu 88
Sibai 79
Taiyi 96
Tianshu 97
Tiaokou 107
Touwei 85
Wailing 98
Wuyi 92
Xiaguan 84
Xiajuxu 108

The Anatomy of Stretching

Brad Walker

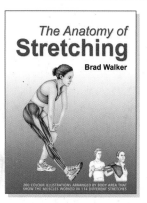

978 1 905367 03 0 (UK)/978 1 55643 596 (US); **£14.99/$24.95**; 176 pages; 265 mm x 194 mm; 320 colour illustrations; paperback

Books on stretching are common, but *The Anatomy of Stretching* takes a more fundamental approach than the others, taking the reader inside the body to show exactly what is happening during a stretch. At the heart of the book are 300 full-colour illustrations that show the primary and secondary muscles worked in 114 key stretches arranged by body area. Author Brad Walker brings years of expertise – he works with elite-level and world-champion athletes, and lectures on injury prevention – to this how-to guide. He looks at stretching from every angle, including physiology and flexibility; the benefits of stretching; the different types of stretching; rules for safe stretching; and how to stretch properly. Aimed at fitness enthusiasts of any level, as well as at fitness pros, *The Anatomy of Stretching* also focuses on which stretches are useful for the alleviation or rehabilitation of specific sports injuries.

Brad Walker, B.Sc. Health Sciences, is a prominent Australian sports trainer with more than 20 years experience in the health and fitness industry. He graduated from the University of New England, and has postgraduate accreditations in athletics, swimming, and triathlon coaching.

The Anatomy of Sports Injuries

Brad Walker

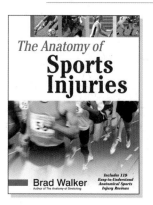

978 1 905367 06 1 (UK)/ 978 1 55643 666 6 (US); **£16.99/$29.95**; 256 pages; 265 mm x 194 mm; 250 colour / black and white illustrations; paperback

The Anatomy of Sports Injuries takes you inside the body to show exactly what is happening when a sports injury occurs. At the heart of *The Anatomy of Sports Injuries* are 300 full-colour illustrations that show the sports injury in detail, along with 200 line drawings of simple stretching, strengthening, and rehabilitation exercises that the reader can use to speed up the recovery process. *The Anatomy of Sports Injuries* is for every sports player or fitness enthusiast who has been injured and would like to know what the injury involves, how to rehabilitate the area, and how to prevent complications or injury in the future. This book is the perfect partner for Brad's other book, *The Anatomy of Stretching*.

Brad Walker, B.Sc. Health Sciences, is a prominent Australian sports trainer with more than 20 years experience in the health and fitness industry. He graduated from the University of New England, and has postgraduate accreditations in athletics, swimming, and triathlon coaching.

Dynamic Bodyuse for Effective, Strain-free Massage

Darien Pritchard

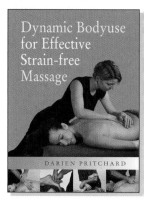

978 0 9543188 9 5 (UK)/ 978 1 55643 655 0 (US); **£24.99/$39.95**; 640 pages; 265 mm x 194 mm; 2000 black and white photographs; paperback

The most significant cause of early retirement from the massage profession is the *cumulative strain* on the body developed in the course of performing massages. The growth of the profession in recent years has been accompanied by an increase in the number of work-induced problems. This book highlights aspects of massage that can lead to these problems and offers guidance for their avoidance. The focus is on how to use your body *safely* and *effectively* in massage sessions. This includes *involving your whole body* to generate the power and movement that supports your working hands, *saving your hands* by using them skilfully, and *conserving them* by using other body areas such as your forearms and elbows whenever possible. This book is essential reading for anyone involved in massage, whether you are a student, a professional massage practitioner or teacher, or sports massage therapist.

Darien Pritchard calls upon over 30 years of training massage professionals. He also teaches bodywork modules in a university degree course, and has written a series of articles for *Massage World* on bodyuse.

The Concise Book of Trigger Points

Simeon Niel-Asher

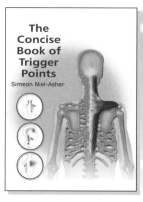

978 0 9543188 5 7 (UK)/ 978 1 55 643 536 2 (US); **£16.99/$29.95**; 208 pages; 275 mm x 212 mm; 260 colour / black and white illustrations; paperback

Written for the student and early practitioner of massage / bodywork, physical therapy, physiotherapy, and any other health-related field. It explains how to treat chronic pain through trigger points. Each two-page spread has colour illustrations of each major skeletal muscle, and text identifying each muscle's origin, insertion, action, and innervation, plus the physiological implications of the trigger points in each muscle, and techniques for treatment.

Simeon Niel-Asher, B. Phil., B.Sc., (Ost.), qualified as an osteopath in 1992. He is involved in treating, research, writing, and teaching throughout Europe, the Middle East, and the USA.

"This book represents an excellent entry level text which will be a powerful learning aid to any student or newly qualified practitioner."
John Sharkey, B.Sc., Neuromuscular Therapist, Director, National Training Centre, Ireland

A Practical Guide
to Acu-points

Chris Jarmey
and Ilaira Bouratinos

Lotus Publishing
Chichester, England

North Atlantic Books
Berkeley, California

First published in 2008 by
Lotus Publishing
3. Chapel Street, Chichester, PO19 1BU and
North Atlantic Books
P O Box 12327
Berkeley, California 94712

Illustrations John Tyropolis, Michael Evdemon and Ilaira Bouratinos
Text Design Wendy Craig, Michael Evdemon and Ilaira Bouratinos
Cover Design Jim Wilkie
Printed and Bound in Singapore by Tien Wah Press

Acknowledgements

The authors would like to thank the teaching staff of the European Shiatsu School and the European Institute of Oriental Medicine, and also the following persons, without whose valuable input and support this project would not have been possible: Vassilis Basios, Emilios Bouratinos, Katia Boustani, Tew Bunnag, George Dellar, Julie Holland, Jonathan Hutchings, Christos Kondis, Christina Kouli, Giorgio Maioletti, Tim Mulvagh, Andrew Parfitt, Vita Revelli, and Peggy Zarrou.

A Practical Guide to Acu-points is sponsored by the Society for the Study of Native Arts and Sciences, a nonprofit educational corporation whose goals are to develop an educational and cross-cultural perspective linking various scientific, social, and artistic fields; to nurture a holistic view of arts, sciences, humanities, and healing; and to publish and distribute literature on the relationship of mind, body, and nature.

British Library Cataloguing in Publication Data

A CIP record for this book is available from the British Library
ISBN 978 0 9543188 4 0 (Lotus Publishing)
ISBN 978 1 55643 696 3 (North Atlantic Books)

Library of Congress Cataloguing-in-Publication Data

Jarmey, Chris.
A practical guide to acu-points / by Chris Jarmey and Ilaira Bouratinos.
    p. ; cm.
Includes bibliographical references and index.
ISBN-13: 978-1-55643-696-3 (pbk. : North Atlantic Books)
ISBN-10: 1-55643-696-3 (pbk. : North Atlantic Books)
ISBN-10: 0-9543188-4-6 (pbk. : Lotus Publishing)
1. Acupuncture points. I. Bouratinos, Ilaira. II. Title.
[DNLM: 1. Acupuncture Points. 2. Acupressure. 3. Acupuncture Therapy.
4. Meridians. WB 369.5.M5 J37c 2006]
RM184.5.J372 2006
615.8'92--dc22
                    2006031085